T0259147

Challenges in Pulmonary Hypertension

Editors

ALBERTO M. MARRA
ALEXANDER E. SHERMAN
PIETRO AMERI

HEART FAILURE CLINICS

www.heartfailure.theclinics.com

Consulting Editor
EDUARDO BOSSONE

Founding Editor
JAGAT NARULA

January 2023 • Volume 19 • Number 1

ELSEVIER

1600 John F. Kennedy Boulevard • Suite 1800 • Philadelphia, Pennsylvania, 19103-2899

http://www.theclinics.com

HEART FAILURE CLINICS Volume 19, Number 1
January 2023 ISSN 1551-7136, ISBN-13: 978-0-323-93877-8

Editor: Joanna Collett
Developmental Editor: Jessica Cañaberal

Heart Failure Clinics (ISSN 1551-7136) is published quarterly by Elsevier Inc., 360 Park Avenue South, New York, NY 10010-1710. Months of publication are January, April, July, and October. Business and editorial offices: 1600 John F. Kennedy Boulevard, Suite 1800, Philadelphia, PA 19103-2899. Periodicals postage paid at New York, NY, and additional mailing offices. Subscription prices are USD 291.00 per year for US individuals, USD 629.00 per year for US institutions, USD 100.00 per year for US students and residents, USD 315.00 per year for Canadian individuals, USD 729.00 per year for Canadian institutions, USD 331.00 per year for international individuals, USD 729.00 per year for international institutions, and USD 100.00 per year for Canadian and foreign students/residents. To receive student and resident rate, orders must be accompanied by name of affiliated institution, date of term, and the *signature* of program/residency coordinator on institution letterhead. Orders will be billed at individual rate until proof of status is received. Foreign air speed delivery is included in all *Clinics* subscription prices. All prices are subject to change without notice. **POSTMASTER:** Send address changes to *Heart Failure Clinics*, Elsevier Health Sciences Division, Subscription Customer Service, 3251 Riverport Lane, Maryland Heights, MO 63043. **Customer Service: 1-800-654-2452 (US and Canada). From outside of the US and Canada, call 314-447-8871. Fax: 314-447-8029. For print support, E-mail: JournalsCustomerService-usa@elsevier.com. For online support, E-mail: JournalsOnlineSupport-usa@elsevier.com.**

Reprints. For copies of 100 or more of articles in this publication, please contact the Commercial Reprints Department, Elsevier Inc., 360 Park Avenue South, New York, NY 10010-1710. Tel.: 212-633-3874; Fax: 212-633-3820; E-mail: reprints@elsevier.com.

Heart Failure Clinics is covered in *MEDLINE/PubMed (Index Medicus)*.

Contributors

CONSULTING EDITOR

EDUARDO BOSSONE, MD, PhD, FCCP, FESC, FACC
Consulting Editor, *Heart Failure Clinics*, Director, Division of Cardiology, AORN Antonio Cardarelli Hospital, Full Professor of Applied Medical Sciences, Department of Public Health, Federico II University, Naples, Italy

EDITORS

ALBERTO MARIA MARRA, MD, PhD, FEFIM
Department of Translational Medical Sciences, Interdepartmental Center for Biomaterials (CRIB), Federico II University, Associate Professor of Internal Medicine, Department of Translational Medical Sciences, Federico II School of Medicine and University Hospital, Naples, Italy; Italian Clinical Outcome Research and Reporting Program (I-CORRP); Centre for Pulmonary Hypertension, Thoraxklinik Heidelberg gGmbH at Heidelberg University Hospital, Translational Lung Research Center Heidelberg (TLRC), German Center for Lung Research (DZL), Heidelberg, Germany

ALEXANDER E. SHERMAN, MD
Clinical Instructor, Division of Pulmonary, Critical Care, Sleep Medicine, Clinical Immunology and Allergy, Health Sciences

Clinical Instructor, Department of Medicine, David Geffen School of Medicine at UCLA, Los Angeles, California, USA

PIETRO AMERI, MD, PhD, FHFA
Associate Professor of Cardiology, Department of Internal Medicine, University of Genova, Cardiovascular Disease Unit, Cardiac, Thoracic and Vascular Department, IRCCS Ospedale Policlinico San Martino - IRCCS Italian Cardiology Network, Genova, Italy

EDUARDO BOSSONE, MD, PhD, FCCP, FESC, FACC
Consulting Editor, *Heart Failure Clinics*, Director, Division of Cardiology, AORN Antonio Cardarelli Hospital, Full Professor of Applied Medical Sciences, Department of Public Health, Federico II University, Naples, Italy

AUTHORS

YALDA AFSHAR, MD, PhD
Assistant Professor, Division of Maternal-Fetal Medicine, Department of Obstetrics and Gynecology, University of California, Los Angeles, Los Angeles, California, USA

PIETRO AMERI, MD, PhD, FHFA
Associate Professor of Cardiology, Department of Internal Medicine, University of Genova, Cardiovascular Disease Unit, Cardiac,

Thoracic and Vascular Department, IRCCS Ospedale Policlinico San Martino - IRCCS Italian Cardiology Network, Genova, Italy

AMANDEEP ANEJA, MD
Department of Pathology, Temple University Hospital, Philadelphia, Pennsylvania, USA

MICHELE ARCOPINTO, MD, PhD
Department of Translational Medical Sciences, Federico II University, Naples, Italy; Italian

Clinical Outcome Research and Reporting Program (I-CORRP)

UMBERTO ATTANASIO, MD
Department of Translational Medical Sciences, Federico II University, Naples, Italy

ROBERTO BADAGLIACCA, MD, PhD
Department of Translational and Precision Medicine, Sapienza University of Rome, Rome, Italy

RIYAZ BASHIR, MD
Department of Interventional Cardiology, Temple University Hospital, Philadelphia, Pennsylvania, USA

STEFANIA BASILI, MD
Department of Translational and Precision Medicine, Sapienza University of Rome, Rome, Italy

NICOLA BENJAMIN, MSC
Centre for Pulmonary Hypertension, Thoraxklinik Heidelberg gGmbH at Heidelberg University Hospital, Translational Lung Research Center Heidelberg (TLRC), Member of the German Center for Lung Research (DZL), Heidelberg, Germany

NADIA BERNARDI, MSC
Department of Internal Medicine, University of Genova, Genova, Italy

EVA BIANCONI, PHD
Cardiovascular Disease Unit, Cardiac, Thoracic and Vascular Department, IRCCS Ospedale Policlinico San Martino - IRCCS Italian Cardiology Network, Genova, Italy

EDUARDO BOSSONE, MD, PhD, FCCP, FESC, FACC
Consulting Editor, *Heart Failure Clinics*, Director, Division of Cardiology, AORN Antonio Cardarelli Hospital, Full Professor of Applied Medical Sciences, Department of Public Health, Federico II University, Naples, Italy

DING CAO, MD
Centre for Pulmonary Hypertension, Thoraxklinik Heidelberg gGmbH at Heidelberg University Hospital, Laboratory for Molecular Genetic Diagnostics, Institute of Human Genetics, Heidelberg University, Heidelberg, Germany

ANTONIO CARANNANTE, MD
Department of Translational Medical Sciences, Federico II University, Naples, Italy

GIUSEPPE CARUSO, MD
AORN Antonio Cardarelli Hospital, Naples, Italy

RICHARD N. CHANNICK, MD
Professor, Division of Pulmonology, University of California, Los Angeles, Los Angeles, California, USA

ANTONIO CITTADINI, MD
Department of Translational Medical Sciences, Interdepartmental Center for Biomaterials (CRIB), Federico II University, Naples, Italy; Italian Clinical Outcome Research and Reporting Program (I-CORRP)

GARY COHEN, MD
Department of Interventional Cardiology, Temple University Hospital, Philadelphia, Pennsylvania, USA

GERARD CRINER, MD
Department of Thoracic Medicine and Surgery, Temple University Hospital, Philadelphia, Pennsylvania, USA

GIULIA CRISCI, MD
Department of Translational Medical Sciences, Federico II University, Naples, Italy; Italian Clinical Outcome Research and Reporting Program (I-CORRP)

ALESSANDRA CUOMO, MD
Department of Translational Medical Sciences, Federico II University, Naples, Italy

ANNA D'AGOSTINO, PhD
IRCCS Synlab SDN, Diagnostic and Nuclear Research Institute, Naples, Italy

MICHELE D'ALTO, MD, PhD
Department of Cardiology, Monaldi Hospital - University "L. Vanvitelli," Naples, Italy

ANDREA D'AMURI, MD
Department of Medicine, University Hospital Sant'Anna, University Internal Medicine Unit, Ferrara, Italy

ROBERTA D'ASSANTE, PhD
Department of Translational Medical Sciences, Federico II University, Naples, Italy; Italian Clinical Outcome Research and Reporting Program (I-CORRP)

PABLO DEMELO-RODRIGUEZ, MD, PhD
Venous Thromboembolism Unit, Internal
Medicine, Hospital General Universitario
Gregorio Marañón, Department of Medicine,
School of Medicine, Universidad Complutense
de Madrid, Sanitary Research Institute
Gregorio Marañón, Madrid, Spain

CHRISTINA A. EICHSTAEDT, PhD
Associate Professor, Centre for Pulmonary
Hypertension, Thoraxklinik Heidelberg gGmbH
at Heidelberg University Hospital, Laboratory for
Molecular Genetic Diagnostics, Institute of
Human Genetics, Heidelberg University,
Translational Lung Research Center Heidelberg
(TLRC), Member of the German Center for Lung
Research (DZL), Heidelberg, Germany

JEAN M. ELWING, MD
Professor of Medicine, Division of Pulmonary,
Critical Care, and Sleep Medicine, University of
Cincinnati, Cincinnati, Ohio, USA

IOANNIS T. FARMAKIS, MD, MSc
Department of Cardiology, AHEPA University
Hospital, Thessaloniki, Greece; Center for
Thrombosis and Hemostasis, University
Medical Center Mainz, Mainz, Germany

NATALIA FERNANDES DA SILVA, MD
Pulmonary Division - Heart Institute (InCor)
Heart Institute (InCor) - Hospital das Clínicas da
Faculdade de Medicina da Universidade de
São Paulo

LUDOVICA FULGIONE, MD
Department of Advanced Biomedical
Sciences, Federico II University, Naples, Italy

FRANCISCO GALEANO-VALLE, MD
Venous Thromboembolism Unit, Internal
Medicine, Hospital General Universitario
Gregorio Marañón, Department of Medicine,
School of Medicine, Universidad Complutense
de Madrid, Sanitary Research Institute
Gregorio Marañón, Madrid, Spain

SHAMEEK GAYEN, MD
Department of Thoracic Medicine and Surgery,
Temple University Hospital, Philadelphia,
Pennsylvania, USA

GEORGE GIANNAKOULAS, MD, PhD
Associate Professor of Cardiology and Adult
Congenital Heart Disease, Center for

Thrombosis and Hemostasis, University
Medical Center Mainz, Mainz, Germany

FEDERICA GIARDINO, MD
Department of Translational Medical Sciences,
Federico II University, Naples, Italy; Italian
Clinical Outcome Research and Reporting
Program (I-CORRP)

EKKEHARD GRÜNIG, MD
Centre for Pulmonary Hypertension,
Thoraxklinik Heidelberg gGmbH at Heidelberg
University Hospital, Translational Lung
Research Center Heidelberg (TLRC), Member
of the German Center for Lung Research (DZL),
Heidelberg, Germany

PAOLA GUINDANI, MD
Department of Medicine, University Hospital
Sant'Anna, University Internal Medicine Unit,
Ferrara, Italy

COURTNEY R. JONES, MD
Associate Professor, Department of
Anesthesiology, University of Cincinnati,
Cincinnati, Ohio, USA

ARUN JOSE, MD, MS
Assistant Professor of Medicine, Division of
Pulmonary, Critical Care, and Sleep Medicine,
University of Cincinnati, Cincinnati, Ohio, USA

MARUTI KUMARAN, MD
Department of Radiology, Temple University
Hospital, Philadelphia, Pennsylvania, USA

VLADIMIR LAKHTER, DO
Department of Interventional Cardiology,
Temple University Hospital, Philadelphia,
Pennsylvania, USA

CHRISTOPHER LEWIS, MD
Department of Internal Medicine, Division of
Cardiovascular Medicine, Henry Ford Hospital,
Detroit, Michigan, USA

ALBERTO MARIA MARRA, MD, PhD, FEFIM
Department of Translational Medical Sciences,
Interdepartmental Center for Biomaterials
(CRIB), Federico II University, Associate
Professor of Internal Medicine, Department of
Translational Medical Sciences, Federico II
School of Medicine and University Hospital,
Italian Clinical Outcome Research and
Reporting Program (I-CORRP), Naples, Italy;

Centre for Pulmonary Hypertension, Thoraxklinik Heidelberg gGmbH at Heidelberg University Hospital, Translational Lung Research Center Heidelberg (TLRC), German Center for Lung Research (DZL), Heidelberg, Germany

JENNY Y. MEI, MD
Maternal-Fetal Medicine Fellow, Division of Maternal-Fetal Medicine, Department of Obstetrics and Gynecology, University of California, Los Angeles, Los Angeles, California, USA

VALENTINA MERCURIO MD, PhD, FISC
Department of Translational Medical Sciences, Interdepartmental Center for Clinical and Translational Research (CIRCET), Federico II University, Naples, Italy

MICHELE MODESTINO, MD
Department of Translational Medical Sciences, Federico II University, Naples, Italy; Italian Clinical Outcome Research and Reporting Program (I-CORRP)

EGLĖ PALEVIČIŪTĖ, MD
Clinic of Cardiac and Vascular Diseases, Institute of Clinical Medicine, Faculty of Medicine, Vilnius University, Vilnius, Lithuania

JOSEPH PANARO, MD
Department of Interventional Cardiology, Temple University Hospital, Philadelphia, Pennsylvania, USA

YURI DE DEUS MONTALVERNE PARENTE, MD
Pulmonary Division - Heart Institute (InCor) Heart Institute (InCor) - Hospital das Clínicas da Faculdade de Medicina da Universidade de São Paulo

LOUISE PILOTE, MD, PhD
Division of Clinical Epidemiology and General Internal Medicine, McGill University Health Centre Research Institute, Montreal, Quebec, Canada

MARCO PROIETTI, MD, PhD
Department of Clinical Sciences and Community Health, University of Milan, Geriatric Unit, IRCCS Istituti Clinici Scientifici Maugeri, Milan, Italy; Liverpool Centre for Cardiovascular Science, University of Liverpool, Liverpool Heart and Chest Hospital, Liverpool, Uinted Kingdom

CARMEN RAINONE, MD
Department of Translational Medical Sciences, Federico II University, Naples, Italy; Italian Clinical Outcome Research and Reporting Program (I-CORRP)

PARTH RALI, MD
Department of Thoracic Medicine and Surgery, Temple University Hospital, Philadelphia, Pennsylvania, USA

BRIGIDA RANIERI, PhD
IRCCS Synlab SDN, Diagnostic and Nuclear Research Institute, Naples, Italy

VALERIA RAPARELLI, MD, PhD
Department of Medicine, University Hospital Sant'Anna, University Internal Medicine Unit, Department of Translational Medicine, University of Ferrara, University Center for Studies on Gender Medicine, University of Ferrara, Ferrara, Italy; Faculty of Nursing, University of Alberta, Edmonton, Canada

SALVATORE REGA, MD
Department of Translational Medical Sciences, Federico II University, Naples, Italy

RAJAN SAGGAR, MD
Director, Pulmonary Hypertension Program, Co-Director, Pulmonary Vascular Disease Program, Lung and Heart-Lung Transplant and Pulmonary Hypertension Programs, Professor of Medicine, Pulmonary and Critical Care Division, David Geffen School of Medicine at UCLA, Los Angeles, California, USA

ANDREA SALZANO, MD, PHD, MRCP(LONDON)
IRCCS Synlab SDN, Diagnostic and Nuclear Research Institute, Naples, Italy

RYAN SANDERSON, MD
Section of Cardiology, The University of Chicago, Chicago, Illinois, USA

GERARDA SCAGLIONE, MD
Department of Medicine, University Hospital Sant'Anna, University Internal Medicine Unit, Ferrara, Italy

CHIARA SEPE
AORN Antonio Cardarelli Hospital, Naples, Italy

ALEXANDER E. SHERMAN, MD
Clinical Instructor, Division of Pulmonary, Critical Care, Sleep Medicine, Clinical Immunology and Allergy, Health Sciences Clinical Instructor, Department of Medicine, David Geffen School of Medicine at UCLA, Los Angeles, California, USA

ROGERIO SOUZA, MD, PhD
Pulmonary Division - Heart Institute (InCor) Heart Institute (InCor) - Hospital das Clínicas da Faculdade de Medicina da Universidade de São Paulo

RICCARDO SPAGGIARI, MD
Department of Medicine, University Hospital Sant'Anna, University Internal Medicine Unit, Ferrara, Italy

SARA TAMASCELLI
Department of Medicine, University Hospital Sant'Anna, University Internal Medicine Unit, Ferrara, Italy

CARLO GABRIELE TOCCHETTI, MD, PhD, FHFA, FISC
Department of Translational Medical Sciences, Center for Basic and Clinical Immunology Research (CISI), Interdepartmental Center for Clinical and Translational Research (CIRCET), Interdepartmental Hypertension Research Center (CIRIAPA), Federico II University, Naples, Italy

VRUKSHA UPADHYAY, MD
Department of Internal Medicine, Temple University Hospital, Philadelphia, Pennsylvania, USA

VALERIA VALENTE, MD
Department of Translational Medical Sciences, Federico II University, Naples, Italy; Italian Clinical Outcome Research and Reporting Program (I-CORRP)

NEKTARIOS VASILOTTOS, MD
Department of Medicine, Division of Cardiovascular Disease, Indiana University, Indianapolis, Indiana, USA

ANDREA VECCHI, MD
Department of Internal Medicine, University of Genova, Genova, Italy

ALESSANDRA DI VINCENZO, MD
Department of Medicine, University Hospital Sant'Anna, University Internal Medicine Unit, Ferrara, Italy

SCOTT VISOVATTI, MA, MD
Associate Professor, Department of Internal Medicine, Division of Cardiovascular Medicine, Davis Heart and Lung Research Institute, The Ohio State University, Columbus, Ohio, USA

CARMINE DARIO VIZZA, MD
Department of Translational and Precision Medicine, Sapienza University of Rome, Rome, Italy

ALEXANDER ZHEUTLIN, MS, MD
Department of Internal Medicine, University of Utah School of Medicine, Salt Lake City, Utah, USA

Contents

During the sixth World Symposium on Pulmonary Hypertension, the threshold of mean pulmonary arterial pressure (mPAP) for the definition of pulmonary hypertension (PH) has been lowered to a value of greater than 20 mmHg, measured by means of right heart catheterization at rest. In this review, we aim at describing the impact of the new definition of PH, analyzing the available data from the latest scientific literature concerning subjects with mPAP between 21 and 24 mmHg (defined as "mildly elevated PH"), discussing the impact of the new threshold for mPAP in the clinical practice, and highlighting the new perspectives in this field.

Biological sex and sociocultural gender are emerging as pivotal modifiers of health and diseases. Sex-based differences exist in the development, pathogenesis, and management of individuals with pulmonary arterial hypertension (PAH). The interplay between gender domains (ie, identity, roles, relations, and institutionalized gender) and PAH has been barely investigated. The aim of this narrative review is to describe up-to-date evidence on the integration of sex and gender in PAH research, highlighting areas for future investigation.

There are several forms of pulmonary hypertension that can be considered unusual not solely due to their prevalence but also due to their geographic distribution. The aim of this review is to highlight some of these forms, most of them classified within group 5 of the current pulmonary hypertension classification. This review also discusses on schistosomiasis-associated pulmonary hypertension, a prevalent form of pulmonary hypertension mostly limited to developing countries.

Cardiopulmonary exercise testing (CPET) is a comprehensive methodology well studied in pulmonary arterial hypertension (PAH) with roles in diagnosis, treatment response, and prognosis. Submaximal and maximal exercise data is a valuable tool in detecting abnormal hemodynamics associated with exercise-induced and resting pulmonary hypertension as well as right ventricular dysfunction. The increased granularity of CPET may help further risk stratify patients to inform prognosis and better individualize treatment decisions. This article reviews the most commonly implicated variables from CPET in PAH literature and summarizes the latest developments in CPET and exercise testing.

High-altitude pulmonary edema (HAPE) is the main cause of nontraumatic death at high altitude. HAPE development is not only related to the mode and speed of ascent and the maximum altitude reached, but also individual susceptibility plays an important role. In susceptible individuals, hypoxic pulmonary vasoconstriction leads to exaggerated elevated pulmonary arterial pressures and capillary leakage in the lungs. Thus, this review provides an overview of studies investigating the genetic background in HAPE susceptibles by focusing on specific variants, entire genes, genome-wide signatures, or family studies.

Pulmonary hypertension (PH), in particular pulmonary arterial hypertension and chronic thromboembolic PH, burdens patients with relevant morbidity and mortality. The use of oral anticoagulants (OACs) seems able to mitigate the risk of adverse outcomes and death in these patients. Despite scarce evidence, the use of OAC is recommended to treat PH patients, mainly based on observational data. So far, data are still unclear about the impact of direct oral anticoagulant (DOACs), whereas vitamin K antagonists are the main drugs recommended. More data are needed to fully clarify the role of OAC and DOACs in PH patients.

In this review, we discuss the evidence regarding the course and management of COVID-19 in patients with pulmonary arterial hypertension (PAH), the challenges in PAH management during the pandemic and, lastly, the long-term complications of COVID-19 in relation to pulmonary vascular disease. The inherent PAH disease characteristics, as well as age, comorbidities, and the patient's functional status act synergistically to define the prognosis of COVID-19 in patients with PAH. Management of COVID-19 should follow the general guidelines, while PAH-targeted therapies should be continued. The pandemic has caused a shift toward telemedicine in the chronic care of patients with PAH. Whether COVID-19 could predispose to the development of chronic pulmonary hypertension is a subject of future investigation.

Anabolic deficiencies play a pivotal role in left-sided heart failure. Little is known about their impact on idiopathic pulmonary arterial hypertension (iPAH). Therefore, the aim of this study was to assess the impact of multiple hormone-metabolic deficiencies on clinical features and outcomes in idiopathic pulmonary arterial hypertension. We have demonstrated that the assessment of anabolic hormone levels in patients with iPAH allows the identification of a subpopulation with worse exercise capacity, pulmonary hemodynamics, right ventricular size, and function generating the hypothesis about the potential role of hormonal replacement therapy. These data should be confirmed by larger studies.

In recent years, several observations reported that intolerance of physical exertion and other cardinal symptoms in heart failure (HF) are closely related to the functionality of the right ventricular (RV), regardless of left heart. It has been demonstrated that the RV dysfunction complicates the course, aggravates the quality of life, and increases the mortality of HF patients. The present review is aimed to report tips physicians about the current therapeutic management of right HF during acute stage and chronic phase, shedding light on the RV and its failure and providing physicians with essential information for everyday clinical practice.

Several microRNAs and long noncoding RNAs contribute to pulmonary arterial hypertension (PAH) pathogenesis by impairing nitric oxide production, enhancing proliferation and migration and decreasing apoptosis of smooth muscle cells, and promoting endothelial-to-mesenchymal transition in pulmonary arteries. These noncoding RNAs (ncRNAs) could serve as both biomarkers and therapeutic targets for PAH. Nonetheless, the knowledge about their role in PAH is still incomplete. Furthermore, ncRNAs may vary across species and often act differently in different tissues and organs, and technical issues currently limit the implementation of ncRNA-based technologies. Additional studies are warranted to finally bring ncRNA into the clinical arena.

HEART FAILURE CLINICS

HEART FAILURE CLINICS

SERIES OF RELATED INTEREST

Cardiology Clinics
http://www.cardiology.theclinics.com
Cardiac Electrophysiology Clinics
https://www.cardiacep.theclinics.com
Interventional Cardiology Clinics
http://www.interventional.theclinics.com

THE CLINICS ARE AVAILABLE ONLINE!
Access your subscription at
www.theclinics.com

Preface
Challenges in Pulmonary Hypertension

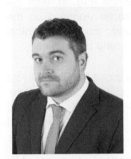
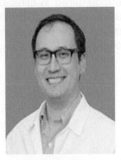
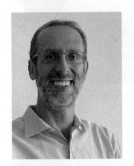
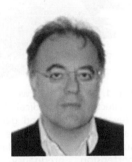

Alberto M. Marra, MD, PhD, FEFIM

Alexander E. Sherman, MD

Pietro Ameri, MD, PhD, FAHA

Eduardo Bossone, MD, PhD, FACC, FESC

Editors

Pulmonary hypertension (PH) is a clinical condition that has gained mounting attention in the last two decades. The development of several effective drugs has led to a remarkable improvement in quality of life and prognosis of patients with pulmonary arterial hypertension (PAH), which in fact is no longer considered an orphan disease as it was in the 1990s. However, there are several outstanding diagnostic and therapeutic issues that need to be addressed by clinical research in PAH and other forms of PH. This issue of *Heart Failure Clinics* includes a series of reviews on burning problems in the field of PH. Moreover, interesting original preliminary data regarding PH diagnosis and therapy are presented. In the opening article, the group of Marra and colleagues discusses the topic of mildly elevated PH, taking into account the new lower threshold of 20 mmHg for the diagnosis of PH. Next, Pilote and collaborators provide an overview on PH in women, bringing gender medicine into PH. Unusual PH forms (such as schistosomiasis, sarcoidosis, veno-occlusive disease, Langerhans cell histiocytosis, and hemoglobinopathies) are addressed by Souza and colleagues in their review. This contribution is of utmost importance considering that these patients are underrepresented in clinical trials. The cardiopulmonary exercise test is an important tool to assess treatment response and prognosis in PH, and Sherman and Saggar describe all the meaningful information that can be gathered by this technique. Visovatti covers the diagnostic and therapeutic issues regarding PAH associated with connective tissue diseases others than systemic sclerosis. Portopulmonary hypertension is another relevant PAH form in which the decision making regarding liver transplant is usually challenging, and this is the object of the article by Jose and colleagues. In their original work, Upadhyay and colleagues report intriguing data on microscopic examination of clots from percutaneous mechanical embolectomies in pulmonary embolism (PE). They analyzed 13 thrombectomy aspirates from patients with acute PE and determined the age of the clots according to histologic characteristics. Patients with "younger" thrombi had higher initial oxygen requirement, while those with "older" PE tended to require long-term oxygen therapy. Mei and colleagues discuss critical aspects of PH during pregnancy, from preconception to risk stratification through pregnancy and postpartum. The German group headed by Eichstaedt and colleagues presents an interesting overview of the genetic background of high-altitude pulmonary edema. Oral anticoagulation has long been a mainstay of supportive therapy in idiopathic PAH, and it is mandatory in chronic thromboembolic PH. This topic is covered by Demelo-Rodriguez and colleagues in their article. The COVID-19 pandemic impacted dramatically on the health care system worldwide. The questions of how to manage PAH patients during COVID-19 and whether COVID-19 may lead to future development of PH are answered by Giannakoulas and Farmakis. A preliminary report regarding the hormonal abnormalities in PAH is

Heart Failure Clin 19 (2023) xv–xvi
https://doi.org/10.1016/j.hfc.2022.10.001

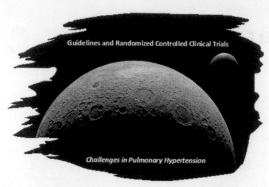

Guidelines and Randomized Controlled Clinical Trials

Challenges in Pulmonary Hypertension

Fig. 1. In this issue, we covered PH topics commonly neglected by medical literature, including mildly elevated PH, sex and gender issues, unusual forms, cardiopulmonary exercise testing, rarer connective tissue diseases, liver transplant and portopulmonary hypertension, pregnancy, high-altitude pulmonary edema, anticoagulation, COVID-19, right-ventricular failure, noncoding RNAs, and novel research regarding embolectomy specimens and hormonal abnormalities in PH. Such issues are like the dark side of the moon, something usually not seen by observers from the earth. (*Modified from* Wright E. The Moon's Far Side. February 12, 2015. https://svs.gsfc.nasa.gov/11747.)

provided by Marra and colleagues. According to this study, patients presenting two or more hormonal deficiencies (testosterone, Dehydroepiandrosterone sulfate, insulin-like growth factor-1, insulin resistance, and thyroid hormones) cluster in a subgroup with worse exercise capacity, pulmonary hemodynamics, and right-ventricular size and function, generating the hypothesis that hormonal replacement therapy may be useful. Cittadini and colleagues overview the occurrence of

right-ventricular failure and its management. In the last article of this issue, Ameri and colleagues address the emerging topic of noncoding RNAs in PH.

In conclusion, this issue brings attention to novel or unsolved aspects of PH that are commonly encountered in clinical practice (**Fig. 1**), with the ambition of keeping the reader updated on the main lines of research and, possibly, clinical changes in the challenging arena of PH.

Alberto M. Marra, MD, PhD, FEFIM
Department of Translational Medical Sciences
"Federico II" School of Medicine and
University Hospital
Naples, Italy

Alexander E. Sherman, MD
Department of Medicine
David Geffen School of Medicine at UCLA
Los Angeles, CA, USA

Pietro Ameri, MD, PhD, FAHA
Cardiovascular Disease Unit
IRCCS Ospedale Policlinico San Martino
Department of Internal Medicine
University of Genova
Genova, Italy

Eduardo Bossone, MD, PhD, FACC, FESC
Department of Public Health
"Federico II" University of Naples
Naples, Italy

E-mail addresses:
alberto_marra@hotmail.it
albertomaria.marra@unina.it

Mildly Elevated Pulmonary Hypertension
Gray Zone or Already a Disease?

Alberto M. Marra, MD, PhD[a,b,1], Umberto Attanasio, MD[a,1],
Alessandra Cuomo, MD[a], Carmen Rainone, MD[a], Anna D'Agostino, PhD[c],
Antonio Carannante, MD[a], Andrea Salzano, MD, PhD[c],
Eduardo Bossone, MD, PhD[d], Antonio Cittadini, MD, PhD[a],
Carlo Gabriele Tocchetti, MD, PhD, FHFA, FISC[a,e,f,g],
Valentina Mercurio, MD, PhD, FISC[a,f,*]

KEYWORDS

- Mildly elevated pulmonary hypertension • Pulmonary arterial hypertension • Hemodynamics
- Pulmonary vascular disease • Pulmonary vasodilators

KEY POINTS

- The sixth World Symposium on Pulmonary Hypertension (WSPH) proposed to lower mean pulmonary arterial pressure (mPAP) threshold from 25 mmHg or greater to greater than 20 mmHg, extending pulmonary vascular resistance (PVR) 3 WU or greater as cutoff for precapillary disease, whereas maintaining pulmonary artery wedge pressure (PAWP) 15 mmHg or lesser threshold for the same purpose.
- The new definition bares a new group of pulmonary arterial hypertension (PAH) patients with a mild elevation of mPAP between 21 and 24 mmHg, which has an increased risk of disease progression and higher mortality but very few/close to no randomized controlled trials' (RCT) validated therapeutic options.
- The sixth WSPH made the choice of reconsidering one of the hemodynamic parameters (mPAP) threshold based on latest evidences but conservatively remaining other parameters untouched. Similarly, we may expect PAWP and PVR thresholds to change in the years to come.
- Despite the changes, thanks to the strict precapillary cut-offs, the incidence of new diagnosis that can be accounted to the new mPAP threshold, within PAH patients, is expected to be modest.
- The decisions discussed during the sixth WSPH animated a vivid and constructive debate within PH scientific community. Despite discordant opinions, there is large consent on the urgent need of interventional RCT on mildly elevated PH patients.

INTRODUCTION

Pulmonary hypertension (PH) is a clinical condition that can have different causes and pathophysiological mechanisms. PH can primarily be caused by a chronic and progressive adverse remodeling of pulmonary arterioles, known as precapillary PH, or can be a

[a] Department of Translational Medical Sciences, Federico II University, Naples, Italy; [b] Centre for Pulmonary Hypertension, Thoraxklinik Heidelberg gGmbH at Heidelberg University Hospital, Translational Lung Research Center Heidelberg (TLRC), German Center for Lung Research (DZL), Heidelberg, Germany; [c] IRCCS SDN Nuclear and Diagnostic Research Institute, Naples, Italy; [d] Division of Cardiology, A Cardarelli Hospital, Naples 80131, Italy; [e] Center for Basic and Clinical Immunology Research (CISI), Federico II University, Naples 80131, Italy; [f] Interdepartmental Center for Clinical and Translational Research (CIRCET), Federico II University, Naples, Italy; [g] Interdepartmental Hypertension Research Center (CIRIAPA), Federico II University, Naples, Italy

[1] These authors share first authorship.

* Corresponding author. Department of Translational Medical Sciences, Federico II University, Via Sergio Pansini, 5, Naples 80131, Italy.

E-mail address: valentina.mercurio@unina.it

Heart Failure Clin 19 (2023) 1–9
https://doi.org/10.1016/j.hfc.2022.08.013

complication of left-sided heart diseases, being in this case postcapillary PH, or it can involve both arterioles and venules, known as combined precapillary and postcapillary PH. According to the current World Health Organization (WHO) classification, PH can be classified into 5 clinical groups: Group 1 PH, precapillary PH, characterized by a primary remodeling of pulmonary arterioles, named "pulmonary arterial hypertension" (PAH); Group 2, postcapillary PH secondary to left heart diseases; Group 3, precapillary PH secondary to lung diseases; Group 4, including chronic thromboembolic PH; and Group 5, comprising a miscellany of underlying diseases, such as hematological disorders, or systemic and metabolic disorders.[1] Despite being the characterization of PH based on several diagnostic tools, its final diagnosis is based on hemodynamics, and right heart catheterization (RHC) is the gold standard for PH classification. The hemodynamic definition of PH has been basically the same since the WHO Meeting of Geneva in 1973[2] but different authors demonstrated that normal mean pulmonary arterial pressure (mPAP) values are far lower than 25 mmHg (the actual cutoff for PH, according to 2015 ESC/ERS guidelines). In 2018, during the sixth World Symposium on Pulmonary Hypertension (WSPH) held in Nice, it has been proposed to redefine the mPAP diagnostic threshold measured by means of RHC at rest to establish the presence of PH, lowering this value from 25 mmHg or greater to less than 20 mmHg.[3] Furthermore, it has also been discussed how to better define and identify the presence of a pulmonary vascular disease, which, beside the mPAP values, should include the measurement of pulmonary vascular resistance (PVR). This new definition implicates the emergence of a cluster of subjects who did not fulfill the previous definition of PH but that show a mild increase of mPAP that may suggest the presence of an initial pulmonary vascular disease.

During the past 2 decades, different studies have led to novel therapeutic approaches for the treatment of PH but it is still burden by limited treatment choices and poor prognosis.[4] PH clinical management differs according to its underlying cause, being the pharmacologic approach with pulmonary vasodilators mostly effective for Group 1 and Group 4 PH. PAH specific treatment focuses on the targeting of NO, endothelin, and prostacyclin pathways, which are widely impaired in PAH patients. Notably, to date, all the clinical trials that led to the commercialization of the drugs for PAH did enroll patients with mPAP 25 mmHg or greater, so there is a lot of uncertainty about how to manage clinically and therapeutically the subjects in the "buffer zone" with abnormal mPAP ranging from 21 to 24 mmHg.

In this review, we aim at describing the impact of the new definition of PH as introduced in 2018 by the sixth WSPH, analyzing the available data from the latest scientific literature concerning subjects with mPAP between 21 and 24 mmHg, discussing the impact of the new threshold for mPAP in the clinical practice, and highlighting the new perspectives in this field.

A Glimpse to the New Definition of Pulmonary Hypertension and Pulmonary Vascular Disease

During the sixth WSPH, held in Nice in 2018, it has been proposed to redefine the mPAP diagnostic threshold measured by means of RHC at rest to determine the presence of PH, lowering this value from 25 mmHg or greater to lesser than 20 mmHg.[3] Such proposal arises as a consequence of the growing evidence that populations presenting even a mild elevation in mPAP are associated with an increased risk of disease progression and higher mortality,[5–8] along with the recent publication of a comprehensive pooled analysis performed by Kovacs *and colleagues* on RHC values obtained from healthy individuals, showing that the normal value of mPAP is 14 ± 3 mmHg. Therefore, considering 2 standard deviations above this mean value, the upper limit of normality (above the 97.5th percentile) would ultimately be placed at 20 mmHg.[9] Such evidence can be considered a milestone in the scientific and clinical approach to the whole spectrum of diseases related directly or collaterally with an increase in pressures of pulmonary circulation, although it is still a matter of intense debate throughout PH research and clinical community.[10–13] This is particularly true since this threshold had remained (almost) untouched since the year 1973, when the limit of mPAP greater than 25 mmHg was arbitrarily stated during the first WSPH, as this decision was originally taken being aware that this value does not normally exceed 20 mmHg.[2] **Table 1** summarizes how the hemodynamic definition of PH has changed over time. This definition created a sort of "buffer zone" that has been accepted through the years in order to protect patients from a premature diagnosis that could have had an immediate and dramatic psychological impact on patients and their families. That zone comprehends subjects with a mPAP of 21 to 24 mmHg, a cluster population with abnormal pulmonary hemodynamics that did not fulfill the older definition of PH. This condition has been often referred in the past as "borderline

Table 1
Summary of the different hemodynamic definitions of pulmonary hypertension over the years

Hemodynamic Definition	First WSPH Geneva 1973	Second WSPH Evian 1998	Third WSPH Venice 2003	Fourth WSPH Dana Point 2008	Fifth WSPH Nice 2013	Sixth WSPH Nice 2018
mPAP	>25 mmHg at rest or >30 mm Hg with exertion	No change	No change	≥25 mmHg at rest (Exercise PH removed)	No change	>20 mm Hg at rest
POST-CAPILLARY PH PAWP THRESHOLD	≥12 mmHg	No change	≥15 mmHg	No change	No change	No change
PVR THRESHOLD	Not mentioned	Not mentioned	>3 WU for PAH definition	Removed	>3 WU for PAH definition	≥3 WU for precapillary PH

PH," and more recently addressed as "mildly elevated PH." When looking at the scientific literature, there is a huge heterogeneity in the definition of this population because different cutoffs have been used for the identification of the lower limit of PAP, varying from 19 to 21 mmHg.[14,15] Of note, it should be considered that a single value of mPAP used alone is not accurate enough to characterize a clinical condition because mPAP could be mildly increased in different conditions that not necessarily refer to a primary pulmonary vascular disease, such as in case of high cardiac output (CO), or left-to-right cardiac shunts, or even left heart diseases.

Given these premises, in the attempt to stick to the new definition of PH, to provide a proper definition of "mildly elevated PH" as an actual pathologic entity, also other hemodynamic measures need to be considered: pulmonary artery wedge pressure (PAWP), CO, and PVR calculated with the following formula: (mPAP − PAWP)/CO. Indeed, the use of mPAP alone cannot define a clinical condition and does not identify a pathologic condition *per se*. Therefore, according to the latest news from the sixth WSPH, PVR of 3 WU or greater is now required to define the presence of a pulmonary vascular disease. Both PAWP and PVR overwent the course of WSPHs as well, being PAWP set as threshold for left heart disease PH indicator when greater than 12 mmHg during the first WSPH in 1973, then increased to greater than 15 mmHg during the third WSPH in 2003, and then remained untouched, and PVR introduced after the third WSPH as an added criterion for definition of PAH when greater than 3 WU, being subsequently removed and then added

back, until lately has been set as an added criterion to all precapillary forms of PH when PVR of 3 WU or greater, during the sixth WSPH in 2018 (see **Table 1**).[3,11] To summarize, with the new definition we can differentiate among mildly elevated (mPAP 21–24 mmHg) precapillary (PAWP 15 mmHg or lesser, PVR 3 WU or greater), isolated postcapillary (PAWP greater than 15 mmHg, PVR lesser than 3 WU), and combined precapillary and postcapillary (PAWP greater than 15 mmHg, PVR 3 WU or greater) PH.

As said, the proposals made during the sixth WSPH, promoted a heated debate, not only about the mPAP cutoff being changed but also about other thresholds not being addressed. Although some appreciated the task-force evidence-based decision about using 20 mmHg as new cutoff of mPAP, others concerned about losing that "buffering zone," warned about the possibility of overdiagnosing PH. However, other experts claimed that including PVR of 3 WU or greater would be a limit to the new definition of PH, considering that evidences show that normal PVR are usually within 2 WU, making the new mPAP threshold only a slight change in the overall diagnosis of PH.[10–13] The assessment of PVR can be quite complex and hardly influenced by the precise and accurate measurement of CO and PAWP, being the latter one of the trickiest to properly obtain during RHC. In addition, although PVR tend to be higher for elevated mPAP, in the context of a mildly elevated PH, where mPAP stands between 21 and 24 mmHg, a combination of low CO and/or low PAWP, it is required to obtain the diagnosis of precapillary mildly elevated PH,[10–12] leading to a very low number of new diagnosis and shifting

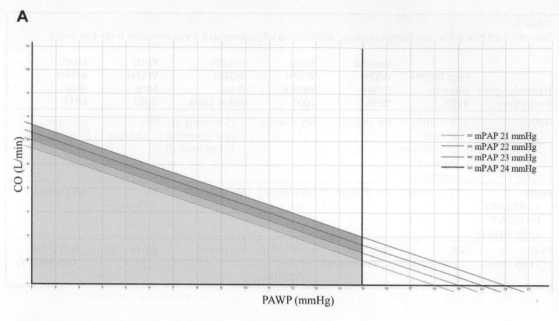

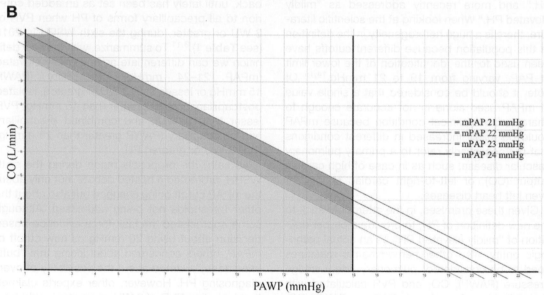

Fig. 1. (*A*) Combinations of CO and PAWP resulting in a PVR of 3 WU or greater for mPAP ranging from 21 to 24 mmHg. (*B*) Combinations of CO and PAWP resulting in a PVR greater than 2 WU for mean mPAP ranging from 21 to 24 mmHg. We drew the lines of **Fig. 1**, based on the equation: PVR= (PAPm − PAWP)/CO that is used to determine PVR for a set of PAWP, mPAP, and CO combinations. By setting a determined mPAP (21, 22, 23, and 24 mmHg, respectively) and a fixed PVR (3 WU for Panel A and 2 WU for Panel B), we obtained a linear function that returns the exact combinations of PAWP (X variable) and CO (Y variable) for fixed values of PVR and mPAP. The area under the curve represents the group of combinations of PAWP and CO for each value of mPAP, which will determine a PVR superior to the set value, whereas the area above the curve represents the group of combinations that will determine a PVR inferior to the set value. The black line corresponds to a PWAP of 15 mmHg. GeoGebra web software was used to draw the graphs.

that "buffering zone" from the mPAP variable to the PVR one.[12,16] The Panel A of **Fig. 1** shows the possible combinations of CO and PAWP resulting in a PVR of 3 WU or greater for mPAP ranging from 21 to 24 mm Hg. Finally, others pointed out the controversial about the task-force of sixth WSPH changing mPAP threshold for the sake of an evidence-based approach, whereas leaving unaltered the cutoffs of PAWP and PVR, because those were originally decided arbitrary as well, and having some evidences of their upper limit of normal being 12 mmHg instead of 15 mmHg[17] and 2 WU instead of 3 WU,[3,9,18] respectively.[10,12,19] The Panel B of **Fig. 1** shows the possible combinations of CO and PAWP resulting in a PVR greater than 2 WU for mPAP ranging from 21 to 24 mmHg. Speaking of PVR, particular attention has been addressed to this parameter because it has been thought to be a key factor that allows to discriminate between an elevation of mPAP due to pulmonary vascular disease from one due to an increase of PAWP.[3] Still, the concern of using an arbitrary cutoff for PVR, summed up to the disappointment of this threshold limiting in efficacy the updated classification on new diagnosis and early recognition of the early stages of this disease[20] and to awareness that Group 1 patients presenting mildly elevated PH and 2 or lesser PVR less than 3 WU retain an increased mortality to the one with PVR of 3 WU or greater, being unlikely that pulmonary vascular disease may drive mortality alone in those patients, especially when RV afterload is not substantially altered.[11,21,22] However, the experts of the task force cleared out that using 3 WU or greater as PVR cutoff was a conservative choice,[3] being already considered a clinically relevant indicator of significant pulmonary vascular disease in different clinical settings such as the decision process of correction of congenital systemic-to-pulmonary shunts[1] or as in the patient prognosis assessment after heart transplantation.[23]

The Clinical Impact of the New Definition of Pulmonary Hypertension

As said, one of the reasons behind the changes proposed during sixth WSPH, was the crescent evidence that, when compared with subjects with normal mPAP (<20 mmHg), patients with mildly elevated PH present an increased mortality[14,15,24,25] and are at higher risk of progression to an mPAP of 25 mmHg or greater. In particular, this has been demonstrated in cohorts of patients at risk of developing PH, such as patients with systemic sclerosis (SSc),[5,26] and in a pooled analysis of mixed population (including the PHARAOS registry, people without left heart or respiratory disease, and SSc patients).[15] In an elegant metanalysis, Xue and colleagues confirmed the increased risk of progression to PH and mortality than those with a normal PAP in subjects with mildly elevated PH analyzing the results from 8 large studies. The selected studies were either retrospective and prospective, enrolling heterogenous groups of patients for a total

of 2015 patients (802 subjects with normal PAP, 880 PH patients, and 333 with mildly elevated PAP). Assad and colleagues,[27] Kovacs and colleagues, [28] and Douschan and colleagues[25] included patients who underwent RHC for clinical indication (including patients with overt heart and lung diseases), Bae and colleagues,[7] Valerio and colleagues,[5] Coghlan and colleagues,[26] and Xanthouli and colleagues[29] included SSc patients at high-risk of developing PAH (including patients in the PHARAOS study), Heresi and colleagues[30] included patients sent to RHC with clinical indication but with no lung or left heart disease, whereas Nemoto and colleagues[31] included patients with overt interstitial lung disease but no PAH associated to connective tissue disease.

Moreover, as claimed by the sixth WSPH task force itself, by including PVR in the novel definition of PH they aimed at changing the definition of pulmonary vascular disease, considering that mPAP alone is not sufficient to identify such complex pathologic entity. Indeed, the task force underlined the need for a revolution in PH definition, considering that recent data suggest that mildly elevated PAP are associated with higher disease progression by means of PH development and higher mortality risk, leading to the recognition of mildly elevated PH as an early stage of the disease.[32] When discussing clinical impact and management options of the potentially new patients diagnosed with mildly elevated PH among all clinical groups of PH classification, it becomes clear that, beyond Group 1 (PAH), no other PH group clinical and therapeutic management will likely be affected by those changes in PH definition.[32] Indeed, Group 2 and Group 3 patients are not eligible for specific PH treatment, and the lower mPAP threshold will not change their standard of care.[1] Similarly, the lower mPAP threshold may indeed lead to a reclassification of patients from chronic thromboembolic disease without PH (CTED) to a new diagnosis of chronic thromboembolic PH (CTEPH) but being the gold standard treatment (pulmonary endarterectomy) recommended both for CTED and CTEPH when operable, revised definition is not expected to change the clinical course of these patients.[1,00,04]

On the contrary, the updated definition might have a consistent impact on the early identification of Group 1 patients. Nevertheless, because initial symptoms of PH are nonspecific, it is more likely that a confirmed diagnosis will eventually be made when the disease is already at advanced stage.[35] Accordingly, the novel PH definition will more likely affect the early diagnosis in population at high-risk of developing PH and therefore already included in screening programs, such as SSc patients and subject at risk of developing heritable PAH.[1]

Concerning the SSc population, which is one of the most explored population at risk of developing different forms of PH,[36] it represents probably the vastest data pool due to the screening algorithms already in use. Bae and coworkers[5] demonstrated that mildly elevated PH is associated with increased lung fibrosis on high-resolution CT (HRCT). In another study from Valerio *and colleagues*, SSc patients with mildly elevated PH are more prone to develop a manifest PH than patients with normal mPAP.[5] A post hoc analysis of the DETECT data showed that patients with SSc and borderline pressures represent a continuum between normal lung circulation and frank PH, with regards to clinical variable (number of telangiectasias), and also in terms of pulmonary vascular resistance. Recently, it was demonstrated in a monocentric retrospective cohort of 4343 patients (not only SSc) that borderline mPAP is associated with an increased risk to develop a manifest PH over time.[37] According to a large retrospective study performed in the United States on all veterans (including 21,727 subjects) undergoing RHC between 2007 and 2012, the presence of mildly elevated PH confers a 23% increased risk of death with respect to normal mPAP values. This finding was recently confirmed by a prospective study performed in Austria on 547 patients. In this study, mildly elevated PH was associated with poor outcome (hazard ratio: 2.37, 95% confidence interval: 1.14–4.97 [$P = .022$]).[25] On the basis of such evidence, mildly elevated PH might be considered as an early stage of disease with initial involvement of pulmonary vessels, with an increased risk to develop PH and consequently poorer outcomes when compared with patients with normal hemodynamics. However, this clinical subgroup needs to be better characterized, in order to implement future therapeutic approach, which in turn might grant beneficial effects and maybe delay the progression of the disease. This concept was also underlined by the fifth world symposium on PH (76), as well as by the ESC/ERS guidelines (103), both emphasizing further research to better phenotype this cluster of patients.

Jaafar *and colleagues*, retrospectively, analyzed the hemodynamic parameters of SSc patients screened for PAH at the University of Michigan, to assess the impact of the updated PH definition, including data on the reclassification of patients from not having PH to having PH according to the novel definition.[25] Interestingly, they found that out of the 131 patients with no PH according to the prior PH classification, only 4 of them were reclassified to precapillary mildly elevated PH (3 with Group 3 PH and 1 with Group 1 PAH, whereas 3 more patients were reclassified as postcapillary mildly elevated PH). Thus, the authors concluded that the impact of the updated definition was insignificant, given that only 5% of non-PH population was reclassified as mildly elevated PH and only 0.7% of said population had PAH. Of note, within the 124 patients that did not meet the PH diagnostic criteria according to the updated classification, 76 presented mPAP greater than 20 mmHg and 45 had mildly elevated PH (mPAP 21–24 mmHg), associated to PAWP 15 mmHg or greater, and PVR less than 3 WU. Moreover, 7 of the latest had 2 or lesser PVR less than 3 WU. Considering that normal PVR do not exceed 2 WU, the authors conclude that lowering PVR threshold at 2 WU or greater would have a greater influence on PH diagnosis.

Similar results come from another study that included 284 SSc patients, where only 1.4% had a combination of mildly elevated PH (present in 19.3% of the whole population when considered alone), PAWP of 15 mmHg or lesser and PVR of 3 WU or lesser. Such percentage grows up to 9.8% when considering PVR 2 WU or lesser as an alternative cutoff for the identification of precapillary mildly elevated PH.[29] However, another study found a greater impact of the updated PH definition, probably due to an overrepresentation of patients with mildly elevated PH due to different screening strategies used by their centers.[38]

Furthermore, data from literature indicate that most of patients presenting with mPAP 21 to 24 mmHg are older and present cardiac or lung comorbidities, suggesting that most of subjects with mildly elevated mPAP might be classified as Group 2 or Group 3 PH.[16]

Finally, the question on whether patients with 21 to 24.9 mmHg mPAP will progress to overt PH, and the latency of such eventual progression, remains unanswered.

Mildly elevated pulmonary hypertension: to treat or not to treat, that is the question

One of the greatest concerns that emerged after sixth WSPH is that currently there is no data suggesting whether treatment in patients with mildly elevated PH could or should be commenced. Because no randomized controlled trials that led to the approvals of what we now acknowledge as the standard of care in PAH treatment included patients with mPAP of 21 to 24 mmHg, some experts are worried about the medical and ethical implications of having to make such an impactful diagnosis of PAH in patients that could not benefit from an approved therapy, until they may worsen to overt PAH or until new RTCs get to be completed.[10,11] Others even speculated that patients and their families may push to start off-label treatments that, in turn, may lead to difficult interpretations of the results (eg, considering therapeutic success at follow-up a patient whose mPAP remains in the 21–24 mmHg range, without having the RTCs rigorous group-control setup[12]). However, the fact that there is no approved therapy for a given condition should not influence *per se* the definition of a disease. Conversely evidence about a harmful condition should drive the diagnostic workup choice and the seek for the therapeutic options in the scientific community.

As said, until now, very little has been explored about the possibility of using PAH standard of care medications' in mildly elevated Group 1 PH. A small prospective, randomized, double-blind, placebo-controlled, investigator-initiated phase IIA clinical trial assessed the efficacy of ambrisentan of mPAP in patients with SSc and mildly elevated PH.[39] The study enrolled 38 patients with SSc and mildly elevated PH defined as rest mPAP 21 to 24 mmHg and PAWP less than 15 mmHg or exercise mPAP greater than 30 mmHg, exercise PAWP less than 18 mmHg, and transpulmonary gradient (calculated as mPAP – PAWP) greater than 15mm Hg. Patients were then randomized 1:1 in 2 groups of 19, and a total of 6 did not complete the study (2 in the ambrisentan arm and 4 in the placebo arm). Of note, 4 patients in the placebo arm and 8 in the ambrisentan arm were included for the exercise mPAP greater than 30 mmHg criteria alone, having a rest mPAP less than 21 mmHg, not meeting the updated definition of PH, that do not consider exercise criteria at all. Furthermore, because during the conduction of the study the PVR criterion was not yet implemented in previous WSPH, it was not used as an inclusion criterion, being mean and standard deviations of the entire population 2.16 ± 0.78 WU. After 6 months, the 2 groups did not show a significant difference mPAP, which was the primary endpoint but significant improvements in cardiac index (CI), CO, and PVR, that were registered within secondary endpoints. Furthermore, 3 patients from the placebo group and none from the ambrisentan arm progressed to SSc-associated PAH, even though, placebo group had a significantly longer duration of SSc disease in respect of ambrisentan arm. Finally, at the end of the study, even though the difference between groups was not significant, the mean length of 6-minute walking distance improved

in the ambrisentan arm, whereas decreased in the placebo group.[39]

At the best of our knowledge, at this moment, apart from this latter study and 2 small uncontrolled open-label reports, exploring the use of ambrisentan and bosentan in patients with exercise PH and rest mPAP less than 25 mmHg,[40,41] reliable data on the effects of PAH standard of care drugs in mildly elevated PH are actually a prominent lack that heavily limits the therapeutic possibilities in this specific and recently introduced condition. However, despite the evidence of mildly elevated PH being an abnormal condition, characterized by worse outcomes was already there, still almost no RCT had explored the therapeutic possibilities in this population of patients until sixth WSPH. Moreover, although the debate on many aspects of the updated classification still divides the PH community, there is a dominant agreement that RCT in those select groups are now extremely needed.[10–12,20,32] The choices made within the sixth WSPH about the updated classification may represent themselves an additional drive to the design and implementations of new interventional RCT on mildly elevated PH populations.

SUMMARY

The heated debate that started at the sixth WSPH in Nice 2018 is far from being set aside. The decision to lower mPAP threshold was significantly questioned but was also made on scientific evidence. Since its first definition in 1973, different experts have argued the 25 mmHg cutoff for being too arbitrary. However, another long question was resolved during the sixth WSPH, considering that PVR are finally part of the definition of precapillary PH. Since 2008, at almost every WSPH, the question on whether PVR should be part of the PH definition was risen but each time experts of the task force decided to leave it aside. It seems that in the last WSPH, PVR 3 WU or greater was included in the precapillary PH definition as part of a "safety net" to avoid overdiagnosis. It is well known that the estimation of PVR during RHC is one of the most sensitive parts of the diagnostic process and PVR might be influenced by left atrial pressure, the anemic status, and heart rate.

As previously discussed, the new definition will not have a significant impact of Group 2 and Group 3 patients, considering that there is no available treatment of such patients. Concerning Group 4 patients, even if some will be reconsidered as having CTEPH instead of CTED, their clinical management will not change from a therapeutic standpoint, considering that thromboendoarterectomy is the treatment gold standard for CTED patients as well. This leaves the question open only for Group 1 PAH patients. On one hand, this new definition might lightly increase PAH diagnosis but should affect mostly patients already in screening for PAH, such as patients with SSc or at risk of developing hereditable PAH. On the other hand, the new definition will be a stimulus for pharmaceutical companies and clinicians to explore whether common PAH-specific drugs might be helpful in this setting. In particular, it is not yet clear if mildly elevated mPAP is an intermediate condition between PH and normal pulmonary pressure, or if it is a condition *per se* with a different progression than PH. This new definition might open a new door for the understanding of pulmonary vascular disease.

CLINICS CARE POINTS

- The new definition from the sixth World Symposium on Pulmonary Hypertension bares a new group of pulmonary arterial hypertension patients with a mild elevation of mean pulmonary arterial pressure between 21 and 24 mmHg, who did not fulfill the previous definition of pulmonary hypertension.
- Such population has an increased risk of disease progression and higher mortality.
- To date, very few/close to no randomized controlled clinical trials on a possible validated therapeutic approach is available.
- The decision whether to treat or not patients with mildly elevated pulmonary hypertension is a matter of debate.
- There is large consent on the urgent need of interventional RTCs on this new population.

REFERENCES

1. Galiè N, Humbert M, Vachiery JL, et al. 2015 ESC/ERS Guidelines for the diagnosis and treatment of pulmonary hypertension: The Joint Task Force for the Diagnosis and Treatment of Pulmonary Hypertension of the European Society of Cardiology (ESC) and the European Respiratory Society (ERS): Endorsed by: Association for European Paediatric and Congenital Cardiology (AEPC), International Society for Heart and Lung Transplantation (ISHLT). Eur Heart J 2016;37(1):67–119.

2. Hatano S, Strasser T, Organization WH. Primary pulmonary hypertension: Report on a WHO meeting. Geneva: World Health Organization; 1975. p. 15.

3. Simonneau G, Montani D, Celermajer DS, et al. Haemodynamic definitions and updated clinical classification of pulmonary hypertension. Eur Respir J 2019;53(1):1801913.

4. Mercurio V, Bianco A, Campi G, et al. New Drugs, Therapeutic Strategies, and Future Direction for the Treatment of Pulmonary Arterial Hypertension. Curr Med Chem 2019;26(16):2844–64.

5. Valerio CJ, Schreiber BE, Handler CE, et al. Borderline mean pulmonary artery pressure in patients with systemic sclerosis: Transpulmonary gradient predicts risk of developing pulmonary hypertension. Arthritis Rheum 2013;65(4):1074–84.

6. Kovacs G, Maier R, Aberer E, et al. Borderline Pulmonary Arterial Pressure Is Associated with Decreased Exercise Capacity in Scleroderma. Am J Respir Crit Care Med 2009;180(9):881–6.

7. Bae S, Saggar R, Bolster MB, et al. Baseline characteristics and follow-up in patients with normal haemodynamics versus borderline mean pulmonary arterial pressure in systemic sclerosis: results from the PHAROS registry. Ann Rheum Dis 2012;71(8):1335–42.

8. Stamm A, Saxer S, Lichtblau M, et al. Exercise pulmonary haemodynamics predict outcome in patients with systemic sclerosis. Eur Respir J 2016;48(6):1658–67.

9. Kovacs G, Berghold A, Scheidl S, et al. Pulmonary arterial pressure during rest and exercise in healthy subjects: a systematic review. Eur Respir J 2009;34(4):888–94.

10. Kovacs G, Olschewski H. Debating the new haemodynamic definition of pulmonary hypertension: Much ado about nothing? Eur Respir J 2019;54(2):10–2.

11. Brusca SB, Zou Y, Elinoff JM. How low should we go? Potential benefits and ramifications of the pulmonary hypertension hemodynamic definitions proposed by the 6th World Symposium. Curr Opin Pulm Med 2020;26(5):384–90.

12. Gibbs JSR, Torbicki A. Proposed new pulmonary hypertension definition: is 4 mm(Hg) worth re-writing medical textbooks? Eur Respir J 2019;53(3):1900197.

13. Hoeper MM, Humbert M. The new haemodynamic definition of pulmonary hypertension: Evidence prevails, finally. Eur Respir J 2019;53(3):3–6.

14. Kolte D, Lakshmanan S, Jankowich MD, et al. Mild pulmonary hypertension is associated with increased mortality: A systematic review and meta-analysis. J Am Heart Assoc 2018;7(18):1–13.

15. Xue L, Yang Y, Sun B, et al. Mildly Elevated Pulmonary Arterial Pressure Is Associated With a High Risk of Progression to Pulmonary Hypertension and Increased Mortality: A Systematic Review and Meta-Analysis. J Am Heart Assoc 2021;10(7):e018374.

16. Jaafar S, Visovatti S, Young A, et al. Impact of the revised haemodynamic definition on the diagnosis

of pulmonary hypertension in patients with systemic sclerosis. Eur Respir J 2019;54(2):1900586.

17. Vachiéry JL, Tedford RJ, Rosenkranz S, et al. Pulmonary hypertension due to left heart disease. Eur Respir J 2019;53(1):1801897.

18. Kovacs G, Olschewski A, Berghold A, et al. Pulmonary vascular resistances during exercise in normal subjects: a systematic review. Eur Respir J 2012; 39(2):319–28.

19. Hoeper MM, Bogaard HJ, Condliffe R, et al. Definitions and Diagnosis of Pulmonary Hypertension. J Am Coll Cardiol 2013;62(25):D42–50.

20. Kovacs G, Zeder K, Rosenstock P, et al. Clinical Impact of the New Definition of Precapillary Pulmonary Hypertension. Chest 2021;159(5):1995–7.

21. Nagel C, Marra AM, Benjamin N, et al. Reduced Right Ventricular Output Reserve in Patients With Systemic Sclerosis and Mildly Elevated Pulmonary Artery Pressure. Arthritis Rheum 2019;71(5):805–16.

22. Torbicki A. Definition of pulmonary hypertension challenged? Nat Rev Cardiol 2016;13(5):250–1.

23. Tedford RJ, Beaty CA, Mathai SC, et al. Prognostic value of the pre-transplant diastolic pulmonary artery pressure–to–pulmonary capillary wedge pressure gradient in cardiac transplant recipients with pulmonary hypertension. J Hear Lung Transpl 2014;33(3):289–97.

24. Maron BA, Hess E, Maddox TM, et al. Association of Borderline Pulmonary Hypertension With Mortality and Hospitalization in a Large Patient Cohort: Insights From the Veterans Affairs Clinical Assessment, Reporting, and Tracking Program. Circulation 2016;133(13):1240–8.

25. Douschan P, Kovacs G, Avian A, et al. Mild elevation of pulmonary arterial pressure as a predictor of mortality. Am J Respir Crit Care Med 2018;197(4):509–16.

26. Coghlan JG, Wolf M, Distler O, et al. Incidence of pulmonary hypertension and determining factors in patients with systemic sclerosis. Eur Respir J 2018; 51(4):1701197.

27. Assad TR, Maron BA, Robbins IM, et al. Prognostic effect and longitudinal hemodynamic assessment of borderline pulmonary hypertension. JAMA Cardiol 2017;2(12):1361–8.

28. Kovacs G, Avian A, Tscherner M, et al. Characterization of Patients With Borderline Pulmonary Arterial Pressure. Chest 2014;146(6):1486–93.

29. Xanthouli P, Jordan S, Milde N, et al. Haemodynamic phenotypes and survival in patients with systemic sclerosis: the impact of the new definition of pulmonary arterial hypertension. Ann Rheum Dis 2020; 79(3):370–8.

30. Heresi GA, Aytekin M, Hammel JP, et al. Plasma interleukin-6 adds prognostic information in pulmonary arterial hypertension. Eur Respir J 2014;43(3): 912–4.

31. Nemoto K, Oh-Ishi S, Akiyama T, et al. Borderline pulmonary hypertension is associated with exercise intolerance and increased risk for acute exacerbation in patients with interstitial lung disease. BMC Pulm Med 2019;19(1):1–7.

32. Simonneau G, Hoeper MM. The revised definition of pulmonary hypertension: Exploring the impact on patient management. Eur Hear J Suppl 2019;21: K4–8.

33. Swietlik EM, Ruggiero A, Fletcher AJ, et al. Limitations of resting haemodynamics in chronic thromboembolic disease without pulmonary hypertension. Eur Respir J 2019;53(1):1801787.

34. Taboada D, Pepke-Zaba J, Jenkins DP, et al. Outcome of pulmonary endarterectomy in symptomatic chronic thromboembolic disease. Eur Respir J 2014;44(6):1635–45.

35. Kiely DG, Lawrie A, Humbert M. Screening strategies for pulmonary arterial hypertension. Eur Heart J Suppl 2019;21(Supplement_K):K9–20.

36. Attanasio U, Cuomo A, Pirozzi F, et al. Pulmonary Hypertension Phenotypes in Systemic Sclerosis: The Right Diagnosis for the Right Treatment. Int J Mol Sci 2020;21(12):4430.

37. Visovatti SH, Distler O, Coghlan JG, et al. Borderline pulmonary arterial pressure in systemic sclerosis patients: a post-hoc analysis of the DETECT study. Arthritis Res Ther 2014;16(6):493.

38. Sarı A, Şener YZ, Armağan B, et al. How did the updated hemodynamic definitions affect the frequency of pulmonary hypertension in patients with systemic sclerosis? Anatol J Cardiol 2021;25(1):30–5.

39. Pan Z, Marra AM, Benjamin N, et al. Early treatment with ambrisentan of mildly elevated mean pulmonary arterial pressure associated with systemic sclerosis: a randomized, controlled, double-blind, parallel group study (EDITA study). Arthritis Res Ther 2019; 21(1):217.

40. Saggar R, Khanna D, Shapiro S, et al. Brief Report: Effect of ambrisentan treatment on exercise-induced pulmonary hypertension in systemic sclerosis: A prospective single-center, open-label pilot study. Arthritis Rheum 2012;64(12):4072–7.

41. Kovacs G, Maier R, Aberer E, et al. Pulmonary arterial hypertension therapy may be safe and effective in patients with systemic sclerosis and borderline pulmonary artery pressure. Arthritis Rheum 2012; 64(4):1257–62.

Sex- and Gender-Related Aspects in Pulmonary Hypertension

Anna D'Agostino, PhD[a], Paola Guindani, MD[b], Gerarda Scaglione, MD[b],
Alessandra Di Vincenzo, MD[b], Sara Tamascelli[b], Riccardo Spaggiari, MD[b],
Andrea Salzano, MD, PhD[a], Andrea D'Amuri, MD[b],
Alberto Maria Marra, MD, PhD[c,d], Louise Pilote, MD, PhD[e],
Valeria Raparelli, MD, PhD[b,f,g,h,*]

KEYWORDS

- Sex • Gender identity • Socioeconomic status • Pulmonary hypertension • Outcomes
- Marital status • Employment • Epidemiology

KEY POINTS

- Sexual dimorphism in pulmonary arterial hypertension (PAH) affects disease prevalence, severity, response to treatment and importantly, survival; however, female individuals have better outcomes than the male counterpart.
- The impact of sociocultural gender (ie, identity, roles, relations, and institutionalized gender) on PAH is often overlooked and requires further investigation.
- Although gender identity has never been explored as a modifier of PAH, depression and anxiety, highly prevalent in patients with PAH, significantly correlated with their perceived quality of life.
- PAH affects not only patients' social and interpersonal relationships (eg, family or partnered roles) but also impairs their working status.
- Socially vulnerable PAH patients have the worst outcomes; low socioeconomic status, mostly related to inappropriate access to health care, is associated with delayed diagnosis of PAH, limited treatment, and worse outcomes.

INTRODUCTION

Pulmonary hypertension (PH) is a clinical condition defined by the presence of an invasively measured resting mean pulmonary arterial pressure (mPAP) $\geq$ 25 mm Hg with right heart catheterization (RHC),[1,2] with a lower threshold proposed during the last World Symposium for Pulmonary Hypertension (20 mm Hg).[3] Various conditions can lead to PH such as chronic respiratory diseases, left heart failure, and chronic thromboembolic disease.[4] PH has been classified into various subforms,[2] but among these the best characterized is pulmonary arterial hypertension (PAH) defined hemodynamically by the presence of precapillary PH, with a pulmonary artery (PA) wedge

[a] IRCCS SYNLAB SDN, Naples, Italy; [b] Department of Medicine, University Hospital Sant'Anna, University Internal Medicine Unit, Ferrara, Italy; [c] Department of Translational Medical Sciences, "Federico II" University of Naples, Naples, Italy; [d] Interdepartmental Center for Biomaterials (CRIB), "Federico II" University of Naples, Naples, Italy; [e] Division of Clinical Epidemiology and General Internal Medicine, McGill University Health Centre Research Institute, Montreal, Canada; [f] Department of Translational Medicine, University of Ferrara, Ferrara, Italy; [g] University Center for Studies on Gender Medicine, University of Ferrara, Ferrara, Italy; [h] Faculty of Nursing, University of Alberta, Edmonton, Canada
* Corresponding author. Department of Translational Medicine, University of Ferrara, Via dei Borsari 46, 44121, Ferrara, Italy.
E-mail address: valeria.raparelli@unife.it

Heart Failure Clin 19 (2023) 11–24
https://doi.org/10.1016/j.hfc.2022.09.002
1551-7136/23/© 2022 Elsevier Inc. All rights reserved.

pressure $\leq$ 15 mm Hg and pulmonary vascular resistance (PVR) greater than 3 Wood units in the absence of other causes of precapillary PH such as lung diseases, chronic thromboembolic PH (CTEPH), or other rare diseases.[5]

Several conditions have been associated with PAH including autoimmune diseases such as connective tissue diseases (CTDs), congenital heart disease, porto-PH, HIV infection, and *Schistosoma mansoni* infection leading to schistosomiasis. In addition, genetic background can also play an important role in the development of PAH along with sex hormones modifications, infections, autoimmune diseases, inflammation, and/or immune complex deposition.[6]

The pulmonary vascular remodeling process is the hallmark of PAH which consists in an abnormal and progressive hyperproliferation that involves all cell types of the PA wall.[7,8] This process progressively generates profound pulmonary vascular remodeling that shares similarities with malignant cell growth. Although it is generally accepted that vasoconstriction is important in the early stages of the disease, the major factor responsible for the high PVR in severe, established PAH is the formation of occlusive neointimal and plexiform lesions in small, peripheral PAs.[6,8] Furthermore, increased PVR may culminate in right ventricle (RV) remodeling and subsequent RV failure. RV failure is a clinical condition characterized by systolic and diastolic dysfunction, alterations in mitochondrial bioenergetics, ischemia, inflammation, oxidative stress, proapoptotic signaling, and cardiomyocyte death.[9,10] Right ventricular remodeling is a severe condition and the leading cause of death in patients with PAH.[11]

Sexual dimorphism in PAH exists in disease prevalence severity of hemodynamic alterations, RV adaptation, treatment responses, and, importantly, survival. Indeed, females are more prone to develop PAH, but exhibit a more favorable hemodynamic profile, better RV function, a better response to treatment with endothelin receptor antagonists (ERAs), and better survival.[12] Although PAH is a pathology with a higher frequency in females, male patients usually have more severe symptoms and poorer clinical outcome.[5] Therefore, understanding sex differences in PAH may provide important information about the pathogenesis of the disease.[13]

In this review, the authors sought to explore the current knowledge on the impact of biological sex and sociocultural differences across the clinical spectrum of PAH. This narrative review follows the principles of the Scale for the Assessment of Narrative Review Articles.[14]

Specifically, in the first section, the authors summarized the sex-based differences in disease development, outcomes, and management; then, the authors focused on the four domains of sociocultural gender reporting the available evidence on the topic underlying areas of gap in evidence. To perform a search strategy able to capture the complexity that gender encompasses, the authors applied the suggested operational framework of O'Neil and colleagues.[15]

From the Pulmonary Arterial Hypertension Epidemiology and Pathogenesis to the Gender/Sex Issue in Pulmonary Arterial Hypertension

According to the REVEAL and the Spanish Registry of Pulmonary Arterial Hypertension, two among the largest epidemiologic registries that enrolled PAH patients, reported relevant sex differences for PAH patients, reporting a female-to-male ratio for CTD-associated PAH of 9:1.[16,17] The Spanish Registry of Pulmonary Arterial Hypertension found that 61% of CTD-associated PAH patients had the autoimmune CTD systemic sclerosis (SSc), also referred to as scleroderma. Other female-dominant autoimmune diseases or syndromes aside from SSc that have been associated with PAH include systemic lupus erythematosus, mixed CTD, myositis, rheumatoid arthritis, Raynaud's syndrome, CREST syndrome, autoimmune hepatitis, Sjögren's syndrome.[17] However, besides CTD, other PAH subgroups report a similar female/male ratio.[5] The sex differences in PAH are likely mediated at least in part by biologically relevant effects of sex hormones.[18] Genetic alterations in estrogen metabolism enzymes and estrogen receptors have been highlighted in various forms of PAH.[12,19] Moreover, estrogen levels have also been correlated with RV function in healthy postmenopausal hormone replacement therapy users[20] and, finally, the absence of hemodynamic differences between male and female PAH patients who are older than 45 years.[21] Lower testosterone levels in female patients that may make the pulmonary vasculature and RV more vulnerable to insults[22] could be one reasonable explanation for this paradox. Indeed, testosterone acts as a pulmonary vasodilator through calcium antagonism, not through classic androgen receptor signaling.[23] Moreover, estrogen vasodilatory properties mediate these effects using a nitric oxide (NO)-dependent mechanism.[24,25] As a matter of fact, even small changes in plasma estrogen levels can have major consequences on vascular function and physiologic fluctuations in estrogen, such during menstruation, and can reduce PA constrictor responses.[26]

Is There a Genetic Background to Explain Sex Difference Among Pulmonary Arterial Hypertension Patients?

Genetic variations in estrogen metabolism and androgen signaling are associated with right ventricular morphology in a sex-specific manner. An increased risk and severity of idiopathic PAH (iPAH) is associated with elevated plasma estradiol in both males and postmenopausal females[27,28] suggesting that estradiol is not ovarian-derived. Aromatase is responsible for the synthesis of estradiol. Remodeled PAs, lesions, and human PA smooth muscle cells from PAH patients have high levels of aromatase.[29] Cytochrome P450 Family 1 Subfamily B Member 1 (CYP1B1) can convert estradiol to mitogenic 16-hydroxy estrogens, and this enzyme is overexpressed in diseased PAs from PAH patients.[30] Moreover, single nucleotide polymorphisms CYP1B1 are linked to PH, suggesting that these pathways may underpin sexual dimorphism in RV failure. In this regard, a decreased expression of CYP1B1 was found in patients with heritable PAH, whereas on the other hand, a common polymorphism in the CYP1B1 gene was suggested to be associated with familial PAH risk.[19]

Taken together this evidence suggests that differences in the estrogen metabolism rather than estrogens themselves may play a crucial role in the prevalence and progression of PAH in female individuals.

Another explanation could lay in the transmission of the mutation in the bone morphogenetic protein receptor type 2 (BMPR2) gene. Mutations in BMPR2, a gene encoding a member of the transforming growth factor family, are present in 70% to 80% of families with PAH and roughly 25% to 30% of patients with iPAH.[31–33] These mutations are transmitted in an autosomal dominant fashion with incomplete penetrance. Female mutation carriers are more than twice as likely to be affected with PAH as male carriers[34]; in a large cohort of individuals with BMPR2 mutations, roughly 70% of the population were females.[35] Another factor that negatively predisposes the female sex to the development of PAH is the increased interleukin-6 (IL-6) cytokine production. Indeed, this pleiotropic cytokine that plays a crucial role in the acute inflammatory response[36] is increased especially in obese females with induced lipolysis.[37] In normal tissues, IL-6 is promptly and transiently produced in response to infections and tissue injuries and immune reactions. After IL-6 is synthesized in a local lesion in the initial stage of inflammation, it moves to the liver through the bloodstream, followed by the rapid induction of an extensive range of acute phase proteins such as C-reactive protein, serum amyloid A, fibrinogen, haptoglobin, and α1-antichymotrypsin.[38]

Gene expression is an important intermediate phenotype for elucidating mechanisms contributing to sex-biased phenotypic differences as they both impact significantly on gene expression levels. Relatively few genome-wide association studies of immune-related traits have included X chromosome variation and, of those, only few significant associations are reported. Genetic differences at genes on the X chromosome or their responses to immune stimulation may induce differences between males and females in immune responses and potentially to risk for immune-mediated diseases. Indeed, genetic regulation of both autosomal and X-linked transcriptional responses to innate immune stimuli differ between males and females and suggest that these genes may lead to sex differences in disease risk.[39]

Therefore, gene expression analysis results are crucial for elucidating mechanisms contributing to sex-biased phenotypic differences. What we currently know is that in women the immune system seems to be more responsive, and this responsiveness could be attributed to the presence of two X-type chromosomes even if one of them is inactive. Interestingly, many genes that have been demonstrated to be crucial for immune response activation and maintenance have been located on the X chromosome.[39] Both high-profile players of the immune response such as forkhead box P3 and transcription factor for Regulatory T cells are located on the X chromosome. Indeed, females generally produce higher levels of antibodies which remain in circulation longer compared with males. Furthermore, immune cell activation seems higher in females than in males and is correlated with the trigger of Toll-like receptor 7 and the production of interferon γ.[40]

Pulmonary Arterial Hypertension in the Two Sexes: Clinical Phenotypes

Regarding the clinical scenario, the situation is not simplified. As already mentioned, on the one side, female individuals are more prone to develop PAH, but on the other side, they have better right ventricular function than their male counterparts.[40,41] Consequently, female patients have better survival rates, considering that RV function is one of the major determinants of prognosis and functional capacity in PAH.[42–44] Moreover, female PAH patients display also better pulmonary hemodynamics, as shown by a pooled analysis of 1211 subjects with iPAH from 11 randomized trials, in which was found that males with PAH show higher right atrial pressure, higher mPAP, lower cardiac index, and higher PVR than females.[21] Therefore, these differences in male patients were sufficient to translate into a 5% to 8% difference in mortality.[45] Currently, we are not able to elucidate the net effects of sexual steroids on PAH and interplay occurs between sex and PAH clinical features. Therefore, more research is needed to elucidate the underpinnings of sex-related differences in PAH (Table 1).

Different Effects of Pulmonary Arterial Hypertension-Targeted Drugs in the Two Sexes

Currently, a total amount of 12 compounds have been approved for PAH management. The available PAH drugs can be divided into three major categories according to their specific mechanisms of action: ERAs, drugs acting on the NO pathway (phosphodiesterase-5 inhibitors and guanylate cyclase stimulators), drugs acting on the prostacyclin (PC) pathway (PC analogues and prostacyclin receptor (IP) receptor agonist). Regarding ERAs group, drugs are focused on the key role played by endothelin-1 (ET-1) in the pathobiology of PAH.[46,47] Indeed, ET-1 exerts vasoconstrictor and mitogen effects on pulmonary vascular smooth muscle cells through two distinct receptors ET-A and ET-B. What we currently know about ET-1 production and effects is that there are differences between sexes. Indeed, it is clear now that males display higher ET-1 levels than females.[48,49] Furthermore, Stauffer and colleagues demonstrated in middle-aged and older healthy adults that males have a higher vasodilation than females under selective ET-A receptor inhibitions, whereas female individuals exhibit higher vasodilation than their male counterpart with the dual ET-A and ET-B receptor blockade.[50] Three ERAs have been approved for the treatment of PAH: bosentan, ambrisentan, and macitentan.[51] Interestingly, no pharmacokinetic and pharmacodynamics differences related to sex were recorded in clinical studies using ERAs in PAH.[52]

For what regards the second group of drugs, drugs acting on the NO pathway (phosphodiesterase-5 inhibitors and guanylate cyclase stimulators), these are based on the role of NO, which is involved in modulating vascular tone and remodeling in the pulmonary vasculature.[53] Important differences have been highlighted between males and females in the NO pathway. Indeed, it has been demonstrated by Chanand colleagues that NO-mediated vasodilatation in murine mesenteric arteries exhibited sex-specific responses to stimulation of the NO-soluble guanylate cyclase (sGC) pathway.[54] Phosphodiesterase-5 inhibitors (PDE5-i) are a class of drugs, currently recommended for PAH treatment.[51] They act enhancing NO signaling by impairing the catabolism of cyclic guanosine monophosphate, whose downstream effects are vasodilation and inhibition of cell proliferation.[4] Currently, two PDE5-i are approved for PAH treatment: sildenafil and tadalafil. A recently published post hoc analysis of the PHIRST trial reported that male participants have significantly greater benefits from using these groups of drugs than female ones.[55] A similar post hoc analysis was performed in the SUPER trial.[56] A possible explanation could be found in NO metabolism with higher NO endogenous biosynthesis in females than in males.[57] Moreover, male NO deficiencies compared with female NO levels may result in a more robust response to PDE5-i than that seen among females.[55] Another molecule was successfully tested and approved for PAH treatment: the sGC stimulator riociguat. This molecule acts in synergism with endogenous NO and directly stimulating sGC independently of NO availability.[58] In the PATENT-1 study, no differences were seen concerning treatment difference between females and males treated with riociguat.[59] This is crucial in dose setting because it means that for riociguat no dose adjustment according to sex is required.[60]

The last group of drugs is the group of the PC pathway (PC analogues and PC IP receptor agonists). The PC pathway was one of the first and best studied pathways in PAH. Therefore, epoprostenol (a PC analogue) was the first PAH-targeted drug approved.[61,62] Currently, many other approved PC analogues (iloprost, beraprost, and treprostinil) are available, but there are no data that elucidate any possible differences in both sexes with regard to PC analogues. However, the clinical use of PC analogues is strongly limited by adverse events (AEs) because of their delivery system which can lead to pump malfunction, local site infection, and sepsis.[1] The approval of selexipag may limit this side effects being an oral selective IP PC receptor agonist. Selexipag is structurally distinct from PC[63] and no differences in treatment efficacy between males and females have been seen (Table 2). An interesting therapeutic perspective is represented by sotatercept, a novel targeted therapy that acts on the BMPR2 pathway restoring the balance between growth-enhancing and growth-inhibiting signaling. These drugs have been successfully tested in the PULSAR trial, which demonstrated a significant improvement of PVR and 6-minutes walking

Table 1
Epidemiologic studies reporting an increased prevalence of pulmonary arterial hypertension among women compared with male pulmonary arterial hypertension patients

Registry	Number of Participants	Inclusion Period	Female%	Age Years	Female/ Male Ratio	1 y Survival by Incident Patients (%)	3 y Survival by Incident Patients (%)
National Institutes of Health (US NIH)[42,95]	187	1981–1988	63	36 ± 15	1.7	68	48
US PHC registry[96]	576	1991–2007	77	48 ± 14	3.3	86	69
Scottish morbidity records[97]	374	1986–2001	70	52 ± 12	2.3		
Columbia University registry[98]	84	1994–2002	81	42 ± 14	4.3	55	30
French registry (FPHN)[98–100]	674	2002–2003	65	50 ± 15	1.9	89	55
REVEAL[99,100]	2967	2006–2007	65	50 ± 15	1.9	89	55
Spanish registry (REHAP)[17]	1028	1998–2008	71	45 ± 17	2.5	89	77
UK and Ireland registry[101]	482	2001–2009	70	50 ± 17	2.3	93	73
Chinese registry	276	2007–2011	71	33 ± 15	2.5	92	75
COMPERA[102]	1283	2007–2011	60	65 ± 15	1.5	68	26
SERAPHIN[103]	742	2008–2012	77	46 + 16	1.3	93	27
GRIPHON[104]	1156	2009–2014	80	47 ± 16	4	76	12DAta

Data are the mean (SD).

Table 2
Sex-related differences in clinical function and pulmonary arterial hypertension-targeted drug administration

Clinical Function	♀	♂	Description
WHO functional class	↑	↓	
Right ventricular function	↑	↓	
Severity (hemodynamics)	↑	↓	
Outcome	↑	↓	3 y survival rate male 70.1% vs female 87.1%
ERAs	↓	↑	Placebo-adjusted response to ERAs of 29.7 m (95% CI, 3.7–55.7 m) greater in women than in men (P = 0.03)
PDE5-1 (PHIRST trail)	↓	↑	More effective in men
Prostanoids (PROSPECT registry)	↑	↓	Freedom from hospitalization lower in male (38.3% ± 5.9% vs 54.6% ± 3.2%, P = 0.015)

Data from Refs.[5,26,51,53,55,60–62]

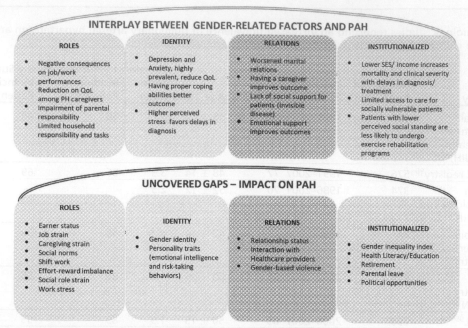

Fig. 1. Gender-related factors affecting pulmonary arterial hypertension and uncovered gaps.

distance in PAH patients without any reported difference regarding to sex.[64]

The Impact of Gender-Related Factors in Pulmonary Hypertension, a Neglected Child

The application of a gender-based lens in the understanding of PH has been rarely pursued, missing an opportunity to better inform our knowledge of the disease. The reasons behind the scarce evidence regarding the impact of sociocultural gender on the development and prognosis of PH are multifactorial. Only recently, the importance of gender as determinant and modifier of health and disease has been recognized in medical science.[65] The complexity and multidimensionality of gender has been an obstacle for the integration of such domains' evaluation in clinical studies. In fact, the collection of gender-related factors is still overlooked, posing challenges in providing the evidence that gender matters when it comes to PH. According to the operational definition of gender which embraces four main domains (ie, identity, roles, relations, and institutionalized gender),[66] hence, the authors reviewed the available literature on the topic (**Fig. 1**).

Gender Identity and Pulmonary Hypertension

Individuals who identify with a gender not associated with their biological sex assigned at birth are a growing population worldwide. Transgender and gender diverse are affected by disparities

across a variety of cardiovascular (CV) risk factors as compared with cisgender people. Thus, the American Heart Association[66] has highlighted the unmet need of addressing the CV health of gender-diverse people. Beyond the different distribution of traditional CV risk factors in gender-diverse people, the excess CV morbidity and mortality is hypothesized to be driven in part by psychosocial stressors across the lifespan at multiple levels, including structural violence (eg, discrimination, affordable housing, and access to health care).

Despite it has previously been reported how gender-diverse people with a pulmonary complaint have unique characteristics when it comes to their lung care,[67] considerations on PH have not been reported suggesting the paucity of specific-disease evidence on the impact of gender identity.

Beyond identity, psychological aspects might be relevant in the management of PH patients.[68] The prevalence of depression and anxiety disorders is higher in patients with PAH than in the general population and it increases with disease progression.[69] Among a cohort of 158 (71% female, mean age 56 year old) patients with PAH or CTEPH, anxiety, and depression significantly correlated with quality of life (QOL), but not with long-term survival.[70]

Among the difficulties faced by patients with PH, living life with uncertainty was reported as a major obstacle in a qualitative observational study suggesting that patients with PAH used different coping styles at various illness trajectory time points.[71] After diagnosis, patients experienced higher levels of anxiety related to the lack of knowledge about PAH.[72] Higher perceived stress was also associated with longer time to PAH diagnosis.[73]

Swedish data from 325 middle-aged adults with PAH (58% female) demonstrated how female patients have a lower coping ability than male counterparts. Moreover, the higher coping ability was associated with the patient' satisfaction about receiving information on the disease.

Finally, attending the PAH-outpatient clinic increased coping ability significantly within 2-year follow-up and those patients who had improved their coping ability also experienced better QOL and exercise capacity over time.[73]

Gender Roles and Pulmonary Hypertension

The domain of "gender roles" includes the behavioral norms applied to men and women in society, which influence individuals' everyday actions, expectations, and experiences. Gender roles are evident in several settings such as at work, within the family or in the educational system.

PAH has a significant impact on the daily lives of patients and of their caregivers. Different areas of life are affected by PAH, including physical activities, employment/work, travel and social opportunities, domestic work/household chores, and relationship issues. An important aspect that often concerns patients is the impact of PAH on their employment status. In fact, most people reported that their work or employment had been affected by PAH.[74] A considerable loss of employment during the disease can be observed.[75] There is limited data discussing how employment status of patients with PAH may be related to patients' outcomes. A better physical QOL among patients with PH has been associated with active employment.[76] The symptoms of PAH impair the ability to perform efficiently at work, maintain a full-time schedule and lead to feelings of loss of independence and purpose.[77] A diminished rate of employment and the educational attainment level were factors strongly associated with overall QOL in PH patients.[78] Patients with PH in physical or manual labor were more likely to be unemployed.[75]

Furthermore, even the work activity of their caregivers was affected. Caring for a patient with PAH can be physically exhausting due to the overwhelmed extra-tasks and responsibilities. This reduction in the job efficiency due to PAH had major consequences on the overall household incomes, with both patients and caregivers reporting a significant reduction in the income below the average.[74]

Clearly all these factors generate changes in many of the social roles that patients had once held, including those as a colleague, friend, and teammate. Around 20% of caregivers reported feelings less close to their spouse and perceived their partner more as a carer than as a lover.[74] Dealing with domestic work/household chores was affected by their disease. Even those patients who are grandfathers complained about difficulties in playing with grandchildren.[74]

Female individuals with PAH often are more likely to turn down the possibility of being mothers. Current international guidelines recommend patients with PAH to avoid pregnancy and, if it should occur, they suggest early termination.[1] The onset of PAH during pregnancy or immediately after childbirth is associated with a significant incidence of clinical worsening and high maternal and fetal mortality.[79] Recently, a retrospective single-center study demonstrates that pro hormone BNP (NT-proBNP), pulmonary arterial systolic pressure (PASP), and serum albumin levels are significant predictors of death among pregnant patients with PAH. These findings may help clinicians in providing better advice on family planning for female individuals of childbearing age with PAH and in offering timely and appropriate medical interventions.[80]

Pulmonary veno-occlusive disease (PVOD), a rare form of PH characterized by predominant remodeling of pulmonary venules, was associated with occupational exposure to organic solvents, with trichloroethylene being the main agent implicated. The most common occupations resulting in trichloroethylene exposure included metal workers, mechanics and repairers, building painters, and cleaners.[81] In the genetic form of PVOD, males and females are equally affected, whereas the sporadic form of PVOD affects more males as they are more likely to have occupations with trichloroethylene exposure, usually ascribed to men.

Within the various subtypes of PAH, the absolute highest percentage of female subjects has been documented in PAH induced by oral anorectics and this is probably related to the use of these drugs significantly higher in the female population. Dexfenfluramine, the main principle involved, was widely used for the treatment of obesity in the 90s, years in which thinness emerged as an esthetic ideal for women.[79] It can be supposed that, although probably only to a lesser extent, the canons of beauty imposed on women have contributed to a greater incidence of PAH.

Gender Relations and Pulmonary Hypertension

Gender relations domain covers all the aspects related to how individuals interact with and are treated by other people (based on their perceived and/or expressed gender identity). Several studies have reported how PH affected not only the life of patients but also their relations with partners, family members, and friends.

The PAH Patient and Carer Survey, a large-scale international survey aimed at exploring four areas affected by PAH (ie, physical and practical, emotional, social, and information needs), provided interesting findings regarding the impact of the disease on patients and carers. Among a total of 455 respondents (72% patients with PAH), social isolation experienced by both patients and carers has emerged as a frequent occurrence, with a notable impact on their QOL.[74] Being confined to their home results in the loss of social roles that patients had once held, including those as a friend, and teammate. Husbands reported the inability to carry out activities traditionally ascribed as their role, including home maintenance and playing football with kids, whereas wives complained about their limited capability of maternal tasks with children and housework.[74]

Social support involves the exchange of assistance through interpersonal relationships; it goes through building new social networks and how patients think the already existing ones.

Participants of a national survey on a Chinese population[82] complained about the lack of understanding of their condition by others, including their community, family members, or spouse, also because they feel like having an "invisible" disease.[82] A study about 108 US outpatients with PH referring to a pulmonary clinic has shown that the length of time as diagnosis was positively associated with greater perceived social support.[73] Otherwise, long-time since PAH diagnosis is also associated with higher perceived stress.[73] These data are consistent with the guidelines of European Society of Cardiology and European Respiratory Society proposing that "psychosocial support should be offered to patients with PAH" with a level I-C recommendation.[1]

The interesting data come from a cross-sectional designed study with 97 participants from the outpatient clinic of a medical center located in southern Taiwan[83]; it showed that emotional support was the only social support factor that played a mediating role between illness concealment and developing depression symptoms, whereas practical support and social networks did not. When participants received emotional support, they were less likely to have depression symptoms, they were more prone to positive thinking, which is a coping strategy, and overall, they had a better health-related QOL.[83]

Institutionalized Gender and Pulmonary Arterial Hypertension

Institutionalized gender is defined as the way that power, resources, and opportunities are distributed in society based on the gender of individuals, examples of gender-related variables included in this domain are socioeconomic status (SES) and education level. It is specific for country and culture, and it represents a relevant modifier of health and outcomes.

SES has been linked to the occurrence of disparities in the access to health care in many diseases, leading to worse disease severity at initial presentation. Components of SES that could lead to disparities in health include the social environment, psychology, behavior, and physical environment. SES also has behavioral components, potentially affecting the likelihood of enacting health-related activities such as exercise and scheduled medication taking. A person's perceptions of risk and severity of disease impact his or her own behavior and subsequently the success of an intervention which can result in disparate outcomes between different socioeconomic groups in PAH.

Data on the impact of SES on the outcomes of PAH population are scarce and conflicting. Some studies reported an association between low SES and worse outcomes in PAH.[84,85] A lower SES (defined as a score obtained from educational level, annual household income, occupation, and medical reimbursement rate) was strongly associated with a higher risk of death in iPAH.[86] Of note, this association was independent of clinical characteristics and therapies received. A low SES has been also reported to have an impact on time of diagnosis. Specifically, in a retrospective study using zip code as surrogate of SES, patients with low SES experienced a delay in the diagnosis of PH and they presented a more clinically severe disease. In fact, the low SES may preclude patients from subspecialized health care. In a review by Taiwar and colleagues, SES has been demonstrated to be related to a worse functional status at first visit and therefore to a more severe disease at presentation, perhaps due to the aforementioned delay in diagnosis secondary to the limited access to advanced diagnostic techniques (eg, RHC) and an increase in time before referring to a specialist center.[84] They concluded that SES should be considered when dealing with PAH patients, in particular for risk stratification, genetic determination, the development of training courses addressing disparities in health, and a legislation of ameliorated government standard.[84] Finally, SES has a strong impact on the prognosis because the 5-year mortality rates doubled among patients with greater functional impairment as compared with those with mild disease.[85]

Increased social deprivation is not associated with worse survival in patients with CTD-associated PH (CTDPH) and CTEPH managed in the Scottish National Health Service.[87] Evidence of referral barriers was evident only in CTEPH, and lower deprivation was associated with worse functional class at presentation.[87] Other US and Chinese studies reported the inverse relationship between survival and lower income and residing in rural areas. These discrepant results might be related to the different health care system which is publicly funded in Scotland. Whereas the high cost of PH therapy in private health care systems (ie, China and the USA) might represent a critical barrier in access to appropriate care.[88] Future research might highlight even more the impact of the income on PAH outcomes. Of note, at international scientific congresses, some interesting data on the abovementioned gaps in evidence have been recently presented; a higher income was associated with lower pulmonary arterial pressure and lung vascular resistances and lower risk for severe disease at follow-up.[89]

Particularly for certain countries, differences in employment state and job types might relate with sex and gender. PAH may have a role in increasing this discrepancy, given the fact that the employment state seems to be affected by PAH, where people suffering from this disease are more prone to be unemployed or retired due to disability, when having a lower educational status at baseline.[75] In addition, COVID-19 pandemic has exacerbated the disparities between minorities in access to health care and respective coping mechanisms, leading to the possibility that discrimination for certain individuals, as might happen for transgender people, could affect PAH prognosis.

The level of education of an individual defines his ability to collect and understand as much information as possible about its disease, an ability defined as health literacy. As educational status might vary based on gender, this could be a significant factor to be considered. In literature, the relationship between health literacy and PAH outcomes seems not to be clearly investigated; however, it seems that for chronic obstructive pulmonary disease, a disease that might evolve into a condition of PH secondary to the pathology involving the lung, patients with inadequate health literacy have a 1.80 chance of developing a more severe form.[90]

Exercise rehabilitation improves the exercise capacity and QOL of individuals with PH, nevertheless, is underutilized. Specifically, PAH and CTEPH patients with low socioeconomic and educational status, as depicted by MacArthur Scale of Subjective Social Status, are less prone to undergo this kind of rehabilitation (39% vs 71%) despite no difference in this cohort has been reported according to sex.[91]

Finally, it should be noticed how the etiology PH might vary across countries based on the different levels of development of the country. In industrialized countries, the main etiologies of PH are chronic ischemic heart disease and heart failure with preserved ejection fraction, whereas in developing countries such as those in Africa, hypertensive heart disease, cardiomyopathy, and rheumatic heart disease are more prevalent.[92] Furthermore, in developed areas, industrial and household air pollution have been claimed as key players in favoring the increased incidence of PH. Interestingly, young children and female adults are at higher risk of PH as they spend more time in the domestic environment.[93,94]

SUMMARY

Females are more affected by PAH compared with males. Despite female patients with PAH having a higher WHO functional class, male PAH patients have a more impaired RV function and hemodynamics compared with females with PAH. For this reason, males affected by PAH have poorer outcomes than females. The effects of estrogens and other sex hormones on the pulmonary vasculature and RV are complex yet highly fascinating because of their direct relevance to clinical manifestations of various forms of PAH.

Beyond sex (biological-based) differences, the interplay between gender domains and PAH has been only partially studied. PAH has a significant impact on daily lives of patients and caregivers. It generates changes in many social roles such as at work (eg, reduction in the job efficiency) and within the family (limited activities as parent or partner). Social isolation affects the QOL of both PAH patients and their careers, resulting in the loss of social roles that patients once held. As patients with PH feel like having an "invisible" disease, lacking the understanding by patients' social network, psychological support should be offered according to guidelines. In fact, emotional support can help to improve the outcome of PAH. Finally, differences in society and opportunities can relate with gender identity, in particular for individuals that are often discriminated such as transgender people. Lower SES and incomes are associated with different etiologies, a delay in diagnosis and treatment, a more severe disease at first visit, and therefore a raise in mortality and a worse prognosis. Even the educational level might play an important role, despite not being still clearly investigated in the literature.

Further studies, aimed at understanding the mechanisms behind the observed sex- and gender-based differences in PAH, may inform the development of novel tailored and personalized approaches for the management of PAH patients.

DISCLOSURE

AD's work was supported by institutional grant from Italian healthcare ministry (Ricerca finalizzata per giovani ricercatori GR-2016-02364727).

CLINICS CARE POINTS

- Be aware of the differences in outcomes when treating a female or male patient with pulmonary arterial hypertension (PAH).

- When managing patients with PAH, do not overlook the impact of gendered factors such as identity, roles and relations, and social norms.

- For the risk stratification of adverse outcomes and consequent therapeutic decision-making of individuals with PAH collect information on gender-related factors.

- Take into consideration how the quality of life among patient with PAH is influenced by both biological and psychosociocultural factors; therefore, an holistic approach should be applied to improve PAH management.

REFERENCES

1. Galiè N, Humbert M, Vachiery JL, et al. [2015 ESC/ERS Guidelines for the diagnosis and treatment of pulmonary hypertension]. Kardiol Pol 2015;73(12): 1127–206.

2. Hoeper MM, Bogaard HJ, Condliffe R, et al. Definitions and diagnosis of pulmonary hypertension. J Am Coll Cardiol 2013;62(25 Suppl):D42–50.

3. Simonneau G, Montani D, Celermajer DS, et al. Haemodynamic definitions and updated clinical classification of pulmonary hypertension. Eur Respir J 2019;53(1). https://doi.org/10.1183/13993003.01913-2018.

4. Galiè N, Corris PA, Frost A, et al. Updated treatment algorithm of pulmonary arterial hypertension. J Am Coll Cardiol 2013;62(25 Suppl):D60–72.

5. Marra AM, Benjamin N, Eichstaedt C, et al. Gender-related differences in pulmonary arterial hypertension targeted drugs administration. Pharmacol Res 2016;114:103–9.

6. Batton KA, Austin CO, Bruno KA, et al. Sex differences in pulmonary arterial hypertension: role of infection and autoimmunity in the pathogenesis of disease. Biol Sex Differ 2018;9(1):15.

7. Rabinovitch M. Molecular pathogenesis of pulmonary arterial hypertension. J Clin Invest Dec 2012; 122(12):4306–13.

8. Lahm T, Tuder RM, Petrache I. Progress in solving the sex hormone paradox in pulmonary hypertension. Am J Physiol Lung Cell Mol Physiol 2014; 307(1):L7–26.

9. Cassady SJ, Ramani GV. Right Heart Failure in Pulmonary Hypertension. Cardiol Clin May 2020;38(2): 243–55.

10. Bogaard HJ, Abe K, Vonk Noordegraaf A, et al. The right ventricle under pressure: cellular and molecular mechanisms of right-heart failure in pulmonary hypertension. Chest Mar 2009;135(3):794–804.

11. Tonelli AR, Arelli V, Minai OA, et al. Causes and circumstances of death in pulmonary arterial hypertension. Am J Respir Crit Care Med 2013;188(3): 365–9.

12. Hester J, Ventetuolo C, Lahm T. Sex, Gender, and Sex Hormones in Pulmonary Hypertension and Right Ventricular Failure. Compr Physiol 2019; 10(1):125–70.

13. Franco V, Ryan JJ, McLaughlin VV. Pulmonary Hypertension in Women. Heart Fail Clin Jan 2019; 15(1):137–45.

14. Baethge C, Goldbeck-Wood S, Mertens S. SANRA-a scale for the quality assessment of narrative review articles. Res Integr Peer Rev 2019;4:5.

15. O'Neill ZR, Raparelli V, Norris CM, et al. Demystifying how to incorporate Sex and Gender into cardiovascular research: a practical guide. Can J Cardiol 2022. https://doi.org/10.1016/j.cjca.2022.05.017.

16. McGoon MD, Miller DP. REVEAL: a contemporary US pulmonary arterial hypertension registry. Eur Respir Rev Mar 01 2012;21(123):8–18.

17. Escribano-Subias P, Blanco I, López-Meseguer M, et al. Survival in pulmonary hypertension in Spain: insights from the Spanish registry. Eur Respir J Sep 2012;40(3):596–603.

18. Sweeney L, Voelkel NF. Estrogen exposure, obesity and thyroid disease in women with severe pulmonary hypertension. Eur J Med Res Sep 28 2009; 14(10):433–42.

19. Austin ED, Cogan JD, West JD, et al. Alterations in oestrogen metabolism: implications for higher penetrance of familial pulmonary arterial hypertension in females. *Eur Respir J* Nov 2009;34(5): 1093–9.

20. Ventetuolo CE, Ouyang P, Bluemke DA, et al. Sex hormones are associated with right ventricular structure and function: The MESA-right ventricle study. *Am J Respir Crit Care Med* Mar 01 2011; 183(5):659–67.

21. Ventetuolo CE, Praestgaard A, Palevsky HI, et al. Sex and haemodynamics in pulmonary arterial hypertension. *Eur Respir J* Feb 2014;43(2):523–30.

22. Memon HA, Park MH. Pulmonary Arterial Hypertension in Women. Methodist Debakey Cardiovasc J 2017;13(4):224–37.

23. Jones RD, English KM, Pugh PJ, et al. Pulmonary vasodilatory action of testosterone: evidence of a calcium antagonistic action. *J Cardiovasc Pharmacol* Jun 2002;39(6):814–23.

24. Lahm T, Crisostomo PR, Markel TA, et al. Selective estrogen receptor-alpha and estrogen receptor-beta agonists rapidly decrease pulmonary artery vasoconstriction by a nitric oxide-dependent mechanism. *Am J Physiol Regul Integr Comp Physiol* Nov 2008;295(5):R1486–93.

25. Lahm T, Patel KM, Crisostomo PR, et al. Endogenous estrogen attenuates pulmonary artery vasoreactivity and acute hypoxic pulmonary vasoconstriction: the effects of sex and menstrual cycle. *Am J Physiol Endocrinol Metab* Sep 2007; 293(3):E865–71.

26. Sun Y, Sangam S, Guo Q, et al. Sex Differences, Estrogen Metabolism and Signaling in the Development of Pulmonary Arterial Hypertension. Front Cardiovasc Med 2021;8:719058.

27. Ventetuolo CE, Baird GL, Barr RG, et al. Higher Estradiol and Lower Dehydroepiandrosterone-Sulfate Levels Are Associated with Pulmonary Arterial Hypertension in Men. Am J Respir Crit Care Med 2016;193(10):1168–75.

28. Baird GL, Archer-Chicko C, Barr RG, et al. Lower DHEA-S levels predict disease and worse outcomes in post-menopausal women with idiopathic, connective tissue disease- and congenital heart disease-associated pulmonary arterial hypertension. Eur Respir J 2018;51(6). https://doi.org/10. 1183/13993003.00467-2018.

29. Mair KM, Wright AF, Duggan N, et al. Sex-dependent influence of endogenous estrogen in pulmonary hypertension. Am J Respir Crit Care Med 2014;190(4):456–67.

30. White K, Johansen AK, Nilsen M, et al. Activity of the estrogen-metabolizing enzyme cytochrome P450 1B1 influences the development of pulmonary arterial hypertension. Circulation 2012; 126(9):1087–98.

31. Deng Z, Morse JH, Slager SL, et al. Familial primary pulmonary hypertension (gene PPH1) is caused by mutations in the bone morphogenetic protein receptor-II gene. *Am J Hum Genet* Sep 2000;67(3):737–44.

32. Soubrier F, Chung WK, Machado R, et al. Genetics and genomics of pulmonary arterial hypertension. J Am Coll Cardiol 2013;62(25 Suppl):D13–21.

33. Morrell NW, Aldred MA, Chung WK, et al. Genetics and genomics of pulmonary arterial hypertension. Eur Respir J 2019;53(1). https://doi.org/10.1183/ 13993003.01899-2018.

34. Best DH, Sumner KL, Smith BP, et al. EIF2AK4 Mutations in Patients Diagnosed With Pulmonary Arterial Hypertension. *Chest.* 04 2017;151(4):821–8.

35. Evans JD, Girerd B, Montani D, et al. BMPR2 mutations and survival in pulmonary arterial hypertension: an individual participant data meta-analysis. *Lancet Respir Med* Feb 2016;4(2):129–37.

36. Akinyemi R, Arnett DK, Tiwari HK, et al. Interleukin-6 (IL-6) rs1800796 and cyclin dependent kinase inhibitor (CDKN2A/CDKN2B) rs2383207 are associated with ischemic stroke in indigenous West African Men. J Neurol Sci 2017;379:229–35.

37. Varghese M, Griffin C, McKernan K, et al. Sex Differences in Inflammatory Responses to Adipose Tissue Lipolysis in Diet-Induced Obesity. Endocrinology 2019;160(2):293–312.

38. Taxy JB. Tubular carcinoma of the male breast: report of a case. *Cancer* Aug 1975;36(2):462–5.

39. Stein MM, Conery M, Magnaye KM, et al. Sex-specific differences in peripheral blood leukocyte transcriptional response to LPS are enriched for HLA region and X chromosome genes. Sci Rep 2021; 11(1):1107.

40. Gemmati D, Bramanti B, Serino ML, et al. COVID-19 and Individual Genetic Susceptibility/Receptivity: Role of ACE1/ACE2 Genes, Immunity, Inflammation and Coagulation. Might the Double X-chromosome in Females Be Protective against SARS-CoV-2 Compared to the Single X-Chromosome in Males? Int J Mol Sci 2020;21(10). https:// doi.org/10.3390/ijms21103474.

41. Jacobs W, van de Veerdonk MC, Trip P, et al. The right ventricle explains sex differences in survival in idiopathic pulmonary arterial hypertension. *Chest* Jun 2014;145(6):1230–6.

42. D'Alonzo GE, Barst RJ, Ayres SM, et al. Survival in patients with primary pulmonary hypertension. Results from a national prospective registry. Ann Intern Med 1991;115(5):343–9.

43. Ryan JJ, Huston J, Kutty S, et al. Right ventricular adaptation and failure in pulmonary arterial hypertension. *Can J Cardiol* Apr 2015;31(4):391–406.

44. Grünig E, Peacock AJ. Imaging the heart in pulmonary hypertension: an update. *Eur Respir Rev* Dec 2015;24(138):653–64.

45. Naeije R, D'Alto M. Sex matters in pulmonary arterial hypertension. *Eur Respir J* Aug 2014;44(2): 553–4.

46. Galié N, Manes A, Branzi A. The endothelin system in pulmonary arterial hypertension. *Cardiovasc Res* Feb 2004;61(2):227–37.

47. Schermuly RT, Ghofrani HA, Wilkins MR, et al. Mechanisms of disease: pulmonary arterial hypertension. Nat Rev Cardiol 2011;8(8):443–55.

48. Miyauchi T, Yanagisawa M, Iida K, et al. Age- and sex-related variation of plasma endothelin-1 concentration in normal and hypertensive subjects. *Am Heart J* Apr 1992;123(4 Pt 1):1092–3.

49. Polderman KH, Stehouwer CD, van Kamp GJ, et al. Influence of sex hormones on plasma endothelin levels. *Ann Intern Med* Mar 15 1993;118(6):429–32.

50. Stauffer BL, Westby CM, Greiner JJ, et al. Sex differences in endothelin-1-mediated vasoconstrictor tone in middle-aged and older adults. *Am J Physiol Regul Integr Comp Physiol* Feb 2010;298(2): R261–5.

51. Galié N, Humbert M, Vachiery JL, et al. 2015 ESC/ ERS Guidelines for the Diagnosis and Treatment of Pulmonary Hypertension. Rev Esp Cardiol 2016; 69(2):177.

52. Dingemanse J, van Giersbergen PL. Clinical pharmacology of bosentan, a dual endothelin receptor antagonist. Clin Pharmacokinet 2004;43(15): 1089–115.

53. Galié N, Ghofrani HA, Torbicki A, et al. Sildenafil citrate therapy for pulmonary arterial hypertension. N Engl J Med 2005;353(20):2148–57.

54. Chan MV, Bubb KJ, Noyce A, et al. Distinct endothelial pathways underlie sexual dimorphism in vascular auto-regulation. Br J Pharmacol Oct 2012;167(4):805–17.

55. Mathai SC, Hassoun PM, Puhan MA, et al. Sex differences in response to tadalafil in pulmonary arterial hypertension. Chest 2015;147(1):188–97.

56. Galié N, Palazzini M, Manes A. Pulmonary arterial hypertension: from the kingdom of the near-dead to multiple clinical trial meta-analyses. Eur Heart J 2010;31(17):2080–6.

57. Forte P, Kneale BJ, Milne E, et al. Evidence for a difference in nitric oxide biosynthesis between healthy women and men. Hypertension 1998; 32(4):730–4.

58. Marra AM, Egenlauf B, Ehlken N, et al. Change of right heart size and function by long-term therapy with riociguat in patients with pulmonary arterial hypertension and chronic thromboembolic pulmonary hypertension. Int J Cardiol 2015;195:19–26.

59. Galié N, Channick RN, Frantz RP, et al. Risk stratification and medical therapy of pulmonary arterial hypertension. Eur Respir J 2019;53(1). https://doi. org/10.1183/13993003.01889-2018.

60. Frey R, Saleh S, Becker C, et al. Effects of age and sex on the pharmacokinetics of the soluble guanylate cyclase stimulator riociguat (BAY 63-2521). Pulm Circ 2016;6(Suppl 1):S58–65.

61. Barst RJ, Rubin LJ, Long WA, et al. A comparison of continuous intravenous epoprostenol (prostacyclin) with conventional therapy for primary pulmonary hypertension. N Engl J Med 1996;334(5): 296–301.

62. Rubin LJ, Mendoza J, Hood M, et al. Treatment of primary pulmonary hypertension with continuous intravenous prostacyclin (epoprostenol). Results of a randomized trial. Ann Intern Med 1990; 112(7):485–91.

63. Sitbon O, Morrell N. Pathways in pulmonary arterial hypertension: the future is here. Eur Respir Rev 2012;21(126):321–7.

64. Humbert M, McLaughlin V, Gibbs JSR, et al. Sotatercept for the Treatment of Pulmonary Arterial Hypertension. N Engl J Med 2021;384(13):1204–15.

65. Mauvais-Jarvis F, Bairey Merz N, Barnes PJ, et al. Sex and gender: modifiers of health, disease, and medicine. Lancet 2020;396(10250):565–82.

66. Johnson JL, Greaves L, Repta R. Better science with sex and gender: Facilitating the use of a sex and gender-based analysis in health research. Int J Equity Health 2009;8:14.

67. Turner GA, Amoura NJ, Strah HM. Care of the Transgender Patient with a Pulmonary Complaint. Ann Am Thorac Soc 2021;18(6):931–7.

68. Mai AS, Lim OZH, Ho YJ, et al. Prevalence, Risk Factors and Intervention for Depression and Anxiety in Pulmonary Hypertension: A Systematic Review and Meta-analysis. Front Med (Lausanne) 2022;9:765461.

69. Löwe B, Gräfe K, Ufer C, et al. Anxiety and depression in patients with pulmonary hypertension. Psychosom Med 2004;66(6):831–6.

70. Harzheim D, Klose H, Pinado FP, et al. Anxiety and depression disorders in patients with pulmonary arterial hypertension and chronic thromboembolic pulmonary hypertension. Respir Res 2013;14:104.

71. Armstrong I, Rochnia N, Harries C, et al. The trajectory to diagnosis with pulmonary arterial hypertension: a qualitative study. BMJ Open 2012;2(2): e000806.

72. Kingman M, Hinzmann B, Sweet O, et al. Living with pulmonary hypertension: unique insights from an international ethnographic study. BMJ Open 2014;4(5):e004735.

73. Von Visger TT, Kuntz KK, Phillips GS, et al. Quality of life and psychological symptoms in patients with pulmonary hypertension. Heart Lung 2018;47(2): 115–21.

74. Guillevin L, Armstrong I, Aldrighetti R, et al. Understanding the impact of pulmonary arterial

hypertension on patients' and carers' lives. Eur Respir Rev 2013;22(130):535–42.

75. Fuge J, Park DH, von Lengerke T, et al. Impact of Pulmonary Arterial Hypertension on Employment, Work Productivity, and Quality of Life - Results of a Cross-Sectional Multi-Center Study. Front Psychiatry 2021;12:781532.

76. Taichman DB, Shin J, Hud L, et al. Health-related quality of life in patients with pulmonary arterial hypertension. Respir Res 2005;6:92.

77. McGoon MD, Ferrari P, Armstrong I, et al. The importance of patient perspectives in pulmonary hypertension. Eur Respir J 2019;53(1). https://doi.org/10.1183/13993003.01919-2018.

78. Matura LA, McDonough A, Carroll DL. Health-related quality of life and psychological states in patients with pulmonary arterial hypertension. J Cardiovasc Nurs 2014;29(2):178–84.

79. Manes A, Palazzini M, Dardi F, et al. [Female gender and pulmonary arterial hypertension: a complex relationship]. G Ital Cardiol (Rome) 2012;13(6):448–60.

80. Dai LL, Jiang TC, Li PF, et al. Predictors of Maternal Death Among Women With Pulmonary Hypertension in China From 2012 to 2020: A Retrospective Single-Center Study. Front Cardiovasc Med 2022;9:814557.

81. Montani D, Lau EM, Descatha A, et al. Occupational exposure to organic solvents: a risk factor for pulmonary veno-occlusive disease. Eur Respir J 2015;46(6):1721–31.

82. Brahams D. Pertussis vaccine: court finds no justification for association with permanent brain damage. Lancet 1988;1(8589):837.

83. Chao HY, Hsu CH, Wang ST, et al. Mediating effect of social support on the relationship between illness concealment and depression symptoms in patients with pulmonary arterial hypertension. Heart Lung 2021;50(5):706–13.

84. Talwar A, Garcia JGN, Tsai H, et al. Health Disparities in Patients with Pulmonary Arterial Hypertension: A Blueprint for Action. An Official American Thoracic Society Statement. Am J Respir Crit Care Med 2017;196(8):e32–47.

85. Talwar A, Sahni S, Kohn N, et al. Socioeconomic status affects pulmonary hypertension disease severity at time of first evaluation. Pulm Circ 2016;6(2):191–5.

86. Wu WH, Yang L, Peng FH, et al. Lower socioeconomic status is associated with worse outcomes in pulmonary arterial hypertension. Am J Respir Crit Care Med 2013;187(3):303–10.

87. McGettrick M, McCaughey P, MacLellan A, et al. Social deprivation in Scottish populations with pulmonary hypertension secondary to connective tissue disease and chronic thromboembolic disease. *ERJ Open Res* Oct 2020;6(4). https://doi.org/10.1183/23120541.00297-2019.

88. Ong MS. Socioeconomic status and survival in patients with pulmonary hypertension. ERJ Open Res 2020;6(4). https://doi.org/10.1183/23120541.00638-2020.

89. Alquraishi 1 JS H, Lee 2 L, Legkaia 2 L, et al, Division of Medicine UoBC, Vancouver, BC, Canada DoR, University of British Columbia, Vancouver, BC, Canada, 3 Centre for Health Evaluation and Outcome Sciences, University of British Columbia, Vancouver, BC, Canada M, University of Alberta, Edmonton, AB, Canada, Respiratory Division,, Vancouver General Hospital V, BC, Canada, Cardiology, University of British Columbia, Vancouver, BC, Canada. The Association Between Median Income and Severity of Pulmonary Hypertension at Diagnosis and Risk at Follow Up in a Public Health Care System. Am J Respir Crit Care Med 2022. https://doi.org/10.1164/ajrccm-conference.2022.205.1_MeetingAbstracts.A5085. Available at:.

90. Azkan Ture D, Bhattacharya S, Demirci H, et al. Health Literacy and Health Outcomes in Chronic Obstructive Pulmonary Disease Patients: An Explorative Study. Front Public Health 2022;10:846768.

91. Cascino TM, Ashur C, Richardson CR, et al. Impact of patient characteristics and perceived barriers on referral to exercise rehabilitation among patients with pulmonary hypertension in the United States. Pulm Circ 2020;10(4). 2045894020974926.

92. Sliwa K, Davison BA, Mayosi BM, et al. Readmission and death after an acute heart failure event: predictors and outcomes in sub-Saharan Africa: results from the THESUS-HF registry. Eur Heart J 2013;34(40):3151–9.

93. Moran-Mendoza O, Pérez-Padilla JR, Salazar-Flores M, et al. Wood smoke-associated lung disease: a clinical, functional, radiological and pathological description. Int J Tuberc Lung Dis 2008;12(9):1092–8.

94. Sandoval J, Salas J, Martinez-Guerra ML, et al. Pulmonary arterial hypertension and cor pulmonale associated with chronic domestic woodsmoke inhalation. Chest 1993;103(1):12–20.

95. Thenappan T, Shah SJ, Rich S, et al. Survival in pulmonary arterial hypertension: a reappraisal of the NIH risk stratification equation. Eur Respir J 2010;35(5):1079–87.

96. Peacock AJ, Murphy NF, McMurray JJ, et al. An epidemiological study of pulmonary arterial hypertension. Eur Respir J 2007;30(1):104–9.

97. Kawut SM, Horn EM, Berekashvili KK, et al. New predictors of outcome in idiopathic pulmonary arterial hypertension. Am J Cardiol 2005;95(2):199–203.

98. Humbert M, Sitbon O, Yaïci A, et al. Survival in incident and prevalent cohorts of patients with pulmonary arterial hypertension. Eur Respir J 2010;36(3): 549–55.

99. Humbert M, Sitbon O, Chaouat A, et al. Pulmonary arterial hypertension in France: results from a national registry. Am J Respir Crit Care Med 2006; 173(9):1023–30.

100. Humbert M, Sitbon O, Chaouat A, et al. Survival in patients with idiopathic, familial, and anorexigen-associated pulmonary arterial hypertension in the modern management era. Circulation 2010;122(2):156–63.

101. Ling Y, Johnson MK, Kiely DG, et al. Changing demographics, epidemiology, and survival of incident pulmonary arterial hypertension: results from the pulmonary hypertension registry of the United

Kingdom and Ireland. Am J Respir Crit Care Med 2012;186(8):790–6.

102. Olsson KM, Delcroix M, Ghofrani HA, et al. Anticoagulation and survival in pulmonary arterial hypertension: results from the Comparative, Prospective Registry of Newly Initiated Therapies for Pulmonary Hypertension (COMPERA). Circulation 2014;129(1):57–65.

103. Pulido T, Adzerikho I, Channick RN, et al. Macitentan and morbidity and mortality in pulmonary arterial hypertension. N Engl J Med 2013;369(9): 809–18.

104. Gaine S, Sitbon O, Channick RN, et al. Relationship Between Time From Diagnosis and Morbidity/Mortality in Pulmonary Arterial Hypertension: Results From the Phase III GRIPHON Study. Chest 2021; 160(1):277–86.

Unusual Forms of Pulmonary Hypertension

Yuri de Deus Montalverne Parente, MD[a], Natalia Fernandes da Silva, MD[a], Rogerio Souza, MD, PhD[a],*

KEYWORDS

- Schistosomiasis • Venoocclusive disease • Sickle cell disease • Sarcoidosis
- Langerhans cell histiocytosis

KEY POINTS

- Although mostly limited to developing regions, schistosomiasis-associated pulmonary arterial hypertension (PAH) is an important form of PAH characterized by a better clinical course and some specific features such as significant pulmonary artery dilations.
- Sarcoidosis-associated pulmonary hypertension (PH) is mostly characterized by lung parenchyma disease although multiple mechanisms might be present such as myocardial involvement, direct pulmonary vascular disease, vascular compression, or even thrombosis.
- Pulmonary veno-occlusive disease represents a rare form of PH characterized by predominant involvement of the pulmonary venous/capillary system but with management similar to other PAH forms.
- Pulmonary Langerhans' cell histiocytosis-associated PH is a rare form of pulmonary hypertension with multiple vascular components involved and not necessarily associated with the severity of the lung parenchyma disease.
- PH associated with hemoglobinopathies, particularly sickle cell disease, is an important form of PH associated with multiple potential pathophysiological mechanisms.

SCHISTOSOMIASIS

Introduction

Pulmonary arterial hypertension (PAH) is a fatal complication of schistosomiasis, a neglected tropical disease, that results from chronic and recurrent infection with the helminthic parasite Schistosoma. The main disease-causing species are *Schistosoma haematobium*, *Schistosoma mansoni*, and *Schistosoma japonicum*. These species present characteristic geographic distribution with *S haematobium* more prevalent in Africa, *S mansoni* in Latin America, and *S japonicum* in Asia. PAH associated with schistosomiasis (Sch-PAH) is currently classified within group 1 of the PH classification, representing one of the major etiologies of PAH.[1,2]

Epidemiology/Etiology

Schistosomiasis is believed to affect about 200 million individuals worldwide and to be underdiagnosed.[3] More than 85% of these patients live in Brazil and sub-Saharan Africa where the prevalence of infected individuals can exceed 50% in the local population.[4] In turn, Sch-PAH is thought to affect up to 5% of those with chronic manifestation of schistosomiasis, mostly hepatosplenic disease in the case of *S mansoni*.[5] The pathophysiological mechanism of PAH is not yet fully elucidated and may influence the actual distribution and prevalence of Sch-PAH worldwide. Infection with *S mansoni*, the species most clearly associated with Sch-PAH, also causes severe preportal liver fibrosis in up to 10% of patients, termed

None of the authors has any conflict of interest related to the content of this article.

[a] Pulmonary Division – Heart Institute (InCor) - Hospital das Clínicas da Faculdade de Medicina da Universidade de São Paulo

* Corresponding author. Av. Dr. Eneas de Carvalho Aguiar, 44 – 5 and – Bl 2 – s.6, São Paulo, São Paulo 05403-900, Brazil.

E-mail address: rogerio.souza@hc.fm.usp.br

Heart Failure Clin 19 (2023) 25–33
https://doi.org/10.1016/j.hfc.2022.08.021

schistosomiasis-associated hepato-splenic disease (SchHSD), which can be diagnosed and staged by abdominal ultrasound through the evaluation of periportal fibrosis.[6] SchHSD causes portal hypertension but not cirrhosis and is thought to be a precursor to the development of Sch-PAH in many individuals. Portal hypertension opens perihepatic shunts, with embolization of eggs in the systemic vena cava and in precapillary pulmonary vessels where they elicit a strong type 2 inflammatory reaction and pathologic Transforming growth factor beta (TGF-β) signaling, the latter likely representing a pathway to PAH that is shared across etiologies.[7] This putative pathway supports the hypothesis that patients with SchHSD are at elevated risk for Sch-PAH.

Individuals with signs and symptoms of progressive right heart failure, history of environmental exposure, earlier treatment of schistosomiasis, or evidence of hepatosplenic abnormalities (hepatosplenomegaly, esophageal varices, gastropathy, and anemia) with portal fibrosis or enlargement of left lobe should be screened for Sch-PAH. Another feature that should raise the suspicion of schistosomiasis is the presence of excessive dilation of the pulmonary arteries, usually larger than idiopathic PAH (IPAH) (**Fig. 1**).[8] Transthoracic echocardiography is the screening modality of choice but right heart catheterization is mandatory not only to confirm the presence of pulmonary hypertension (PH) but also to ensure precapillary pattern because postcapillary PH can also be present.[5]

Treatment

Despite the similarities with IPAH (histologic and hemodynamics),[9] Sch-PAH has a distinct, more benign course. However, Sch-PAH still presents 36 month mortality of 15%, in the absence of therapy.[10] Small case series suggested that the use of an inhibitor of phosphodiesterase 5 or endothelin-receptor antagonists led to improvements in

functional class, distance in the 6-min walking distance, and hemodynamics (cardiac index and pulmonary vascular resistance).[11] More recently, the use of specific PAH therapy in patients with Sch-PAH was associated with improved survival, in comparison with a historical control group of untreated patients.[12] These data suggest that Sch-PAH should follow the same recommendations of other causes of PAH, concerning specific PAH treatment.[13] It is important to remember that some of these patients may have an increased bleeding risk due to the presence of esophageal varices.

SARCOIDOSIS
Introduction

Sarcoidosis is an inflammatory granulomatous disease of unknown cause, characterized by inflammation, lymphadenopathy, and the presence of sterile granulomas in one or more organs.[14] More than 90% of people with sarcoidosis have lung or intrathoracic lymph node involvement.[15] Sarcoidosis-associated PH (SAPH) is a significant cause of morbidity and mortality in patients with advanced sarcoidosis, with studies reporting up to a seven-fold increase in the risk of death compared with patients without PH.[16] It can be caused by different and sometimes overlapping mechanisms such as direct vascular involvement, cardiac infiltration, compression of pulmonary vessels due to lymphadenopathy and lung parenchyma disease. Owing to these multiple potential mechanisms, it is classified within group 5 of the clinical classification of PH (unclear or multifactorial mechanisms).[17] Exertional dyspnea is the most common presentation of SAPH. Chest pain, exertional syncope, and palpitations are also observed and must be distinguished from cardiac sarcoidosis. Patients with SAPH often have a disproportionately low gas transfer (diffusion capacity of carbon monoxide [DLCO]) to the degree

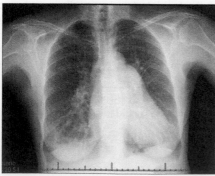
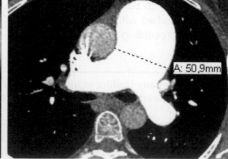

Fig. 1. Pulmonary artery enlargement in Sch-PAH.

of pulmonary fibrosis and a reduction in forced vital capacity (FVC). Oxygen desaturation to less than 90% during the 6 min walk distance (6MWD) test has been shown to predict PH.[18] A recent international registry evidenced that reduced DLCO and 6MWD were the main factors associated with a worse prognosis.[19] In addition, the presence of PH is associated with greater oxygen demand and a worsening of quality of life.[20]

Epidemiology/Etiology

The reported incidence of SAPH has been around 5% in studies from across the world. A recent Dutch registry of SAPH estimated a prevalence of 2.9%.[21] Pabst and colleagues showed a similar prevalence (3.6%) in a German cohort.[22] The true incidence of SAPH is unknown, and prevalence is dependent on the stage at which the patients are assessed for PH.[23] For instance, the prevalence can be as high as 73% in patients listed for lung transplantation.[24]

Among the multiple mechanisms associated with SAPH, lung parenchymal disease seems to be the most prevalent one.[25] In patients with fibrotic lung disease, SAPH is attributed to the destruction of the distal capillary bed by fibrotic processes or to the resultant chronic hypoxemia. In some patients, the degree of PH and right ventricular dysfunction is not compatible with fibrotic changes in the parenchyma, leading to the recognition of phenotypes of SAPH characterized by a lack of parenchymal involvement. Previous pathologic studies have demonstrated noncaseating granulomas in the walls of the pulmonary vasculature; this form of granulomatous inflammation can affect the entire pulmonary vasculature including the pulmonary veins. The granulomas can also be found in the lymphatics and postcapillary venules, which can mimic pulmonary venoocclusive disease (PVOD).

Cardiac sarcoidosis leading to left heart disease is an important differential diagnosis to exclude in patients with suspected SAPH. Cardiac involvement in sarcoidosis most often presents with conduction disease and heart failure; however, silent cardiac involvement with subclinical diastolic dysfunction in sarcoidosis is increasingly being recognized. There is also early evidence to suggest isolated involvement of the right ventricle (RV) in cardiac sarcoid resulting in severe RV strain without evidence of other organ system involvement.[26]

It is well known that patients with sarcoidosis are also at increased risk of thromboembolic events. Some series report a 3-fold increased risk of pulmonary embolism in patients with sarcoidosis.[27] Therefore, patients with sarcoidosis are clearly at higher risk of developing chronic thromboembolic PH.

Extrapulmonary factors can also contribute to SAPH. Extrinsic compression of the large pulmonary arteries by enlarged hilar lymph nodes or fibrosing mediastinitis leading to architectural distortion of vessels may lead to increased pulmonary resistance. Furthermore, sarcoidosis-related liver disease can also be associated with PH (porto-PH).

Treatment

The treatment of SAPH is based on the correct diagnosis and, for this, a multidisciplinary approach in service with experience in PAH and interstitial lung diseases is recommended. It is important to follow the diagnostic algorithm of PH, performing a transthoracic echocardiogram, pulmonary function test, and pulmonary ventilation-perfusion scintigraphy. High-resolution computed tomographic (CT) scans should be performed to assess parenchymal involvement and the presence of mediastinal lymphadenopathy that may contribute to PH. Other noninvasive imaging modalities such as cardiac MRI and PET scans are commonly used to detect cardiac involvement in sarcoidosis; however, their utility in early detection of SAPH is unclear.

Right heart catheterization will be necessary to define the hemodynamic pattern of precapillary or postcapillary PH. It should be performed in patients with moderate (especially if FVC > 50%) to high probability of PH by transthoracic echocardiography.[28]

There is no strong evidence for the use of pulmonary vasodilators in SAPH. A recent statement suggests that treatment decisions and followups should be made by a multidisciplinary team with a sarcoidosis and a PH expert. Concurrent causes of PH, such as thromboembolic disease, resting hypoxemia, and mechanical obstruction of the pulmonary artery, should also be evaluated and treated appropriately. Offlabel use of PAH therapy may be considered for symptomatic patients on a case-by-case basis.[29] Uncontrolled studies have provided evidence of response to PAH-targeted therapies in SAPH.[30,31] Recently, a small randomized trial reinforced these findings.[32] For those with moderate-to-severe parenchymal lung disease (FVC <50% predicted value), PH-specific treatment may not be as effective, and it is not indicated. However, a recently published study did demonstrate that treatment of mild PH with inhaled treprostinil in idiopathic interstitial lung disease was associated with a positive response.[33]

The extrapolation of these results to SAPH should be done with caution given the heterogeneity that can be related to the elevation in pulmonary artery pressures.

Combination therapy with both PAH therapies and immunosuppressants is common and is an attractive approach in SAPH, although the evidence to justify its use is weak. The rationale would be to improve vascular granulomatous inflammatory activity, lymphadenopathy, and possible associated parenchymal involvement.

PULMONARY VENO-OCCLUSIVE DISEASE
Introduction

PVOD represents a rare form of PH characterized by the predominant involvement of the pulmonary venous/capillary system. Like PVOD, pulmonary capillary hemangiomatosis (PCH) also affects this pulmonary vascular territory and, currently, both are considered a spectrum of the same process. Both conditions are classified within group 1 of the current PH classification as 1.6-PAH with overt features of venous/capillaries involvement.[1] The histopathological hallmarks of PVOD/PCH are abnormal alveolar capillary proliferation, intimal fibrosis and luminal narrowing, arterialization or obliteration of the septal veins and venules. Fresh hemorrhage and hemosiderin-laden macrophages in the alveolar spaces are usually present in PVOD/PCH. Arterial lesions in PVOD resemble that of PAH with eccentric intimal fibrosis and medial hypertrophy. However, plexiform lesions characteristic of severe PAH is not present.[34]

Epidemiology/Etiology

Prevalence and incidence rates of PVOD/PCH can only be estimated as accurate diagnosis is challenging without histologic (or genetic) confirmation and many cases of PVOD/PCH remain misclassified as PAH.

PVOD/PCH can occur sporadically or heritable, related to the eukaryotic translation initiation factor 2 α kinase 4 (EIF2AK4) gene. EIF2AK4 mutations are found in nearly all PCH/PVOD patients with a family history, but are also identified in 8.6% to 25% of sporadic cases of PCH/PVOD. Risk factors and associated conditions with PVOD/PCH are chemotherapy (especially with alkylating agents), occupational exposures (organic solvents such as trichloroethylene), tobacco exposure, and autoimmunity conditions (particularly systemic sclerosis).[34]

In practice, differentiating PVOD/PCH from PAH could be quite difficult. The signs and symptoms of PH are present in both situations; however, some points must be highlighted: (1) hypoxemia is more marked in PCH/PVOD than in PAH, and DLCO is markedly reduced, to a greater degree than in PAH[35]; (2) a history of occupational exposures to solvents like trichloroethylene or chemotherapeutic agents is much more frequent in patients with PCH/PVOD than PAH[36]; and (3) cardiopulmonary exercise testing may be useful as exercise capacity is lower and dyspnea intensity during exercise is more severe in patients with PCH/PVOD compared with matched patients with PAH due to higher ventilatory demand, higher minute ventilation/exhaled carbon dioxide and physiologic dead space (dead space/tidal volume), more severe gas exchange impairment and earlier onset of lactic acidosis.[37]

The features of PVOD/PCH on chest CT include (1) hilar and mediastinal lymphadenopathy; (2) poorly circumscribed centrilobular ground glass nodular opacities; and (3) smooth thickening of the interlobular septae (**Fig. 2**). Having two or three of these CT features has a sensitivity of 75% and specificity of 84.6% for PCH/PVOD. These features correspond to the lymph node congestion, capillary infiltration/proliferation, and venous remodeling in the interalveolar septae and focal alveolar hemorrhage observed on histology.[35]

Most of sporadic PCH/PVOD cases do not carry EIF2AK4 mutations, so the sensitivity of genetic testing is likely to be low, especially in older patients. Therefore, negative genetic testing does not exclude PVOD/PCH but identification of biallelic EIF2AK4 mutations is highly supportive of the diagnosis.[38]

Genetic testing can be helpful to distinguish PCH/PVOD from PAH, particularly when there is a supportive family history, as EIF2AK4 mutations are uncommon in heritable PAH and BMPR2 mutations uncommon in PCH/PVOD.

Treatment

Data on the natural history of PVOD are limited, but the disease is usually characterized by inexorable progression. Prognosis is considered significantly worse than other forms of PAH. A recent study found that the survival time of patients with PVOD/PCH is reported to be approximately 2 years after initial reported symptoms and the mean time from diagnosis to death or lung transplantation was 11.8 months.

The differentiation of PCH/PVOD from PAH is of utmost therapeutic importance, as the prognosis is poor in PCH/PVOD and the use of PAH-targeted therapies in PCH/PVOD is usually less effective and can result in pulmonary edema. A systematic review of 64 patients treated with pulmonary vasodilators, despite some improvement

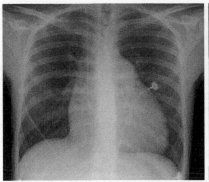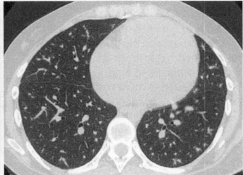

Fig. 2. Radiographic features of PVOD/PCH.

in the 6MWD test and pulmonary vascular resistance (PVR), evidenced pulmonary edema in almost 50% of them.[39]

In a French study,[40] 90% of the 94 patients with PCH/PVOD had received PAH medical therapies but only 3 out of 47 patients with a follow-up assessment had achieved satisfactory clinical responses, despite statistically significant improvements in 6MWD, cardiac index, and pulmonary vascular resistance. The results were similar in EIF2AK4 mutation carriers and noncarriers in that study. Patients with underlying connective tissue disease and suspected PAH are also prone to developing pulmonary edema with prostacyclin therapy. As such, patients with known or suspected PCH/PVOD lung transplantation should be promptly considered.

PULMONARY LANGERHANS' CELL HISTIOCYTOSIS
Introduction

Pulmonary Langerhans' cell histiocytosis (PLCH) is an uncommon cystic lung disease that affects primarily young adults, between 20 and 40 years, related with smoking in greater than 90% of the cases, suggesting a strong relation with tobacco use. PLCH is characterized by micronodules and cysts, predominantly in the upper lobes and sparing costophrenic angle (>90%). It can be asymptomatic or associated with dyspnea, dry cough, weight loss, chest pain, night sweats, or recurrent pneumothorax.[41] PH and dynamic hyperinflation are the most important factors that limit exercise capacity in patients with PLCH.[42,43]

Epidemiology/Etiology

PLCH has an estimated prevalence in adults of 1 to 2 out of 1 million. In Japanese hospitalized patients, the prevalence rates of PLCH were reported to be 0.07 of 100,000 in women and 0.27 of 100,000 in

men. Moderate or severe PH (mean pulmonary artery pressure [PAPm] > 35 mm Hg) might be present in up to 92% of the patients with PLCH who presented for lung transplantation.[44]

The pathogenesis of PH in PLCH is not completely understood and might be multifactorial. When patients with advanced PLCH and severe PH were compared with patients with chronic obstructive pulmonary disease (COPD) or idiopathic pulmonary fibrosis, the degree of PH was not related to pulmonary function in patients with PLCH in contrast to patients with COPD or idiopathic pulmonary fibrosis and seems to be more severe.[45] Radiographic features of PH in PLCH are similar to those seem in other forms (**Fig. 3**).

Vasculopathy in PLCH can involve pulmonary arteries and veins. In a study of 12 patients with PLCH and severe PH, vascular changes included mild-to-severe intimal fibrosis and medial hypertrophy of pulmonary arteries and mild-to-severe intimal fibrosis and moderate-to-severe muscularization of pulmonary veins. Veno-occlusive-like disease with venular obliteration, hemosiderosis, and capillary dilatation was also observed[45].

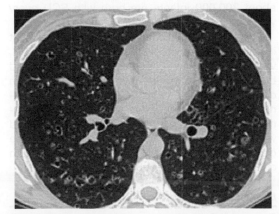

Fig. 3. Radiographic features of PH associated with PLCH.

Treatment

Prognosis of PLCH in adults is greatly affected by the response to treatment and the occurrence of relapses. Prognosis can range from an absence of sequelae to severe organ (liver, lung) dysfunction.

The treatment of PLCH is multimodal, the main measure being smoking cessation. By itself, it can lead to injury reduction and disease stabilization in up to 50% of cases. Drug therapy is indicated for patients with extensive disease or that affects other organs and consists of several drug classes, from glucocorticoids to chemotherapy and targeted therapy (such as BRAF inhibitors). Patients with PLCH also have a higher risk of infections; therefore, influenza and pneumococcal vaccines are recommended.

Regarding the treatment of PH, oxygen therapy should be offered to all hypoxemic patients. The use of specific therapy for PAH has been reported to cause pulmonary edema, similar to what can occur in PVOD.[45] However, a small cohort of patients with PLCH treated with different PAH therapies reported improvement in hemodynamics without causing worsening of oxygenation.[46] In this sense, patients should be evaluated for the use of PAH-targeted therapies, especially those awaiting lung transplantation; nevertheless, the risk of pulmonary edema has to be considered throughout the treatment.

SICKLE CELL DISEASE
Introduction

Sickle cell disease (SCD) is autosomal recessive hemoglobinopathy leading to the formation of hemoglobin S that polymerizes when deoxygenated forming sickle-shaped erythrocytes. These abnormal red cells are the basis for the two main pathophysiological events in the disease: hemolysis and vaso-occlusive crisis.[47] It is estimated that about 300,000 infants are born with SCD every year, worldwide.[48]

Pulmonary complications are among the most important causes of death in SCD, including PH, venous thromboembolic disease, sleep-disordered breathing, and acute chest pain.[49] These multiple complications also highlight the potential mechanisms that could be associated with the development of PH in SCD; for this reason, PH associated with SCD is currently classified into group 5 of the classification proposed at the 6th World Symposium on Pulmonary Hypertension.[1]

Epidemiology/Etiology

As within other clinical conditions that predispose to the development of PH, it is of utmost importance to identify the predominant pathophysiological mechanism driving the elevation of pulmonary artery pressures. Therefore, the complete diagnostic approach is mandatory.[50] The increased risk of thrombotic complications due to hemolysis associated with functional asplenia, for instance, highlight the potential for chronic thromboembolic disease in SCD. This is just an example to reinforce that PH should not be considered as a sole clinical condition associated with SCD.

Echocardiogram remains as the main noninvasive tool for the initial investigation of PH; however, potentially due to the presence of anemia and high cardiac output, the use of a tricuspid regurgitant jet velocity (TRV) of 2.5 m/s as a cutoff for pulmonary artery systolic pressure elevation has low specificity, with only about 25% of individuals confirming the presence of PH.[51–53] Nevertheless, even this mild elevation of the TRV is associated with a worse prognosis.[54]

Similarly, right heart catheterization remains the main tool for the appropriate diagnosis. Three different studies using invasive hemodynamics for the diagnosis of PH in patients with SCD evidenced a prevalence of PH ranging from 6% to 10%.[51–53] Moreover, these studies allowed the recognition of different hemodynamic patterns, such as high cardiac output state, precapillary, and postcapillary PH (**Table 1**).

More recently, the significant prevalence of postcapillary PH in SCD has been better approached. An autopsy study from Brazil[55] evidenced abnormalities in the whole pulmonary vascular tree of patients with SCD. Beyond the well-known prevalence of acute and chronic thrombotic lesions, the study described a significant proliferation of capillaries. This finding had been already described in chronic congestion secondary to left heart disease.[56] In fact, the role of left ventricular dysfunction in SCD is a matter of growing concern.[57] Chronic anemia leading to a high cardiac output state, hemolysis interfering with nitric oxide bioavailability, inflammation, vasoocclusive events, all these mechanisms can lead to increased left ventricular wall stress than can result in fibrosis and hypertrophy to a lower or greater degree. This can result in the development of diastolic dysfunction that could explain, at least in part, the postcapillary pattern evidence in the previously mentioned studies.

Treatment

Although there is no robust evidence regarding PH management in SCD, some strategies have been proposed for better clinical control. The first

Table 1
Hemodynamic profile in pulmonary hypertension associated with sickle cell disease

	French Cohort	Brazilian Cohort	US Cohort
Patients enrolled	385	80	531
RHC – n	96	26	84
PH – n (%)	24 (6%)	8 (10%)	55 (10%)
PH hemodynamic pattern			
Precapillary	11 (46%)	3 (37%)	31 (56%)
Postcapillary	13 (54%)	5 (63%)	24 (44%)
Mortality in the PH group	12.5%	38%	36%

Abbreviation: RHC, right heart catheterization.

approach is based on the intensification of SCD-directed therapy. The American Thoracic Society guidelines propose the use of hydroxyurea, a fetal hemoglobin inducer, to all patients with SCD with increased mortality risk and chronic transfusion therapy for those without response to hydroxyurea.[58] Gene therapy and stem cell transplantation still have limited application although represent important perspectives in the setting of better treating SCD.

Data are also limited regarding the use of PAH-targeted therapies for PH-SCD. A large trial using sildenafil for SCD with echocardiographic findings of PH was stopped due to an increased rate of hospitalization due to pain crises.[59] More recently, a retrospective cohort of 36 patients with PH-SCD diagnosed through right heart catheterization and treated with long-term use of sildenafil reported improvement in symptoms with an increased rate of hospitalization. Noteworthy, the study did not demonstrate improvement in exercise capacity or hemodynamics.[60] Two trials addressing the potential role of endothelin receptor antagonists were stopped due to slow enrollment.[61] Altogether, these findings highlight the need for appropriate evidence in the use of targeted therapies. Although there are case series suggesting the use of PAH therapies in this setting, their use should be individualized[58] with close monitoring of the patients not only for assessing response but mostly for safety monitoring, preferentially at a PH reference center.

CLINICS CARE POINTS

- Patients with significant pulmonary artery enlargement in evaluation for pulmonary hypertension (PH) should always have their epidemiology to schistosomiasis checked
- Chest computed tomography scans should always be checked for the presence of pulmonary veno-occlusive disease features during PH diagnosis
- There is growing evidence of left ventricular disease in patients with sickle cell disease.
- PH diagnostic algorithm should be followed in all patients with sarcoidosis, regardless of the severity of lung parenchyma disease

REFERENCES

1. Simonneau G, Montani D, Celermajer DS, et al. Haemodynamic definitions and updated clinical classification of pulmonary hypertension. Eur Respir J 2019;53(1). https://doi.org/10.1183/13993003.01913-2018.
2. Gavilanes F, Fernandes CJ, Souza R. Pulmonary arterial hypertension in schistosomiasis. Curr Opin Pulm Med 2016;22(5):408–14.
3. Gryseels B, Polman K, Clerinx J, et al. Human schistosomiasis. Lancet 2006;368(9541):1106–18.
4. Colley DG, Bustinduy AL, Secor WE, et al. Human schistosomiasis. Lancet 2014;383(9936):2253–64.
5. Lapa M, Dias B, Jardim C, et al. Cardiopulmonary Manifestations of Hepatosplenic Schistosomiasis. Circulation 2009;119(11):1518–23.
6. Hatz C, Jenkins JM, Ali QM, et al. A review of the literature on the use of ultrasonography in schistosomiasis with special reference to its use in field studies. 2. Schistosoma mansoni. Acta Trop 1992; 51(1):15–28.
7. Sibomana JP, Campeche A, Carvalho Filho RJ, et al. Schistosomiasis Pulmonary Arterial Hypertension. Front Immunol 2020;11:608883.
8. Hoette S, Figueiredo C, Dias B, et al. Pulmonary artery enlargement in schistosomiasis associated pulmonary arterial hypertension. BMC Pulm Med 2015; 15:118.
9. Mauad T, Pozzan G, Lancas T, et al. Immunopathological aspects of schistosomiasis-associated pulmonary arterial hypertension. J Infect 2014;68(1): 90–8.

10. dos Santos Fernandes CJ, Jardim CV, Hovnanian A, et al. Survival in schistosomiasis-associated pulmonary arterial hypertension. J Am Coll Cardiol 2010; 56(9):715–20.

11. Fernandes C, Dias BA, Jardim CVP, et al. The role of target therapies in schistosomiasis-associated pulmonary arterial hypertension. *Chest* Apr 2012; 141(4):923–8.

12. Fernandes CJC, Piloto B, Castro M, et al. Survival of patients with schistosomiasis-associated pulmonary arterial hypertension in the modern management era. Eur Respir J 2018;51(6). https://doi.org/10. 1183/13993003.00307-2018.

13. Fernandes CJ, Calderaro D, Assad APL, et al. Update on the Treatment of Pulmonary Arterial Hypertension. Arq Bras Cardiol 2021;117(4):750–64. Atualizacao no Tratamento da Hipertensao Arterial Pulmonar.

14. Baughman RP, Field S, Costabel U, et al. Sarcoidosis in America. Analysis Based on Health Care Use. Ann Am Thorac Soc 2016;13(8):1244–52.

15. Belperio JA, Shaikh F, Abtin FG, et al. Diagnosis and Treatment of Pulmonary Sarcoidosis: A Review. JAMA 1 2022;327(9):856–67.

16. Kirkil G, Lower EE, Baughman RP. Predictors of Mortality in Pulmonary Sarcoidosis. Chest 2018;153(1): 105–13.

17. Jeny F, Uzunhan Y, Lacroix M, et al. Predictors of mortality in fibrosing pulmonary sarcoidosis. *Respiratory medicine*. Aug 2020;169:105997. https://doi. org/10.1016/j.rmed.2020.105997.

18. Bourbonnais JM, Samavati L. Clinical predictors of pulmonary hypertension in sarcoidosis. *Eur Respir J* Aug 2008;32(2):296–302.

19. Shlobin OA, Kouranos V, Barnett SD, et al. Physiological predictors of survival in patients with sarcoidosis-associated pulmonary hypertension: results from an international registry. Eur Respir J 2020;55(5). https://doi.org/10.1183/13993003.01747-2019.

20. Shorr AF, Helman DL, Davies DB, et al. Pulmonary hypertension in advanced sarcoidosis: epidemiology and clinical characteristics. Eur Respir J 2005;25(5):783–8.

21. Huitema MP, Bakker ALM, Mager JJ, et al. Prevalence of pulmonary hypertension in pulmonary sarcoidosis: the first large European prospective study. Eur Respir J 2019;54(4). https://doi.org/10. 1183/13993003.00897-2019.

22. Pabst S, Hammerstingl C, Grau N, et al. Pulmonary arterial hypertension in patients with sarcoidosis: the Pulsar single center experience. Adv Exp Med Biol 2013;755:299–305.

23. Bandyopadhyay D, Humbert M. An update on sarcoidosis-associated pulmonary hypertension. Curr Opin Pulm Med 2020;26(5):582–90.

24. Nunes H, Humbert M, Capron F, et al. Pulmonary hypertension associated with sarcoidosis: mechanisms, haemodynamics and prognosis. Thorax 2006;61(1): 68–74.

25. Baughman RP, Shlobin OA, Wells AU, et al. Clinical features of sarcoidosis associated pulmonary hypertension: Results of a multi-national registry. Respir Med 2018;139:72–8.

26. Ozyilmaz E, Akilli R, Berk I, et al. The frequency of diastolic dysfunction in patients with sarcoidosis and it's relationship with HLA DRB1* alleles. Sarcoidosis Vasculitis Diffuse Lung Dis 2019;36(4): 285–93.

27. Ungprasert P, Crowson CS, Matteson EL. Association of Sarcoidosis With Increased Risk of VTE: A Population-Based Study, 1976 to 2013. Chest 2017;151(2):425–30.

28. Savale L, Huitema M, Shlobin O, et al. WASOG statement on the diagnosis and management of sarcoidosis-associated pulmonary hypertension. Eur Respir Rev 2022;(163):31. https://doi.org/10. 1183/16000617.0165-2021.

29. Perlman DM, Sudheendra MT, Furuya Y, et al. Clinical Presentation and Treatment of High-Risk Sarcoidosis. Ann Am Thorac Soc 2021;18(12):1935–47.

30. Keir GJ, Walsh SL, Gatzoulis MA, et al. Treatment of sarcoidosis-associated pulmonary hypertension: A single centre retrospective experience using targeted therapies. Sarcoidosis Vasculitis Diffuse Lung Dis 2014;31(2):82–90.

31. Boucly A, Cottin V, Nunes H, et al. Management and long-term outcomes of sarcoidosis-associated pulmonary hypertension. Eur Respir J 2017;50(4). https://doi.org/10.1183/13993003.00465-2017.

32. Baughman RP, Shlobin OA, Gupta R, et al. Riociguat for Sarcoidosis-Associated Pulmonary Hypertension: Results of a 1-Year Double-Blind, Placebo-Controlled Trial. Chest 2022;161(2):448–57.

33. Waxman A, Restrepo-Jaramillo R, Thenappan T, et al. Inhaled Treprostinil in Pulmonary Hypertension Due to Interstitial Lung Disease. N Engl J Med 2021; 384(4):325–34.

34. Gunther S, Perros F, Rautou PE, et al. Understanding the Similarities and Differences between Hepatic and Pulmonary Veno-Occlusive Disease. Am J Pathol 2019;189(6):1159–75.

35. Montani D, Achouh L, Dorfmuller P, et al. Pulmonary veno-occlusive disease: clinical, functional, radiologic, and hemodynamic characteristics and outcome of 24 cases confirmed by histology. Medicine (Baltimore) 2008;87(4):220–33.

36. Montani D, Lau EM, Descatha A, et al. Occupational exposure to organic solvents: a risk factor for pulmonary veno-occlusive disease. Eur Respir J 2015; 46(6):1721–31.

37. Laveneziana P, Montani D, Dorfmuller P, et al. Mechanisms of exertional dyspnoea in pulmonary veno-occlusive disease with EIF2AK4 mutations. Eur Respir J 2014;44(4):1069–72.

38. Weatherald J, Dorfmuller P, Perros F, et al. Pulmonary capillary haemangiomatosis: a distinct entity? Eur Respir Rev : official J Eur Respir Soc 2020;(156):29. https://doi.org/10.1183/16000617.0168-2019.

39. Ogawa A, Sakao S, Tanabe N, et al. Use of vasodilators for the treatment of pulmonary veno-occlusive disease and pulmonary capillary hemangiomatosis: A systematic review. Respir Investig 2019;57(2): 183–90.

40. Montani D, Girerd B, Jais X, et al. Clinical phenotypes and outcomes of heritable and sporadic pulmonary veno-occlusive disease: a population-based study. Lancet Respir Med 2017;5(2):125–34.

41. Emile JF, Cohen-Aubart F, Collin M, et al. Histiocytosis. Lancet 2021;398(10295):157–70.

42. Radzikowska E. Update on Pulmonary Langerhans Cell Histiocytosis. Front Med (Lausanne) 2020;7: 582581.

43. Heiden GI, Sobral JB, Freitas CSG, et al. Mechanisms of Exercise Limitation and Prevalence of Pulmonary Hypertension in Pulmonary Langerhans Cell Histiocytosis. Chest 2020;158(6):2440–8.

44. Dauriat G, Mal H, Thabut G, et al. Lung transplantation for pulmonary langerhans' cell histiocytosis: a multicenter analysis. Transplantation 2006;81(5): 746–50.

45. Fartoukh M, Humbert M, Capron F, et al. Severe pulmonary hypertension in histiocytosis X. Am J Respir Crit Care Med 2000;161(1):216–23.

46. Le Pavec J, Lorillon G, Jais X, et al. Pulmonary Langerhans cell histiocytosis-associated pulmonary hypertension: clinical characteristics and impact of pulmonary arterial hypertension therapies. Chest 2012;142(5):1150–7.

47. Kavanagh PL, Fasipe TA, Wun T. Sickle Cell Disease: A Review. JAMA 2022;328(1):57–68.

48. Piel FB, Hay SI, Gupta S, et al. Global burden of sickle cell anaemia in children under five, 2010-2050: modelling based on demographics, excess mortality, and interventions. Plos Med 2013;10(7): e1001484.

49. Mehari A, Klings ES. Chronic Pulmonary Complications of Sickle Cell Disease. Chest 2016;149(5): 1313–24.

50. Alves JL, Oleas FG, Souza R. Pulmonary Hypertension: Definition, Classification, and Diagnosis. Semin Respir Crit Care Med 2017;38(5):561–70.

51. Parent F, Bachir D, Inamo J, et al. A hemodynamic study of pulmonary hypertension in sickle cell disease. N Engl J Med 2011;365(1):44–53.

52. Fonseca GH, Souza R, Salemi VM, et al. Pulmonary hypertension diagnosed by right heart catheterisation in sickle cell disease. Eur Respir J 2012;39(1): 112–8.

53. Mehari A, Gladwin MT, Tian X, et al. Mortality in adults with sickle cell disease and pulmonary hypertension. JAMA 2012;307(12):1254–6.

54. Gladwin MT, Sachdev V, Jison ML, et al. Pulmonary hypertension as a risk factor for death in patients with sickle cell disease. N Engl J Med 2004;350(9): 886–95.

55. Carstens GR, Paulino BBA, Katayama EH, et al. Clinical relevance of pulmonary vasculature involvement in sickle cell disease. Br J Haematol 2019;185(2): 317–26.

56. Ribeiro de Campos PT, Lopes AA, Issa VS, et al. Morphologic and immunohistochemical features of pulmonary vasculopathy in end-stage left ventricular systolic failure. J Heart Lung Transplant 2018;37(3): 422–5.

57. Wood KC, Gladwin MT, Straub AC. Sickle cell disease: at the crossroads of pulmonary hypertension and diastolic heart failure. Heart 2020;106(8):562–8.

58. Klings ES, Machado RF, Barst RJ, et al. An official American Thoracic Society clinical practice guideline: diagnosis, risk stratification, and management of pulmonary hypertension of sickle cell disease. Am J Respir Crit Care Med 2014;189(6):727–40.

59. Machado RF, Barst RJ, Yovetich NA, et al. Hospitalization for pain in patients with sickle cell disease treated with sildenafil for elevated TRV and low exercise capacity. Blood 2011;118(4):855–64.

60. Cramer-Bour C, Ruhl AP, Nouraie SM, et al. Long-term tolerability of phosphodiesterase-5 inhibitors in pulmonary hypertension of sickle cell disease. Eur J Haematol 2021;107(1):54–62.

61. Barst RJ, Mubarak KK, Machado RF, et al. Exercise capacity and haemodynamics in patients with sickle cell disease with pulmonary hypertension treated with bosentan: results of the ASSET studies. Br J Haematol 2010;140(3):126–36.

Cardiopulmonary Exercise Testing in Pulmonary Arterial Hypertension

Alexander E. Sherman, MD[a],*, Rajan Saggar, MD[a,b]

KEYWORDS

- Pulmonary arterial hypertension • Pulmonary hypertension • Cardiopulmonary exercise test • CPET

KEY POINTS

- Cardiopulmonary exercise testing (CEPT) is a safe, noninvasive method of evaluating for pulmonary arterial hypertension with roles in assessing treatment response and prognosis.
- Reduced oxygen uptake and ventilatory inefficiency are hallmarks of a pulmonary vascular limitation and should prompt further evaluation.
- The greater diagnostic resolution of CPET allows for potential earlier detection of disease progression compared with resting studies.

INTRODUCTION

Cardiopulmonary exercise testing (CPET) is a noninvasive method of assessing functional capacity and characterizing exercise limitation.[1,2] Precapillary pulmonary arterial hypertension (PAH), defined by a mean pulmonary artery pressure (mPAP) of greater than 20 mm Hg and pulmonary vascular resistance (PVR) 3 or greater Wood units, is a disease characterized by elevated pulmonary artery pressures and PVR leading to impaired right ventricular function and heart failure.[3,4] PAH causes a multitude of downstream effects affecting cardiac function and pulmonary gas exchange leading to exercise intolerance and shortness of breath.[5] CPET has been used to investigate PAH at each stage of clinical progression including detection in high-risk populations, diagnosis, treatment response, and prognosis.[6,7]

Early in disease development, symptoms of PAH are nonspecific and include impaired exercise tolerance. Since the first treatment of PAH, epoprostenol, was shown to improve mortality, subsequent therapies have targeted exercise capacity as an endpoint from regulatory agencies for approval.[8–12] Although submaximal exercise testing such as the six-minute walk test (6MWT) remain a central parameter in treatment response and risk assessment, parameters derived from CPET have been shown to aid in diagnosis, treatment response, and have prognostic significance in PAH and remains a critical and underutilized test.[13,14]

This review summarizes developments and evidence on the application of CPET in the field of PAH. Changes in exercise physiology and gas exchange reflecting the pathophysiology of pulmonary hypertension include reduction in oxygen uptake ($\dot{V}O_2$) at anaerobic threshold (AT) and at peak exercise, ventilatory inefficiency, arterial hypoxemia, and altered kinetics of $\dot{V}O_2$.

Reduction in Oxygen Uptake

Reduced $\dot{V}O_2$ is a key abnormality seen in multiple cardiopulmonary processes with exercise

a Division of Pulmonary, Critical Care, Sleep Medicine, Clinical Immunology and Allergy, David Geffen School of Medicine at UCLA, 650 Charles East Young Drive South 43-229 CHS, Los Angeles, CA 90095-1690, USA;
b Pulmonary Hypertension Program, Pulmonary Vascular Disease Program, Lung & Heart-Lung Transplant and Pulmonary Hypertension Programs, Pulmonary and Critical Care Division, David Geffen School of Medicine at UCLA, Los Angeles, CA, USA
* Corresponding author. Division of Pulmonary, Critical Care, & Sleep Medicine, 650 Charles East Young Drive South 43-229 CHS, Los Angeles, CA 90095-1690.
E-mail address: asherman@mednet.ucla.edu

Heart Failure Clin 19 (2023) 35–43
https://doi.org/10.1016/j.hfc.2022.08.015
1551-7136/23/© 2022 Elsevier Inc. All rights reserved.

intolerance. $\dot{V}O_2$ is a complex variable affected by pulmonary, cardiovascular, pulmonary vascular, and skeletal muscle systems, and is practically used to quantify exercise capacity. Reductions in peak $\dot{V}O_2$ have been associated repeatedly with increased mortality, and improvement in peak $\dot{V}O_2$ have been associated with an improved survival.[15] The AT, the highest $\dot{V}O_2$ one can achieve without the accumulation of lactic acid, is often reduced in PAH.[16] The earlier reliance on anaerobic metabolism coupled with ventilatory inefficiency leads to sooner cessation of exercise and increased sensation of dyspnea.[17]

Minute ventilation relative to carbon dioxide production, ventilatory inefficiency, defined by an abnormal increase in minute ventilation relative to carbon dioxide production ($\dot{V}E/\dot{V}CO_2$) slope, is a key abnormality seen in PAH and also in heart failure, regardless of ejection fraction.[18] In the absence of shunting through a patent foramen ovale, an elevated $\dot{V}E/\dot{V}CO_2$ slope in PAH is thought to be caused by either an increase in dead space fraction (V_D/V_T) or a change in the set point of CO_2 regulation.[19] The method to report $\dot{V}E/\dot{V}CO_2$ data (nadir value, value at AT, slope between onset of ramped exercise and either AT, respiratory compensation point, or peak exercise) varies across institutions but has repeatedly demonstrated prognostic value when elevated.[20,21] A $\dot{V}E/\dot{V}CO_2$ value at AT greater than 33 along with other compatible CPET parameters may identify patients with a pulmonary vascular limitation to exercise.[22] The main factors contributing to the abnormal $\dot{V}E/\dot{V}CO_2$ in PAH are regional ventilation/perfusion (V/Q) mismatching, impaired cardiac output (CO), and deranged chemosensitivity.[23] Vascular remodeling in PAH leads to increased physiologic dead space.[19] Commonly estimated using the Enghoff modification of the Bohr equation [$V_D/V_T = (P_aCO_2 - P_ECO_2)/P_aCO_2$], which substitutes the arterial partial pressure of CO_2 (P_aCO_2) for the alveolar partial pressure of CO_2 (P_ACO_2), physiologic dead space is vulnerable to overestimation in patients with pathophysiology affecting gas diffusion, thus increasing the arterial-alveolar CO_2 difference, $P(_{a-A}CO_2)$.[24] P_ECO_2, the partial pressure of expired CO_2, is typically determined by breath-by-breath analysis during CPET resulting in instantaneous measurements of CO_2 output and ventilation. This is contrasted to $P_{ET}CO_2$, measured at the end of a tidal breath and generally more affected by V/Q mismatching and expiratory time.[25] Alveoli displaying shunt physiology increase the $P(_{A-a}CO_2)$ leading to higher P_aCO_2, and regional V/Q heterogeneity increases physiological dead space. Evidenced by arterial hypocapnia, changes in dead space do not entirely explain ventilatory inefficiency in PAH and reduced CO leading to reduced pulmonary perfusion may result in ventilatory overstimulation.[26] Parallels to mechanisms in heart failure causing altered chemosensitivity including sympathetic nervous system overactivation from right atrial distension have been implicated.[27]

Arterial hypoxemia

Arterial hypoxemia is present during exercise in more advanced PAH. Increased rates of blood flow through pulmonary vasculature limit diffusion time available for oxygen to saturate hemoglobin leading to hypoxia. Frequently only present during exercise, significant exercise-induced arterial hypoxemia can lead to earlier reliance on anaerobic metabolism and subsequent lactate accumulation. Supplemental oxygen during oxygen has been shown to improve maximal work rate, endurance during constant load exercise, and decrease $\dot{V}E/\dot{V}CO_2$ in patients with PAH or chronic thromboembolic pulmonary hypertension (CTEPH).[28] The accumulation of lactic acid signals central and peripheral chemoreceptors to increased respiration, contributing to the sensation of dyspnea.

Oxygen uptake kinetics

Although not traditionally included in CPET analysis, the relationship between $\dot{V}O_2$ and the logarithmic transformation of minute ventilation ($\dot{V}E$) during incremental exercise, the $\dot{V}O_2$ efficiency slope (OUES), has been analyzed as a submaximal parameter correlating with peak $\dot{V}O_2$.[29,30] In 84 patients with mixed pulmonary hypertension, patients with OUES 0.56 L/min or lesser per log VE had significantly worse rates of PAH-related death or need for atrial septostomy (hazard ratio [HR]) 4.63 (95% confidence interval [CI]: 1.38–15.5) when adjusting for peak $\dot{V}O_2$, $\dot{V}E/\dot{V}CO_2$ slope, and $\dot{V}O_2$/WR slope.[31] OUES can be affected by any systemic derangements affecting $\dot{V}O_2$ and is intrinsically linked to $\dot{V}E/\dot{V}CO_2$.

DISCUSSION
Cardiopulmonary Exercise Testing in Pulmonary Arterial Hypertension Diagnosis

Exertional dyspnea and exercise intolerance are symptoms common to multiple pathophysiological processes. Although many causes can be identified through standard evaluation, CPET is a valuable tool in noninvasively identifying patients more likely to have pulmonary hypertension. **Fig. 1** includes CPET results of a representative patient demonstrating findings consistent with a pulmonary vascular limitation to exercise in a traditional 9-plot layout (see **Fig. 1**).

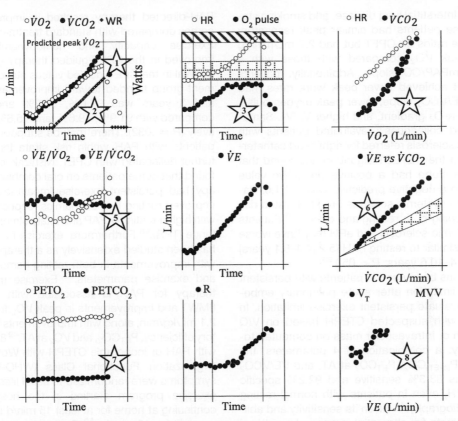

Fig. 1. CPET results for 57-year-old female patient with PAH. Findings supportive of a pulmonary vascular limitation to exercise: (1) low peak $\dot{V}O_2$, (2) low $\dot{V}O_2$/WR slope, (3) early plateau and low peak O_2 pulse, (4) early AT, (5) high nadir $\dot{V}E/\dot{V}CO_2$, (6) high $\dot{V}E/\dot{V}CO_2$ slope, (7) low PETCO$_2$ that does not increase with exertion, (8) No pulmonary mechanical limitation. $\dot{V}CO_2$, carbon dioxide output; $\dot{V}E$, minute ventilation; $\dot{V}O_2$, oxygen uptake; AT, anaerobic threshold; CPET, cardiopulmonary exercise test; HR, heart rate; MVV, maximum voluntary ventilation; O$_2$ pulse, oxygen pulse - $\dot{V}O_2$/heart rate; PAH, pulmonary arterial hypertension; PETCO$_2$, end-tidal carbon dioxide partial pressure; PETO$_2$, end-tidal oxygen partial pressure; R, respiratory exchange ratio; WR, work rate.

Multiple CPET parameters are associated with PAH and can aid in diagnosis in patients with shortness of breath. Although many noninvasive parameters are nonspecific, such as a reduced peak $\dot{V}O_2$, peak work rate, peak $\dot{V}O_2$/work rate (WR) slope, others such as elevated $\dot{V}E/\dot{V}CO_2$ slope or reduced end-tidal CO$_2$ tension (P$_{ET}$CO$_2$) at AT or peak reflect the pathophysiology of pulmonary hypertension and have identified patients at risk for PAH.[32] Oxygen pulse, the relationship between $\dot{V}O_2$ and heart rate (HR), has differentiated patients with normal hemodynamics and patients with mild pulmonary hypertension (mPAP 21–24 mm Hg).[33] P$_{ET}$CO$_2$ represents an intriguing parameter as a correlate with V$_D$/V$_T$, although its utility has limitations due to alterations in V/Q matching, altered chemosensitivity, and changes in CO$_2$ exchange in different lung regions.[19] Still, P$_{ET}$CO$_2$ at AT has been shown to predict mPAP 25 mm Hg or greater, and along with $\dot{V}O_2$, $\dot{V}E/\dot{V}CO_2$, had 91.6% positive predictive value for differentiating patients with connective

tissue disease (CTD) and CTD-associated pulmonary hypertension.[34,35] When using invasive hemodynamics to define a pulmonary vascular limitation to exercise, noninvasive CPET parameters including a peak $\dot{V}O_2$ and $\dot{V}E/\dot{V}CO_2$ at AT had specificity and accuracy to identify a pulmonary vascular limitation to exercise of 88% and 85%, respectively.[22]

Due to a lack of reliable data, exercise-induced pulmonary hypertension (ePH) remains a controversial field.[36] Still, patients with mPAP/CO slope of greater than 3 mm Hg/L/min during exercise have demonstrated differences in cardiac event-free survival and even response to therapy. In a study of 714 patients with preserved ejection fraction and chronic exertional dyspnea who underwent invasive CPET, 296 patients with ePH had a greater than 2-fold higher risk of cardiovascular hospitalization or death (HR 2.03; 95%CI 1.48–2.78) when controlling for age, sex, hypertension, prior heart failure, chronic obstructive pulmonary disease, interstitial lung disease, and smoking status. These patients had similar peak respiratory exchange ratios on CPET but had 2.7 mL/min/kg lower peak $\dot{V}O_2$ compared with those with a normal mPAP/CO slope. Additionally, patients with ePH achieved lower peak work rates, had higher $\dot{V}E/\dot{V}CO_2$ slope, lower peak oxygen pulse, higher A-a-O_2 gradient, and higher V_D/V_T. Santaniello and colleagues[37] evaluated patients with systemic sclerosis referred for right heart catheterization via the DETECT algorithm and found that $\dot{V}E/\dot{V}CO_2$ slope had a positive predictive value 0.636 and a negative predictive value of 1.0. Patients with systemic sclerosis are at elevated risk of developing both resting and ePH.[38,39] Patients with systemic sclerosis and ePH may have worse survival, similar to resting PAH (5.2 [4.4–6.1 years] vs 9.5 [8.4–10.6 years; $P < .05$]).[39]

CPET has been used in patients with persistent exercise limitation after acute pulmonary embolism to evaluate persistent exercise limitation. In patients with suspected CTEPH based on V/Q mismatch or intravascular mass on computed tomography, a combination of 4 parameters, the $P_{(A-a)}O_2$, $P_{(c-ET)}CO_2$, $P_{ET}CO_2$ at AT, and $\dot{V}E/\dot{V}CO_2$ slope was 83.3% sensitive and 92.2% specific for CTEPH, even in patients with normal resting echocardiography.[40] Given its sensitivity and ability to evaluate for alternative causes of exertional dyspnea, CPET has a central role when evaluating exertional dyspnea after acute pulmonary embolism.[41,42] In patients with CTEPH, CPET may be able to help predict severity of disease, as peak $\dot{V}O_2$ and $\dot{V}E$ at AT have been associated with mPAP 45 mm Hg or greater.[43]

Cardiopulmonary Exercise Testing to Evaluate Pulmonary Arterial Hypertension Treatment Response

Exercise tolerance has a central role in risk stratification and therefore guiding treatment in PAH.[44] Although the submaximal exercise test 6MWT is widely accepted for assessing response to therapy, CPET allows for more greater discriminant ability. Although CPET parameters such as peak $\dot{V}O_2$ have been used as outcome measures previously in clinical trials, it is not currently recommended as a primary endpoint in multicenter trials due to variation in CPET interpretation between centers, which may be addressed by central adjudication.[45,46] The GOODEYE trial examined 42 newly diagnosed PAH patients compared with historical controls and found that using peak $\dot{V}O_2$ of 15 mL/min/kg or greater and peak exercise systolic blood pressure greater than 120 mm Hg assessed at 3, 6, and 12 months to determine the need for additional PAH-directed therapy resulted in improved outcomes compared with standard treatment goals.[47] Exercise capacity and hemodynamics were improved in the CPET-guided therapy group and survival in the CPET-guided versus standard treatment group trended toward improvement at 1, 2, and 3 years was 97.6%, 95.2% and 86.0%, compared with 91.9%, 79.6%, and 75.8%, respectively ($P = .082$). There may be subpopulations of patients with PAH within risk strata that can be further delineated with CPET. Nishizaki and others found that some patients on oral combination therapy had persistent exercise impairment despite improved resting hemodynamics, especially those with higher resting mPAP and total pulmonary resistance (TPR).[48] Furthermore, exercise training itself has been studied extensively as a therapy for PAH with improvements in both resting hemodynamics and exercise parameters.[49] Exercise training as therapy for PAH is associated with improved 6MWT and improvements in peak $\dot{V}O_2$ from 1.1 to 2.1 mL/kg/min, along with improvements in ventilatory efficiency, $P_{ET}CO_2$, and $\dot{V}O_2$ at AT.[49] 87 patients with PAH or inoperable CTEPH with World Health Organization Functional Class (WHO-FC) III/IV symptoms were randomized to usual lifestyle or an exercise program starting in the hospital and continuing at home for at least 15 min/d for 5 days a week for 12 weeks.[50] Patients in the exercise group had improvements in peak $\dot{V}O_2$ (3.1 ± 2.7 vs −0.2 ± 2.3 mL/min/kg; $P < .001$) and cardiac index (+9.3% vs −6.5%; $P = .08$) and reduction in mPAP (−7.3% vs +16.1%; $P = .002$) and PVR (−19.3% vs +34.5%; $P = .06$). Quality of life by the Short Form 36 (SF-36) questionnaire improved in patients assigned to exercise training in the vitality subscore.

CPET has been examined extensively in patients with CTEPH. Derangements in exercise physiology and gas exchange are similar in CTEPH and are reflected by CPET findings similar to those in PAH.[51] CPET has been used to evaluate the response to medical, interventional, and surgical treatment of CTEPH.[52,53] Balloon pulmonary angioplasty (BPA) has been increasing used in patients deemed poor surgical candidates for pulmonary thromboendarterectomy or in patients with residual disease. BPA has been shown to improve peak work rate, peak $\dot{V}O_2$, with persistent effects after multiple sessions.[54] There is currently no guidance for determining how many BPA attempts should be made and CPET represents an intriguing methodology of evaluating interventional efficacy.[55] Diffusion capacity of carbon monoxide is frequently used as a marker of pulmonary vascular disease; however, it may not serve as a sensitive marker of treatment response post-BPA.[52]

Prognosis

Despite guidelines risk stratifying PAH patients, determining prognosis in PAH remains a challenge, particularly in intermediate-risk patients.[36] Various attempts to improve personalized risk stratification have been made using various hemodynamic and CPET parameters.

Peak $\dot{V}O_2$ has shown prognostic significance with New York Heart Association class III patients with PAH where those with $\dot{V}O_2$ of 10.4 mL/kg/min or lesser and peak systolic blood pressure of 120 mm Hg or lesser had poorer 12-month survival compared with others.[56] Retrospective studies in patients with PAH undergoing CPET have shown correlation between lower peak $P_{ET}CO_2$, higher $\dot{V}E/\dot{V}CO_2$ slope, and higher mPAP and PVR.[57,58] Badagliacca and colleagues[59] developed a novel risk assessment tool in PAH patients deemed "intermediate risk" by European Society of Cardiology/European Respiratory society criteria and demonstrated the ability of peak $\dot{V}O_2$ (<10 mL/min/kg) and stroke volume index (>30 mL/m^2) to define additional risk groups.

One of the most significant challenges in cardiopulmonary exercising testing is the use of maximal exercise parameters. Although CPET is safe even in patients with advanced PAH, patients with more advanced disease may not be able to participate in maximal effort testing.[60] Submaximal CPET parameters such as anaerobic threshold determination and $\dot{V}E/\dot{V}CO_2$ slope, baseline and exercise $P_{ET}CO_2$ correlate with the REVEAL registry risk score.[61] Even during unloaded exercise, $P_{ET}CO_2$ is abnormal in PAH patients and may correlate with mixed venous oxygen saturation.[62] 6MWT remains central in current risk stratification models but its ability to prognosticate in clinical trials is limited.[63] In a study of 226 idiopathic or familial PAH patients, both peak $\dot{V}O_2$ and PVR were predictive of survival, whereas 6MWT lacked significance.[64] Peak $\dot{V}O_2$ has outperformed both 6MWT and quality-of-life questionnaires in predicting 2-year mortality in PAH.[65] In a study of 210 idiopathic PAH patients, a decrease in the oxygen efficiency uptake slope (slope of the relationship between log($\dot{V}E$) and $\dot{V}O_2$) during exercise was associated with poorer prognosis and correlated with peak $\dot{V}O_2$.[66]

Future Directions and Novel Applications

Despite its well-explored uses, CPET continues to have novel uses in PAH. A recent study used exercise hemodynamics to identify PAH patients with WHO-FC I symptoms and resting mPAP less than 25 mm Hg and PVR less than 3 on a steady dose of intravenous epoprostenol to wean off parenteral therapy. Those without evidence of exercise pulmonary hypertension were successfully weaned off parenteral therapy after initiating oral combination therapy.[67] This combination of CPET data and invasive hemodynamics has been used to investigate ePH. Multiple studies have leveraged the increased granularity of CPET to identify earlier features of PAH and right ventricular dysfunction. The provocative nature of exercise testing can unmask early right ventricular (RV) dysfunction and diminished RV contractile reserve even at submaximal exercise.[68] Impaired RV lusitropy, the ability to relax in diastole, and increased afterload have been associated with higher $\dot{V}E/\dot{V}CO_2$, further strengthening the mechanistic link between ventilatory inefficiency and PAH.[69] Examining rest-to-peak exercise RV-PA uncoupling in both ePH and PAH suggests that RV dysfunction is compromised early in the disease process, before the appearance of resting adaptations.[70] Even during unloaded and submaximal exercise (50% peak $\dot{V}O_2$), reduced RV stroke volume index correlated with lower peak $\dot{V}O_2$, potentially identifying thresholds for exercise strategies that would avoid worsened RV function during exercise.[71] Resting hypocapnia in a group of patients with PAH, CTEPH, and pulmonary venoocclusive disease was associated with worse cardiac index and higher $\dot{V}E/\dot{V}CO_2$, although peak exercise $P_{ET}CO_2$ did outperform this resting measurement.[72]

ePH has been associated with shorter cardiovascular event-free survival in patients with chronic dyspnea evaluated with invasive CPET.[73] There are limited data that treatment of ePH may improve exercise hemodynamics and survival.[74] CPET parameters along with exercise hemodynamics may further uncover groups of PAH patients where optimal management remains to be seen. Should a patient with normal exercise capacity by CPET, and WHO-FC I symptoms be started on treatment if they have abnormal hemodynamics or an elevated $\dot{V}E/\dot{V}CO_2$? Patients with chronic thromboembolic disease without resting pulmonary hypertension have similar CPET findings to patients with CTEPH; however, optimal management of this emerging patient population has not been determined.[40,75]

Although not directly evaluated in standard CPET, decreased skeletal muscle and impaired oxygen extraction have been found to decrease aerobic capacity in PAH.[76] Near-infrared spectroscopy to evaluate myoglobin–deoxyhemoglobin levels during exercise correlate with peak $\dot{V}O_2$ and quadriceps strength in PAH patients. Exercise training increases muscle capillarization and oxidative enzyme activity of slow muscle fibers, which may increase achieved workload at AT.[77] Diaphragm muscle in patients undergoing PTE for CTEPH have impaired contractility, which may contribute to respiratory muscle weakness. The persistent loss of strength leads to difficulty with exercise and a cycle of progressive deconditioning and loss of functional status.

HR recovery remains an intriguing and easily obtainable marker; however, its lack of specificity has limited its utility.[78] A reduction of less than 16 beats per minute at 1 minute rest after a 6MWT has been associated with increased risk of clinical worsening (HR: 6.4, 95% 95%CI: 2.6–19.2), increased risk of hospitalization (HR: 6.6, 95%CI: 2.4–23), and increased risk of death (HR: 4.5, 95%CI: 1.6–15.7).[79] HR expenditure, an integral of HR adjusted for distance during 6MWT, has correlated with improvements in stroke volume with increases in PAH therapy.[80]

Despite its many uses in PAH, CPET remains underutilized.[81] This may be due to limited availability and perceived challenges in interpretation. Yet, the stresses from physical activity remain a valuable tool in identifying patients at risk of disease or disease progression. Assessment of physical activity using wearable devices has been evaluated to predict risk of hospitalization in pulmonary hypertension patients.[82]

SUMMARY

CPET provides a comprehensive assessment of the body's exercise capacity related to the pathophysiology of PAH. Advances in complementary testing including concurrent invasive hemodynamic testing, pressure-volume testing, and imaging provide additional insights and may assist in earlier identification of disease before resting adaptations become apparent. Maximal and submaximal exercise testing remain central to monitoring treatment response and informing prognosis. Future efforts on increasing accessibility and novel uses of exercise data in the management of patients with PAH is warranted.

CLINICS CARE POINTS

- CPET can differentiate a pulmonary vascular limitation to exercise and aid diagnosis in patients with exertional dyspnea, especially in high-risk patient populations.
- High $\dot{V}E/\dot{V}CO_2$ slope, low $P_{ET}CO_2$ at anaerobic threshold, and adequate breathing reserve are hallmarks of pulmonary vascular limitation on CPET. Blood gas analysis may further support the diagnosis demonstrating low P_aCO_2 (hypocapnia) and a high $P_{(a-ET)}CO_2$ gradient.

- CPET may enhance individualized risk assessment in intermediate-risk PAH patients.
- CPET has a role along with echocardiography when evaluating patients with persistent exercise intolerance after acute pulmonary embolism.
- ePH remains under investigation and its presence is currently supported by a mean pulmonary artery pressure to CO slope of less than 3 mm Hg/L/min

---

DISCLOSURE STATEMENT:

AES has no relevant financial disclosures. RS has no relevant financial disclosures.

REFERENCES

1. Sun XG, Hansen JE, Oudiz RJ, et al. Exercise pathophysiology in patients with primary pulmonary hypertension. Circulation 2001;104(4):429–35.
2. ATS/ACCP statement on cardiopulmonary exercise testing. Am J Respir Crit Care Med 2003;167(2):211–77.
3. Simonneau G, Montani D, Celermajer DS, et al. Haemodynamic definitions and updated clinical classification of pulmonary hypertension. Eur Respir J 2019;53(1):1801913.
4. Hassoun PM. Pulmonary arterial hypertension. N Engl J Med 2021;385(25):2361–76.
5. D'Alonzo GE, Gianotti LA, Pohil RL, et al. Comparison of progressive exercise performance of normal subjects and patients with primary pulmonary hypertension. Chest 1987;92(1):57–62.
6. Laveneziana P, Weatherald J. Pulmonary vascular disease and cardiopulmonary exercise testing. Front Physiol 2020;11:964.
7. Weatherald J, Farina S, Bruno N, et al. Cardiopulmonary exercise testing in pulmonary hypertension. Ann ATS 2017;14(Supplement_1):S84–92.
8. Barst RJ, Rubin LJ, Long WA, et al. A comparison of continuous intravenous epoprostenol (prostacyclin) with conventional therapy for primary pulmonary hypertension. N Engl J Med 1996;334(5):296–301.
9. McLaughlin VV, Benza RL, Rubin LJ, et al. Addition of inhaled treprostinil to oral therapy for pulmonary arterial hypertension: a randomized controlled clinical trial. J Am Coll Cardiol 2010;55(18):1915–22.
10. Galiè N, Ghofrani HA, Torbicki A, et al. Sildenafil citrate therapy for pulmonary arterial hypertension. N Engl J Med 2005;353(20):2148–57.
11. Galiè N, Brundage BH, Ghofrani HA, et al. Tadalafil therapy for pulmonary arterial hypertension. Circulation 2009;119(22):2894–903.
12. Sitbon O, Gomberg-Maitland M, Granton J, et al. Clinical trial design and new therapies for pulmonary

arterial hypertension. Eur Respir J 2019;53(1). https://doi.org/10.1183/13993003.01908-2018.

13. Farina S, Correale M, Bruno N, et al. The role of cardiopulmonary exercise tests in pulmonary arterial hypertension. Eur Respir Rev 2018;27(148). https://doi.org/10.1183/16000617.0134-2017.

14. Galiè N, Channick RN, Frantz RP, et al. Risk stratification and medical therapy of pulmonary arterial hypertension. Eur Respir J 2019;53(1): 1801889.

15. Ross R, Blair SN, Arena R, et al. Importance of assessing cardiorespiratory fitness in clinical practice: a case for fitness as a clinical vital sign: a scientific statement from the american heart association. Circulation 2016;134(24):e653–99.

16. Deboeck G, Niset G, Lamotte M, et al. Exercise testing in pulmonary arterial hypertension and in chronic heart failure. Eur Respir J 2004;23(5): 747–51.

17. Wasserman K, Casaburi R. Dyspnea: physiological and pathophysiological mechanisms. Annu Rev Med 1988;39:503–15.

18. Weatherald J, Philipenko B, Montani D, et al. Ventilatory efficiency in pulmonary vascular diseases. Eur Respir Rev 2021;30(161). https://doi.org/10.1183/16000617.0214-2020.

19. Weatherald J, Sattler C, Garcia G, et al. Ventilatory response to exercise in cardiopulmonary disease: the role of chemosensitivity and dead space. Eur Respir J 2018;51(2). https://doi.org/10.1183/13993003.00860-2017.

20. Arena R, Humphrey R, Peberdy MA. Prognostic ability of VE/VCO2 slope calculations using different exercise test time intervals in subjects with heart failure. Eur J Cardiovasc Prev Rehabil 2003;10(6): 463–8.

21. Schwaiblmair M, Faul C, von Scheidt W, et al. Ventilatory efficiency testing as prognostic value in patients with pulmonary hypertension. BMC Pulm Med 2012;12:23.

22. Markowitz DH, Systrom DM. Diagnosis of pulmonary vascular limit to exercise by cardiopulmonary exercise testing. J Heart Lung Transplant 2004;23(1): 88–95.

23. Dantzker DR, D'Alonzo GE. Pulmonary gas exchange and exercise performance in pulmonary hypertension. CHEST 1985;88(4):255S–7S.

24. Robertson HT. Dead space: the physiology of wasted ventilation. Eur Respir J 2015;45(6): 1704–16.

25. Hansen JE, Ulubay G, Chow BF, et al. Mixed-expired and end-tidal CO 2 distinguish between ventilation and perfusion defects during exercise testing in patients with lung and heart diseases. Chest 2007; 132(3):977–83.

26. Hoeper MM, Pletz MW, Golpon H, et al. Prognostic value of blood gas analyses in patients with idiopathic pulmonary arterial hypertension. Eur Respir J 2007;29(5):944–50.

27. Ciarka A, Vachièry JL, Houssière A, et al. Atrial septostomy decreases sympathetic overactivity in pulmonary arterial hypertension. Chest 2007;131(6): 1831–7.

28. Ulrich S, Hasler ED, Saxer S, et al. Effect of breathing oxygen-enriched air on exercise performance in patients with precapillary pulmonary hypertension: randomized, sham-controlled cross-over trial. Eur Heart J 2017;38(15):1159–68.

29. Baba R, Nagashima M, Goto M, et al. Oxygen uptake efficiency slope: a new index of cardiorespiratory functional reserve derived from the relation between oxygen uptake and minute ventilation during incremental exercise. J Am Coll Cardiol 1996; 28(6):1567–72.

30. Tan X, Yang W, Guo J, et al. Usefulness of decrease in oxygen uptake efficiency to identify gas exchange abnormality in patients with idiopathic pulmonary arterial hypertension. PLoS One 2014;9(6): e98889.

31. Ramos RP, Ota-Arakaki JS, Alencar MC, et al. Exercise oxygen uptake efficiency slope independently predicts poor outcome in pulmonary arterial hypertension. Eur Respir J 2014;43(5):1510–2.

32. Luo Q, Yu X, Zhao Z, et al. The value of cardiopulmonary exercise testing in the diagnosis of pulmonary hypertension. J Thorac Dis 2021;13(1):178–88.

33. Jiang R, Liu H, Pudasaini B, et al. Characteristics of cardiopulmonary exercise testing of patients with borderline mean pulmonary artery pressure. Clin Respir J 2019;13(3):148–58.

34. Higashi A, Dohi Y, Yamabe S, et al. Evaluation of end-tidal CO2 pressure at the anaerobic threshold for detecting and assessing pulmonary hypertension. Heart Vessels 2017;32(11):1350–7.

35. Bellan M, Giubertoni A, Piccinino C, et al. Cardiopulmonary exercise testing is an accurate tool for the diagnosis of pulmonary arterial hypertension in scleroderma related diseases. Pharmaceuticals 2021;14(4):342.

36. Galiè N, Humbert M, Vachiery JL, et al. 2015 ESC/ERS Guidelines for the diagnosis and treatment of pulmonary hypertension: The Joint Task Force for the Diagnosis and Treatment of Pulmonary Hypertension of the European Society of Cardiology (ESC) and the European Respiratory Society (ERS): Endorsed by: Association for European Paediatric and Congenital Cardiology (AEPC), International Society for Heart and Lung Transplantation (ISHLT). Eur Heart J 2016;37(1):67–119.

37. Santaniello A, Casella R, Vicenzi M, et al. Cardiopulmonary exercise testing in a combined screening approach to individuate pulmonary arterial hypertension in systemic sclerosis. Rheumatology 2020; 59(7):1581–6.

38. Saggar R, Khanna D, Furst DE, et al. Exercise-induced pulmonary hypertension associated with systemic sclerosis: four distinct entities. Arthritis Rheum 2010;62(12):3741–50.

39. Stamm A, Saxer S, Lichtblau M, et al. Exercise pulmonary haemodynamics predict outcome in patients with systemic sclerosis. Eur Respir J 2016; 48(6):1658–67.

40. Held M, Grün M, Holl R, et al. Cardiopulmonary exercise testing to detect chronic thromboembolic pulmonary hypertension in patients with normal echocardiography. RES 2014;87(5):379–87.

41. Klok FA, Ageno W, Ay C, et al. Optimal follow-up after acute pulmonary embolism: a position paper of the European Society of Cardiology Working Group on Pulmonary Circulation and Right Ventricular Function, in collaboration with the European Society of Cardiology Working Group on Atherosclerosis and Vascular Biology, endorsed by the European Respiratory Society. Eur Heart J 2022;43(3):183–9.

42. Klok FA, Couturaud F, Delcroix M, et al. Diagnosis of chronic thromboembolic pulmonary hypertension after acute pulmonary embolism. Eur Respir J 2020; 55(6). https://doi.org/10.1183/13993003.00189-2020.

43. Zhu H, Sun X, Cao Y, et al. Cardiopulmonary exercise testing and pulmonary function testing for predicting the severity of CTEPH. BMC Pulm Med 2021;21(1):324.

44. Frost A, Badesch D, Gibbs JSR, et al. Diagnosis of pulmonary hypertension. Eur Respir J 2019;53(1): 1801904.

45. Barst RJ, Langleben D, Frost A, et al. Sitaxsentan therapy for pulmonary arterial hypertension. Am J Respir Crit Care Med 2004;169(4):441–7.

46. Hoeper MM, Oudiz RJ, Peacock A, et al. End points and clinical trial designs in pulmonary arterial hypertension: clinical and regulatory perspectives. J Am Coll Cardiol 2004;43(12, Supplement):S48–55.

47. Hirashiki A, Kondo T, Adachi S, et al. Goal-oriented sequential combination therapy evaluated using cardiopulmonary exercise parameters for the treatment of newly diagnosed pulmonary arterial hypertension - goal-oriented therapy evaluated by cardiopulmonary exercise testing for pulmonary arterial hypertension (GOOD EYE). Circ Rep 2019;1(7):303–11.

48. Nishizaki M, Ogawa A, Matsubara H. Response to exercise in patients with pulmonary arterial hypertension treated with combination therapy. ERJ Open Res 2021;7(1):00725–2020.

49. Babu AS, Padmakumar R, Maiya AG, et al. Effects of exercise training on exercise capacity in pulmonary arterial hypertension: a systematic review of clinical trials. Heart Lung Circ 2016;25(4):333–41.

50. Ehlken N, Lichtblau M, Klose H, et al. Exercise training improves peak oxygen consumption and haemodynamics in patients with severe pulmonary arterial hypertension and inoperable chronic thrombo-embolic pulmonary hypertension: a prospective, randomized, controlled trial. Eur Heart J 2016;37(1):35–44.

51. Scheidl SJ, Englisch C, Kovacs G, et al. Diagnosis of CTEPH versus IPAH using capillary to end-tidal carbon dioxide gradients. Eur Respir J 2012;39(1): 119–24.

52. Blanquez-Nadal M, Piliero N, Guillien A, et al. Exercise hyperventilation and pulmonary gas exchange in chronic thromboembolic pulmonary hypertension: Effects of balloon pulmonary angioplasty. J Heart Lung Transplant 2022;41(1):70–9.

53. Aoki T, Sugimura K, Terui Y, et al. Beneficial effects of riociguat on hemodynamic responses to exercise in CTEPH patients after balloon pulmonary angioplasty – A randomized controlled study. IJC Heart & Vasculature 2020;29:100579.

54. Jin Q, Luo Q, Yang T, et al. Improved hemodynamics and cardiopulmonary function in patients with inoperable chronic thromboembolic pulmonary hypertension after balloon pulmonary angioplasty. Respir Res 2019;20(1):250.

55. Puente-Maestu L, Palange P, Casaburi R, et al. Use of exercise testing in the evaluation of interventional efficacy: an official ERS statement. Eur Respir J 2016;47(2):429–60.

56. Wensel R, Opitz CF, Anker SD, et al. Assessment of survival in patients with primary pulmonary hypertension. Circulation 2002;106(3):319–24.

57. Pezzuto B, Badagliacca R, Muratori M, et al. Role of cardiopulmonary exercise test in the prediction of hemodynamic impairment in patients with pulmonary arterial hypertension. Pulm Circ 2022;12(1): e12044.

58. Welch CE, Brittain EL, Newman AL, et al. End-tidal carbon dioxide as a prognostic feature in pulmonary arterial hypertension. Ann ATS 2017;14(6):896–902.

59. Badagliacca R, Rischard F, Giudice FL, et al. Incremental value of cardiopulmonary exercise testing in intermediate-risk pulmonary arterial hypertension. J Heart Lung Transpl 2022. https://doi.org/10.1016/j.healun.2022.02.021. S1053-2498(22)01844-01847.

60. Skalski J, Allison TG, Miller TD. The safety of cardiopulmonary exercise testing in a population with high-risk cardiovascular diseases. Circulation 2012; 126(21):2465–72.

61. Khatri V, Neal JE, Burger CD, et al. Prognostication in pulmonary arterial hypertension with submaximal exercise testing. Diseases 2015;3(1):15–23.

62. Sayegh ALC, Silva BM, Ferreira EVM, et al. Clinical utility of ventilatory and gas exchange evaluation during low-intensity exercise for risk stratification and prognostication in pulmonary arterial hypertension. Respirology 2021;26(3):264–72.

63. Gaine S, Simonneau G. The need to move from 6-minute walk distance to outcome trials in pulmonary

arterial hypertension. Eur Respir Rev 2013;22(130): 487–94.

64. Wensel R, Francis DP, Meyer FJ, et al. Incremental prognostic value of cardiopulmonary exercise testing and resting haemodynamics in pulmonary arterial hypertension. Int J Cardiol 2013;167(4): 1193–8.

65. Chen YJ, Tu HP, Lee CL, et al. Comprehensive exercise capacity and quality of life assessments predict mortality in patients with pulmonary arterial hypertension. Acta Cardiol Sin 2019;35(1):55–64.

66. Tang Y, Luo Q, Liu Z, et al. Oxygen uptake efficiency slope predicts poor outcome in patients with idiopathic pulmonary arterial hypertension. J Am Heart Assoc 2017;6(7):e005037.

67. Takeuchi K, Goda A, Ito J, et al. Successful epoprostenol withdrawal and termination with an aid of the exercise stress test in pulmonary arterial hypertension. Int J Cardiol 2022;346:80–5.

68. Jaijee S, Quinlan M, Tokarczuk P, et al. Exercise cardiac MRI unmasks right ventricular dysfunction in acute hypoxia and chronic pulmonary arterial hypertension. Am J Physiology-Heart Circulatory Physiol 2018;315(4):H950–7.

69. Tello K, Dalmer A, Vanderpool R, et al. Impaired right ventricular lusitropy is associated with ventilatory inefficiency in pulmonary arterial hypertension. Eur Respir J 2019;54(5). https://doi.org/10.1183/13993003.00342-2019.

70. Singh I, Rahaghi FN, Naeije R, et al. Dynamic right ventricular–pulmonary arterial uncoupling during maximum incremental exercise in exercise pulmonary hypertension and pulmonary arterial hypertension. Pulm Circ 2019;9(3). 2045894019862435.

71. Singh I, Oliveira RKF, Heerdt P, et al. Dynamic right ventricular function response to incremental exercise in pulmonary hypertension. Pulm Circ 2020; 10(3). 2045894020950187.

72. Weatherald J, Boucly A, Montani D, et al. Gas exchange and ventilatory efficiency during exercise in pulmonary vascular diseases. Archivos de Bronconeumología. 2020;56(9):578–85.

73. Ho JE, Zern EK, Lau ES, et al. Exercise pulmonary hypertension predicts clinical outcomes in patients with dyspnea on effort. J Am Coll Cardiol 2020; 75(1):17–26.

74. Kusunose K, Yamada H, Nishio S, et al. Pulmonary artery hypertension-specific therapy improves exercise tolerance and outcomes in exercise-induced pulmonary hypertension. JACC: Cardiovasc Imaging 2019;12(12):2576–9.

75. McGuire WC, Alotaibi M, Morris TA, et al. Chronic thromboembolic disease: epidemiology, assessment with invasive cardiopulmonary exercise testing, and options for management. Struct Heart 2021;5(2):120–7.

76. Marra AM, Arcopinto M, Bossone E, et al. Pulmonary arterial hypertension-related myopathy: An overview of current data and future perspectives. Nutr Metab Cardiovasc Dis 2015;25(2):131–9.

77. de Man FS, Handoko ML, Groepenhoff H, et al. Effects of exercise training in patients with idiopathic pulmonary arterial hypertension. Eur Respir J 2009;34(3):669–75.

78. Jin Q, Li X, Zhang Y, et al. Heart rate recovery at 1 min after exercise is a marker of disease severity and prognosis in chronic thromboembolic pulmonary hypertension. RES 2022;101(5):455–64.

79. Minai OA, Nguyen Q, Mummadi S, et al. Heart rate recovery is an important predictor of outcomes in patients with connective tissue disease–associated pulmonary hypertension. Pulm Circ 2015;5(3): 565–76.

80. Lachant DJ, Light A, Offen M, et al. Heart rate monitoring improves clinical assessment during 6-min walk. Pulm Circ 2020;10(4). 2045894020972572.

81. Sabbahi A, Severin R, Ozemek C, et al. The role of cardiopulmonary exercise testing and training in patients with pulmonary hypertension: making the case for this assessment and intervention to be considered a standard of care. Expert Rev Respir Med 2020;14(3):317–27.

82. Marvin-Peek J, Hemnes A, Huang S, et al. Daily step counts are associated with hospitalization risk in pulmonary arterial hypertension. Am J Respir Crit Care Med 2021;204(11):1338–40.

Pulmonary Arterial Hypertension in Connective Tissue Diseases Beyond Systemic Sclerosis

Christopher Lewis, MD[a], Ryan Sanderson, MD[b], Nektarios Vasilottos, MD[c], Alexander Zheutlin, MS, MD[d], Scott Visovatti, MA, MD[e],*

KEYWORDS

• Connective tissue disease • Pulmonary hypertension • Associated pulmonary arterial hypertension
• Scleroderma • Systemic lupus erythematosus • Mixed connective tissue disease • Epidemiology
• Screening

KEY POINTS

- Pulmonary arterial hypertension (PAH) associated with connective tissue disease (CTD) is a syndrome with high morbidity and mortality.
- The prevalence of PAH in specific types of CTD varies geographically. Scleroderma-associated PAH is most common in the Western world, whereas systemic lupus erythematosus-associated PAH is more common in the Asia-Pacific region.
- Current guidelines recommend formalized PAH screening of asymptomatic patients with scleroderma spectrum disease. Evidence supporting PAH screening in other CTDs is currently lacking.

INTRODUCTION

Pulmonary hypertension (PH) is a syndrome characterized by elevated pressures in the pulmonary circulation resulting from a variety of conditions, as defined by the World Health Organization (WHO), including left heart disease (Group 2 PH), chronic lung disease (Group 3 PH), thromboembolic disease (Group 4), or systemic and metabolic disorders (Group 5 PH).[1] Pulmonary arterial hypertension (PAH) (Group 1 PAH) is a rare, devastating PH subgroup characterized by increased pulmonary vascular resistance, severe vascular remodeling, endothelial dysfunction, complex vascular lesions, and dysregulation of the innate and adaptive immune system.[2] Patients with connective tissue disease (CTD) are at increased risk for the development of PH,[3] making it an important consideration for practitioners caring for this patient population. Because CTD has such widespread systemic effects, patients with CTD may develop PH associated with one or more of the WHO groups.[3]

The definitive diagnosis of PH requires a right heart catheterization,[1] and hemodynamic profiles including precapillary PH, postcapillary PH, and combined precapillary and postcapillary PH help define the WHO PH groups (**Table 1**). The diagnosis of Group 1 PAH-CTD requires a comprehensive, multimodality evaluation aimed at excluding

[a] Department of Internal Medicine, Division of Cardiovascular Medicine, Henry Ford Hospital, Detroit, MI, USA; [b] Section of Cardiology, The University of Chicago, 5841 South Maryland Avenue, Chicago, IL 60637, USA; [c] Department of Medicine, Division of Cardiovascular Disease, Indiana University, 1800 North Capitol Avenue, Indianapolis, IN 46202, USA; [d] Department of Internal Medicine, University of Utah School of Medicine, 30 North 1900 East, Room 4C104, Salt Lake City, UT 84132, USA; [e] Department of Internal Medicine, Division of Cardiovascular Medicine, Davis Heart and Lung Research Institute, The Ohio State University, 473 West 12th Avenue, Columbus, OH 43210-1252, USA
* Corresponding author. Davis Heart and Lung Research Institute, The Ohio State University, 473 West 12th Avenue, Columbus, OH 43210-1252.
E-mail address: Scott.visovatti@osumc.edu

Heart Failure Clin 19 (2023) 45–54
https://doi.org/10.1016/j.hfc.2022.08.016
1551-7136/23/© 2022 Elsevier Inc. All rights reserved.

Table 1
Hemodynamic definitions of pulmonary hypertension

	Pulmonary Hypertension		
	Precapillary Pulmonary Hypertension	Postcapillary Pulmonary Hypertension	Combined Precapillary and Postcapillary Pulmonary Hypertension
Clinical example	Group 1 PAH	Group 2 PH due to left heart disease	Group 5 PH due to multifactorial mechanisms
mPAP, mm Hg	>20	>20	>20
PAWP, mm Hg	≤15	>15	>15
PVR, Wood units	≥3	<3	>3

Abbreviations: mPAP, mean pulmonary arterial pressure; PAWP, pulmonary arterial wedge pressure; PVR, pulmonary vascular resistance.

Adapted from Simonneau G, Montani D, Celermajer DS, et al. Haemodynamic definitions and updated clinical classification of pulmonary hypertension. *Eur Respir J.* 2019;53(1):1801913. Published 2019 Jan 24.

other PH groups (**Fig. 1**).[4] In addition to evaluating all patients with suspected PH for history and physical examination findings suggestive of CTD, guidelines recommend anti-nuclear antibody testing using immunofluorescence if CTD is suspected.[5] Additional serologic testing and referral to a rheumatologist can be considered if there is a high index of suspicion for CTD-PAH. A thorough evaluation is especially important in the CTD population because CTD-PAH has a distinct natural history with the potential to progress rapidly, resulting in significant morbidity and mortality due to right heart failure. In addition, clinical trials have demonstrated the efficacy of pulmonary vasodilator therapies in ameliorating the increased pulmonary vascular resistance characteristic of PAH.[6]

A challenge for practitioners caring for patients with CTD is that not all CTDs predispose patients to the same PH groups with the same frequency. For example, patients with rheumatoid arthritis (RA) and systemic sclerosis (SSc) have an increased frequency of Group 2 PH secondary to left heart disease (such as diastolic dysfunction or valvular disease), whereas the frequency is less clear in patients with dermatomyositis (DM), polymyositis (PM), and eosinophilic granulomatosis with polyangiitis.[7] Patients with DM, PM, and SSc more frequently have Group 3 PH secondary to chronic lung disease.[7] Group 4 PH due to chronic thromboembolic disease is more common in patients with SLE and antiphospholipid syndrome,[7] whereas Group 5 PH (PH due to multifactorial mechanisms) is more common in patients with SLE and possibly SSc.[7] The frequency of Group 1 CTD-PAH is also known to vary by CTD subtype.[8] In addition, there is a growing awareness of geographic differences in PAH prevalence in CTDs, with notable differences between Eastern and Western countries.[8,9] Owing to the potential for rapid progression and high morbidity and mortality, PAH associated with SSc (SSc-PAH) has been the subject of intense research aimed at better understanding the pathophysiology, strategies for early diagnosis, optimal treatment, and natural history of this disease. The large body of work generated through these efforts have both greatly improved our understanding of SSc-PAH and emphasized how much less we know about PAH associated with other CTDs. The aim of this review is to explore what is known and what remains to be learned about CTD-PAH beyond SSc.

EPIDEMIOLOGY

Much of what is known about the prevalence of CTD-PAH is based on registries based in the Western world, and that the overall prevalence of CTD-PAH as well as the prevalence of PAH within specific types of CTD likely differs in other parts of the world (**Fig. 2**). The reported prevalence of CTD-PAH also varies depending on how the condition is diagnosed (echocardiographic criteria as opposed to the gold-standard right heart catheterization[1]). Group 1 PAH is estimated to have a prevalence of 15 cases per 1 million people in the Western world,[10] and CTD-PAH accounts for 15% to 25% of PAH.

Scleroderma (Systemic Sclerosis)

SSc is the most common cause of CTD-PAH in the Western world,[8,10–12] and it accounts for 62% to 76% of CTD-PAH cases in the United States and

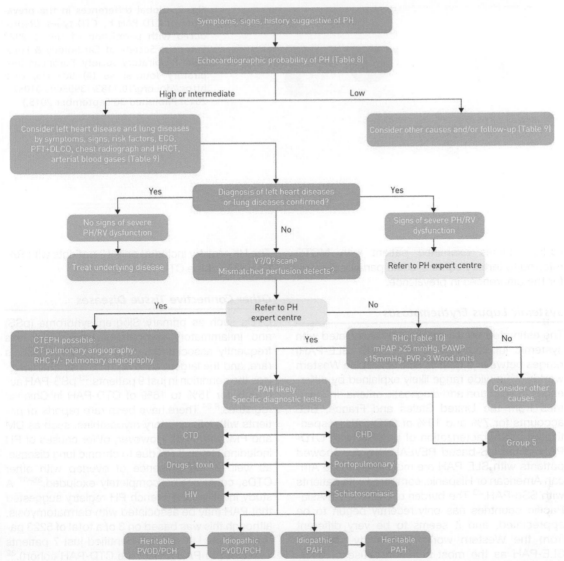

Fig. 1. Diagnostic algorithm for PH. CHD, congenital heart diseases; CT, computed tomography; CTEPH, chronic thromboembolic pulmonary hypertension; D$_{LCO}$, carbon monoxide diffusing capacity; ECG, electrocardiogram; HIV, human immunodeficiency virus; HRCT, high-resolution CT; mPAP, mean pulmonary arterial pressure; PA, pulmonary angiography; PAWP, pulmonary artery wedge pressure; PFT, pulmonary function tests; PVOD/PCH, pulmonary veno-occlusive disease or pulmonary capillary hemangiomatosis; PVR, pulmonary vascular resistance; RHC, right heart catheterization; RV, right ventricular; $\dot{V}/\dot{Q}$, ventilation/perfusion. [a]CT pulmonary angiography alone may miss diagnosis of chronic thromboembolic pulmonary hypertension. Please note: the definition of PH now includes an mPAP greater than 20 mm Hg rather than greater than or equal to 25 mm Hg. Tables 8–10 are found in the ESC/ERS Guidelines for the diagnosis and treatment of pulmonary hypertension. (Reproduced with permission of the © ERS 2022: European Respiratory Journal 2015 46: 903-975; https://doi.org/10.1183/13993003.01032-2015.)

Europe.[8,10,13] The prevalence of PAH in SSc is estimated at 7% to 12%.[14–16] Multiple studies suggest that PAH is more common in limited SSc compared with diffuse SSc.[7]

Mixed Connective Tissue Disease

Mixed connective tissue disease (MCTD) shares signs and symptoms with other CTDs, including

SSc, PM, and SLE. International registries suggest that MCTD accounts for roughly 9% of CTD-PAH.[8–10] Hospital-based studies show a PAH prevalence ranging from 17% to 29% in patients with MCTD, although registry data suggest a lower prevalence.[17–20] Changes in diagnostic criteria for MCTD and PAH and differences in the examined patient populations, including the fact that the

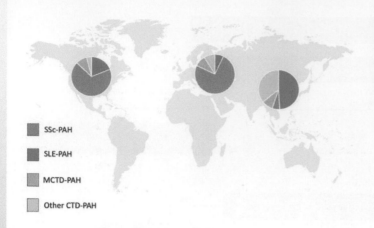

SSc-PAH

SLE-PAH

MCTD-PAH

Other CTD-PAH

Fig. 2. Global differences in the prevalence of CTD-PAH by CTD types. (*Reproduced* with permission of the © 2022 European Society of Cardiology & European Respiratory Society. European Respiratory Journal 46 (4) 903-975; DOI: https://doi.org/10.1183/13993003.01032-2015. Published 30 September 2015.)

earlier studies examined patient with MCTD referred to tertiary centers, could partially account for the differences in prevalence.

Systemic Lupus Erythematosus

The estimated prevalence of PAH associated with systemic lupus erythematosus (SLE) (SLE-PAH) ranges between 0.0005% and 14% in the Western world,[21,22] a wide range likely explained by differences in selection and diagnostic criteria. In registries from the United States and France, SLE accounts for 7% and 19% of CTD-PAH, respectively.[8,10] Characterization of patients with CTD-PAH in the US-based REVEAL Registry showed patients with SLE-PAH are more likely to be African American or Hispanic, compared with patients with SSc-PAH.[23] The burden of SLE-PAH in Asia-Pacific countries has only recently begun to be appreciated, and it seems to be very different from the Western world. One study identified SLE-PAH as the most common cause of CTD-PAH in China, accounting for 59% of cases; SSc was the second most common cause of CTD-PAH.[9] The predominance of SLE-PAH in CTD-PAH has also been shown in Japan and Korea.[24–26] A study based on a Taiwan nationwide database revealed a PAH prevalence of 2.13% in 15,783 patients with SLE.[27]

Rheumatoid Arthritis

The global prevalence of RA is thought to be higher in northern Europe and the United States (0.72%)[28] compared with the rest of the world (0.24%).[29] In the US-based REVEAL and Korean REOPARD registries, RA-PAH made up 8% to 9% of patients with CTD-PAH.[8,30] The prevalence of RA-PAH in the French PH Registry was found to be 0.35%, similar to the general French population and thus not supportive of a specific association.[31]

The UK registry included only 12 patients with RA-PAH (3% of the CTD-PAH cohort).[32]

Other Connective Tissue Diseases

CTDs such as primary Sjögren syndrome (pSS) and inflammatory myopathies have been less frequently associated with PAH. PAH in pSS is rare, and the largest case report series characterizes the condition in just 9 patients.[33] pSS-PAH accounts for 15% to 16% of CTD-PAH in Chinese registries.[9,34] There have been rare reports of patients with inflammatory myopathies, such as DM and PM, with PAH. However, other causes of PH including Group 3 PH due to chronic lung disease, as well as the presence of overlap with other CTDs, could not be completely excluded.[35–37] A study involving the French PH registry suggested that PAH may be associated with dermatomyosis, although this was based on 3 of a total of 5223 patients.[38] The UK registry identified just 7 patients with DM/PM-PAH (2% of the CTD-PAH cohort).[32]

Natural history of pulmonary arterial hypertension associated with connective tissue disease and screening strategies

Given the high morbidity and mortality, SSc-PAH has been the focus of intense research efforts aimed at elucidating its triggers, pathophysiology, diagnosis, clinical course, response to therapy, and outcomes. This work has made SSc-PAH the best characterized cohort within CTD-PAH, and it is this insight that makes SSc-PAH the comparator for other types of CTD-PAH. For example, outcomes in patients with SSc-PAH are worse than those with other types of CTD-PAH, with 1-year survival rates in SSc-PAH of 82% compared with 94% in SLE, 88% in MCTD, and 96% in RA.[23] It is also known that patients with CTD-PAH are not diagnosed with PAH until relatively late in their clinical course.[18,39] These findings emphasize the importance of developing strategies for both screening asymptomatic patients with CTD and early detection of CTD-PAH. The strongest evidence for formalized screening and early detection is in the scleroderma spectrum diseases,[5] where early diagnosis and treatment of SSc-PAH has been shown to improve outcomes.[40] Current guidelines emphasize annual screening in patients with SSc and SSc spectrum (SSc, MCTD, and other CTDs with prominent scleroderma features such as sclerodactyly, nail fold capillary abnormalities, and SSc-specific antibodies) with an uncorrected diffusing capacity of the lung for carbon monoxide (DLCO) less than 80% of predicted.[5] Sufficient data to support standardized screening for PAH in other CTDs is currently lacking (Table 2).

Scleroderma

SSc-PAH is a major cause of morbidity and mortality. Estimates of 1- and 3-year survival in the era between 1960 and 2012 were dismal, with an estimated 1- and 3-year survival rate of 81% and 52%, respectively.[41] These survival estimates have improved in the modern PAH treatment era, although outcomes for SSc-PAH remain worse compared with idiopathic PAH. Late diagnosis and the severity of disease at the time of diagnosis are recognized as significant contributors to the poor prognosis.[42–44] For example, a French study showed that 79% are New York Heart Association (NYHA) functional class III or IV at the time of diagnosis.[42] It is now recognized that formalized early detection programs for SSc-PAH result in improved long-term survival.[40] DETECT was a prospective study that evaluated the performance of an SSc-PAH early detection algorithm for patients with SSc of at least 3 years duration and a DLCO less than 60%. A 2-step approach uses noninvasive biomarkers including the ratio of forced vital capacity % predicted to DLCO % predicted, telangiectasias (current/past), anticentromere antibody, serum N-Terminal (NT)-prohormone of the B-type natriuretic peptide (NT-proBNP), serum urate, and electrocardiographic evidence right axis deviation. Crossing a threshold based on their cumulative score from the aforementioned biomarkers indicates the need for echocardiography (Step 1). Based on echocardiographic findings, calculation of a second risk score indicates appropriate referral for right heart catheterization, the gold-standard test for PAH diagnosis.[45] This algorithm resulted in a false-negative rate of only 4%, which compares favorably to a false-negative rate of 29% using the 2009 ESC/ESR screening recommendations.[45]

Although the DETECT study enrolled high-risk patients with SSc, evidence suggests that the DETECT algorithm is effective in an unselected SSc population.[46] The efficacy of the DETECT algorithm contrasts with efforts to screen patients with other CTDs, for which guidelines currently advise evaluation only after the development of symptoms concerning for PAH.[47,48] Of note, MCTD and CTDs with prominent scleroderma features are considered scleroderma spectrum diseases, and thus guidelines recommend annual screening for PAH associated with these disorders.[5]

Pulmonary Arterial Hypertension Associated with Systemic Lupus Erythematosus

The natural history of SLE-PAH seems to be different from that of SSc-PAH. For example, studies performed in the Western world indicate that most new SLE-PAH cases may be mild and symptomatic,[49] and the prognosis with modern therapies may be significantly better in SLE-PAH compared with SSc-PAH.[32] An analysis of 69 patients with SLE-PAH in the French Pulmonary Hypertension Registry found a mean delay of 4.9 years between the diagnosis of SLE and SLE-PAH.[39] Three-quarters of patients with SLE-PAH endorsed an NYHA functional class of III or IV at the time of diagnosis, and the 5-year survival was 83.9%.[39] The presence of anti-SSA/SSB antibodies were identified as potential risk factors for SLE-PAH, and the presence of anti-U1-RNP antibodies appeared to be protective. may be a protective factor with regard to survival.[39] Despite these insights into the burden and characterization of SLE-PAH early detection algorithms have not proven to be beneficial in the Western world and screening of asymptomatic individuals is not currently recommended in guidelines.[5,47] For example, one echocardiography-based study found no new cases of SLE-PAH, and a low prevalence of other PH groups, after implementing a screening program for asymptomatic patients with SLE in Spain over a 5-year period.[22] Pérez-Peñate and colleagues[50] found similar results in patients with SLE screened prospectively for PAH, in which no new cases of SLE-PAH were discovered through screening. Given the increased prevalence of SLE-PAH in the Eastern world, there is a critical need to evaluate the potential impact of formalized SLE-PAH early detection and screening programs in this region. A study based on the Chinese CSTAR registry concluded that early screening using echocardiography should be performed in patients with SLE with serositis, anti-RNP antibodies, or a DLCO,[51]

Table 2
Screening recommendations for pulmonary arterial hypertension associated with connective tissue

CTD	PAH Screening Recommended?
Scleroderma	Yes
MCTD	Yes
Other CTDs with prominent scleroderma features	Yes
Systemic lupus erythematosus	No
Rheumatoid arthritis	No
Primary Sjögren syndrome	No
Inflammatory myopathies (dermatomyositis and polymyositis)	No

Current recommendations for screening asymptomatic patients with CTD.

although the effectiveness of this approach has not been proven. The Screening of Pulmonary Hypertension in Systemic Lupus Erythematosus (SOPHIE) study is an ongoing prospective study applying PAH screening measures, similar to the DETECT study, to patients with SLE in China.[52]

Pulmonary Arterial Hypertension Associated with Rheumatoid Arthritis

Based on the 28 patients with RA-PAH in the US-based REVEAL Registry, 1-year survival was much better (96%) compared with that of patients with SSc-PAH (82%).[23] Routine PAH screening of asymptomatic patients with RA is not currently endorsed by guidelines.

Other Connective Tissue Diseases

Current data do not support routine programs for the early diagnosis of, or screening of, asymptomatic patients for PAH associated with other CTDs (see **Table 2**). Nevertheless, PAH may develop in this population, and studies suggest that aggressive upfront therapy may improve outcomes.[53,54] Thus, practitioners must remain vigilant for the earliest signs and symptoms of CTD-PAH and pursue further evaluation on a case-by-case basis.

Treatment of pulmonary arterial hypertension associated with connective tissue disease

All 14 currently available PAH-specific therapies are treatment options for patients diagnosed with CTD-PAH, and the same treatment algorithms are used for all patients with Group 1 PAH.[47] Oral options are the endothelin receptor antagonists (ERAs) bosentan, ambrisentan, and macitentan; the phosphodiesterase 5 inhibitors (PDE5is) sildenafil and tadalafil; oral treprostinil; the guanylate cyclase stimulator riociguat; and the selective prostacyclin (IP) receptor agonist selexipag. Iloprost and inhaled treprostinil are inhaled treatment options. Parenteral options are subcutaneous treprostinil, intravenous treprostinil, intravenous epoprostenol, and temperature-stable epoprostenol. Although these medications have been shown to be effective in CTD-PAH, the magnitude of the treatment response may be lower than in idiopathic PAH.[47,55] As is the case with all patients on PAH-specific therapies, patients with CTD-PAH must be followed closely and treatment decisions must be based on baseline and follow-up risk assessments using predictive models.[47] A comprehensive overview of the use of PAH-specific medications approved for treatment of CTD-PAH is beyond the scope of this article, but subgroup analyses of patients with CTD-PAH included in clinical trials involving Group 1 PAH have revealed some important insights.

Selexipag

Selexipag is an oral, selective IP prostacyclin agonist.[56] Subgroup analysis of patients with CTD-PAH included in the GRIPHON trial demonstrated that the treatment effect of selexipag on the primary composite end point of morbidity and mortality in the CTD-PAH subgroup was consistent with the effect in the overall Group 1 PAH study population.[54] Overall, selexipag reduced the risk of composite morbidity/mortality events of patients with CTD-PAH by 41%.[54] No difference in the magnitude of treatment response was seen in SLE-PAH compared with other CTD-PAH. Of note, more rapid progression of PAH was noted in the SSc-PAH cohort compared with the SLEPAH cohort in both the selexipag and placebo groups.

Riociguat

Riociguat is a soluble guanylate cyclase stimulator that acts to increase nitric oxide and promote vascular smooth muscle relaxation. Of the 443 patients with PAH included in the PATENT-1 trial 111 had CTD-PAH.[57] This study showed a significant improvement in exercise and functional capacities in the treatment group, including the CTD-PAH cohort, over a period of 12 weeks. The PATENT-2 open-label extension study showed that these benefits persisted for up to a year.[58]

Combination Therapy (Ambrisentan Plus Tadalafil)

The AMBITION trial showed a significantly lower risk of clinical-failure events (a composite of death, hospitalization for worsening PAH, disease progression, or unsatisfactory long-term clinical response) in patients treated with combination therapy involving the ERA ambrisentan plus the PDE5i tadalafil compared with patients on monotherapy with either of these medications.[59] A post-hoc subgroup analysis of AMBITION confirmed that patients with CTD-PAH and SSc-PAH benefit from combination therapy involving these medications.

Immunosuppression

Limited data are available on the impact of immunosuppression in CTD-PAH. One retrospective analysis involving 23 cases suggested that patients with less severe SLE-PAH or MCTD-PAH might respond to immunosuppression alone, whereas cohorts with more severe PAH likely benefit from combination therapy involving immunosuppressants and PAH-specific medications.[60] Randomized controlled trials are still needed to confirm these results.

SUMMARY AND FUTURE DIRECTIONS

CTD-PAH is a devastating condition that all too often results in disability and even death due to increased pulmonary vascular resistance and right ventricular dysfunction. Patients with CTD are at risk for all 5 WHO PH groups; a right heart catheterization is the pivotal test for diagnosis of PH and, combined with each patient's specific clinical presentation, is the basis for determining which PH groups are present. Current epidemiologic and clinical trial data support the use of standardized, routine early detection and screening programs for PAH in patients with scleroderma spectrum disease. Screening this vulnerable population and early, guideline-directed treatment with PAH-specific therapies has been shown to alter the clinical course and outcomes of SSc-PAH. Efforts to better understand the global impact of, and appropriate screening strategies for, other forms of CTD-PAH have not been as successful. Addressing these knowledge gaps is especially important in the Asia-Pacific region where SLE-PAH, rather than SSc-PAH, is the most common CTD-PAH.

All PAH-specific medications are options for patients with CTD-PAH, and decisions regarding therapy should integrate formalized risk assessments at baseline and reassessments during frequent follow-up clinic visits. Study designs for PAH clinical trials should continue to include prespecified subgroups, which helps to better characterize CTD-PAH types and potential variations in response to therapy.

CLINICS CARE POINTS

- PAH is 1 of 5 WHO PH groups that commonly complicates CTD.
- Routine PAH screening is recommended for with scleroderma spectrum disease (scleroderma, MCTD, and other CTDs with prominent scleroderma features such as sclerodactyly, nail fold capillary abnormalities, and SSc-specific antibodies). The DETECT algorithm is recommended for screening this population due to its low false-negative rate (4%).
- Although PAH screening is not currently recommended for asymptomatic patients with other CTDs, practitioners caring for these patients should consider PAH evaluation on a case-by-case basis.

DISCLOSURE

The authors have nothing to disclose.

REFERENCES

1. Simonneau G, Montani D, Celermajer DS, et al. Haemodynamic definitions and updated clinical classification of pulmonary hypertension. Eur Respir J 2019;53(1). https://doi.org/10.1183/13993003.01913-2018.
2. Humbert M, Guignabert C, Bonnet S, et al. Pathology and pathobiology of pulmonary hypertension: state of the art and research perspectives. Eur Respir J 2019;53(1). https://doi.org/10.1183/13993003.01887-2018.
3. Mathai SC, Hassoun PM. Pulmonary arterial hypertension in connective tissue diseases. Heart Fail Clin 2012;8(3):413–25.
4. McLaughlin VV, Archer SL, Badesch DB, et al. ACCF/AHA 2009 expert consensus document on pulmonary hypertension a report of the American College of Cardiology Foundation Task Force on Expert Consensus Documents and the American

Heart Association developed in collaboration with the American College of Chest Physicians; American Thoracic Society, Inc.; and the Pulmonary Hypertension Association. J Am Coll Cardiol 2009; 53(17):1573–619.

5. Frost A, Badesch D, Gibbs JSR, et al. Diagnosis of pulmonary hypertension. Eur Respir J 2019;53(1). https://doi.org/10.1183/13993003.01904-2018.

6. Sitbon O, Gomberg-Maitland M, Granton J, et al. Clinical trial design and new therapies for pulmonary arterial hypertension. Eur Respir J 2019;53(1). https://doi.org/10.1183/13993003.01908-2018.

7. Fayed H, Coghlan JG. Pulmonary Hypertension Associated with Connective Tissue Disease. Semin Respir Crit Care Med 2019;40(2):173–83.

8. McGoon MD, Miller DP. REVEAL: a contemporary US pulmonary arterial hypertension registry. Eur Respir Rev 2012;21(123):8–18.

9. Zhao J, Wang Q, Liu Y, et al. Clinical characteristics and survival of pulmonary arterial hypertension associated with three major connective tissue diseases: A cohort study in China. Int J Cardiol 2017; 236:432–7.

10. Humbert M, Sitbon O, Chaouat A, et al. Pulmonary arterial hypertension in France: results from a national registry. Am J Respir Crit Care Med 2006; 173(9):1023–30.

11. Ranque B, Mouthon L. Geoepidemiology of systemic sclerosis. Autoimmun Rev Mar 2010;9(5): A311–8.

12. Jansa P, Jarkovsky J, Al-Hiti H, et al. Epidemiology and long-term survival of pulmonary arterial hypertension in the Czech Republic: a retrospective analysis of a nationwide registry. BMC Pulm Med 2014; 14:45. https://doi.org/10.1186/1471-2466-14-45.

13. Coghlan JG, Handler C. Connective tissue associated pulmonary arterial hypertension. Lupus 2006; 15(3):138–42.

14. Mukerjee D, St George D, Coleiro B, et al. Prevalence and outcome in systemic sclerosis associated pulmonary arterial hypertension: application of a registry approach. Ann Rheum Dis 2003;62(11): 1088–93.

15. Avouac J, Airo P, Meune C, et al. Prevalence of pulmonary hypertension in systemic sclerosis in European Caucasians and metaanalysis of 5 studies. J Rheumatol 2010;37(11):2290–8.

16. Hachulla E, Gressin V, Guillevin L, et al. Early detection of pulmonary arterial hypertension in systemic sclerosis: a French nationwide prospective multicenter study. Arthritis Rheum 2005;52(12): 3792–800.

17. Sullivan WD, Hurst DJ, Harmon CE, et al. A prospective evaluation emphasizing pulmonary involvement in patients with mixed connective tissue disease. Medicine (Baltimore) 1984;63(2):92–107.

18. Burdt MA, Hoffman RW, Deutscher SL, et al. Long-term outcome in mixed connective tissue disease: longitudinal clinical and serologic findings. Arthritis Rheum 1999;42(5):899–909.

19. Alpert MA, Goldberg SH, Singsen BH, et al. Cardiovascular manifestations of mixed connective tissue disease in adults. Circulation 1983;68(6):1182–93.

20. Gunnarsson R, Andreassen AK, Molberg O, et al. Prevalence of pulmonary hypertension in an unselected, mixed connective tissue disease cohort: results of a nationwide, Norwegian cross-sectional multicentre study and review of current literature. Rheumatology (Oxford) 2013;52(7):1208–13.

21. Arnaud L, Agard C, Haroche J, et al. [Pulmonary arterial hypertension in systemic lupus erythematosus]. Rev Med Interne 2011;32(11):689–97. Hypertension arterielle pulmonaire associee au lupus systemique.

22. Ruiz-Irastorza G, Garmendia M, Villar I, et al. Pulmonary hypertension in systemic lupus erythematosus: prevalence, predictors and diagnostic strategy. Autoimmun Rev 2013;12(3):410–5.

23. Chung L, Liu J, Parsons L, et al. Characterization of connective tissue disease-associated pulmonary arterial hypertension from REVEAL: identifying systemic sclerosis as a unique phenotype. Chest 2010;138(6):1383–94.

24. Shirai Y, Yasuoka H, Okano Y, et al. Clinical characteristics and survival of Japanese patients with connective tissue disease and pulmonary arterial hypertension: a single-centre cohort. Rheumatology (Oxford) 2012;51(10):1846–54.

25. Chung WJ, Park YB, Jeon CH, et al. Baseline Characteristics of the Korean Registry of Pulmonary Arterial Hypertension. J Korean Med Sci 2015;30(10): 1429–38.

26. Song S, Lee SE, Oh SK, et al. Demographics, treatment trends, and survival rate in incident pulmonary artery hypertension in Korea: A nationwide study based on the health insurance review and assessment service database. PLoS One 2018;13(12): e0209148.

27. Chen HA, Hsu TC, Yang SC, et al. Incidence and survival impact of pulmonary arterial hypertension among patients with systemic lupus erythematosus: a nationwide cohort study. Arthritis Res Ther 2019; 21(1):82.

28. Myasoedova E, Davis JM 3rd, Crowson CS, et al. Epidemiology of rheumatoid arthritis: rheumatoid arthritis and mortality. Curr Rheumatol Rep 2010; 12(5):379–85.

29. Cross M, Smith E, Hoy D, et al. The global burden of rheumatoid arthritis: estimates from the global burden of disease 2010 study. Ann Rheum Dis 2014;73(7):1316–22.

30. Jeon CH, Chai JY, Seo YI, et al. Pulmonary hypertension associated with rheumatic diseases: baseline

characteristics from the Korean registry. Int J Rheum Dis 2012;15(5):e80–9.

31. Montani D, Henry J, O'Connell C, et al. Association between Rheumatoid Arthritis and Pulmonary Hypertension: Data from the French Pulmonary Hypertension Registry. Respiration 2018;95(4):244–50.

32. Condliffe R, Kiely DG, Peacock AJ, et al. Connective tissue disease-associated pulmonary arterial hypertension in the modern treatment era. Am J Respir Crit Care Med 2009;179(2):151–7.

33. Launay D, Hachulla E, Hatron PY, et al. Pulmonary arterial hypertension: a rare complication of primary Sjogren syndrome: report of 9 new cases and review of the literature. Medicine (Baltimore) 2007;86(5):299–315.

34. Hao YJ, Jiang X, Zhou W, et al. Connective tissue disease-associated pulmonary arterial hypertension in Chinese patients. Eur Respir J 2014;44(4):963–72.

35. Taniguchi Y, Horino T, Kato T, et al. Acute pulmonary arterial hypertension associated with anti-synthetase syndrome. Scand J Rheumatol 2010;39(2):179–80.

36. Grateau G, Roux ME, Franck N, et al. Pulmonary hypertension in a case of dermatomyositis. J Rheumatol 1993;20(8):1452–3.

37. Bunch TW, Tancredi RG, Lie JT. Pulmonary hypertension in polymyositis. Chest 1981;79(1):105–7.

38. Sanges S, Yelnik CM, Sitbon O, et al. Pulmonary arterial hypertension in idiopathic inflammatory myopathies: Data from the French pulmonary hypertension registry and review of the literature. Medicine (Baltimore). Sep 2016;95(39):e4911.

39. Hachulla E, Jais X, Cinquetti G, et al. Pulmonary Arterial Hypertension Associated With Systemic Lupus Erythematosus: Results From the French Pulmonary Hypertension Registry. Chest 2018;153(1):143–51.

40. Humbert M, Yaici A, de Groote P, et al. Screening for pulmonary arterial hypertension in patients with systemic sclerosis: clinical characteristics at diagnosis and long-term survival. Arthritis Rheum 2011;63(11):3522–30.

41. Lefevre G, Dauchet L, Hachulla E, et al. Survival and prognostic factors in systemic sclerosis-associated pulmonary hypertension: a systematic review and meta-analysis. Arthritis Rheum 2013;65(9):2412–23.

42. Launay D, Sitbon O, Hachulla E, et al. Survival in systemic sclerosis-associated pulmonary arterial hypertension in the modern management era. Ann Rheum Dis 2013;72(12):1940–6.

43. Kawut SM, Taichman DB, Archer-Chicko CL, et al. Hemodynamics and survival in patients with pulmonary arterial hypertension related to systemic sclerosis. Chest 2003;123(2):344–50.

44. Tyndall AJ, Bannert B, Vonk M, et al. Causes and risk factors for death in systemic sclerosis: a study from the EULAR Scleroderma Trials and Research (EUSTAR) database. Ann Rheum Dis 2010;69(10):1809–15.

45. Coghlan JG, Denton CP, Grunig E, et al. Evidence-based detection of pulmonary arterial hypertension in systemic sclerosis: the DETECT study. Ann Rheum Dis 2014;73(7):1340–9.

46. Vandecasteele E, Drieghe B, Melsens K, et al. Screening for pulmonary arterial hypertension in an unselected prospective systemic sclerosis cohort. Eur Respir J 2017;49(5). https://doi.org/10.1183/13993003.02275-2016.

47. Galie N, Humbert M, Vachiery JL, et al. 2015 ESC/ERS Guidelines for the diagnosis and treatment of pulmonary hypertension: The Joint Task Force for the Diagnosis and Treatment of Pulmonary Hypertension of the European Society of Cardiology (ESC) and the European Respiratory Society (ERS): Endorsed by: Association for European Paediatric and Congenital Cardiology (AEPC), International Society for Heart and Lung Transplantation (ISHLT). Eur Respir J 2015;46(4):903–75.

48. Kato M, Atsumi T. Pulmonary arterial hypertension associated with connective tissue diseases: A review focusing on distinctive clinical aspects. Eur J Clin Invest 2018;48(2). https://doi.org/10.1111/eci.12876.

49. Prabu A, Patel K, Yee CS, et al. Prevalence and risk factors for pulmonary arterial hypertension in patients with lupus. Rheumatology (Oxford) 2009;48(12):1506–11.

50. Perez-Penate GM, Rua-Figueroa I, Julia-Serda G, et al. Pulmonary Arterial Hypertension in Systemic Lupus Erythematosus: Prevalence and Predictors. J Rheumatol 2016;43(2):323–9.

51. Zhang N, Li M, Qian J, et al. Pulmonary arterial hypertension in systemic lupus erythematosus based on a CSTAR-PAH study: Baseline characteristics and risk factors. Int J Rheum Dis 2019;22(5):921–8.

52. Huang D, Cheng YY, Chan PH, et al. Rationale and design of the screening of pulmonary hypertension in systemic lupus erythematosus (SOPHIE) study. ERJ Open Res 2018;4(1). https://doi.org/10.1183/23120541.00135-2017.

53. Coghlan JG, Galie N, Barbera JA, et al. Initial combination therapy with ambrisentan and tadalafil in connective tissue disease-associated pulmonary arterial hypertension (CTD PAH): subgroup analysis from the AMBITION trial. Ann Rheum Dis 2017;76(7):1219–27.

54. Gaine S, Chin K, Coghlan G, et al. Selexipag for the treatment of connective tissue disease-associated pulmonary arterial hypertension. Eur Respir J 2017;50(2). https://doi.org/10.1183/13993003.02493-2016.

55. Avouac J, Wipff J, Kahan A, et al. Effects of oral treatments on exercise capacity in systemic

sclerosis related pulmonary arterial hypertension: a meta-analysis of randomised controlled trials. Ann Rheum Dis 2008;67(6):808–14.

56. Noel ZR, Kido K, Macaulay TE. Selexipag for the treatment of pulmonary arterial hypertension. Am J Health Syst Pharm 2017;74(15):1135–41.

57. Ghofrani HA, Galie N, Grimminger F, et al. Riociguat for the treatment of pulmonary arterial hypertension. N Engl J Med 2013;369(4):330–40.

58. Rubin LJ, Galie N, Grimminger F, et al. Riociguat for the treatment of pulmonary arterial hypertension: a

long-term extension study (PATENT-2). Eur Respir J 2015;45(5):1303–13.

59. Galie N, Barbera JA, Frost AE, et al. Initial Use of Ambrisentan plus Tadalafil in Pulmonary Arterial Hypertension. N Engl J Med 2015;373(9):834–44.

60. Jais X, Launay D, Yaici A, et al. Immunosuppressive therapy in lupus- and mixed connective tissue disease-associated pulmonary arterial hypertension: a retrospective analysis of twenty-three cases. Arthritis Rheum 2008;58(2):521–31.

Struggling Between Liver Transplantation and Portopulmonary Hypertension

Arun Jose, MD, MS[a],*, Courtney R. Jones, MD[b], Jean M. Elwing, MD[a]

KEYWORDS

- Portopulmonary hypertension • Liver transplantation • Pulmonary arterial hypertension
- Pulmonary vascular resistance • Reperfusion syndrome

KEY POINTS

- Portopulmonary hypertension (PoPH) is associated with among the worst long-term survival of all pulmonary arterial hypertension subtypes.
- Targeted pulmonary vascular therapy is the mainstay of management in PoPH, improving cardiac function and lowering pulmonary vascular resistance.
- Liver transplantation (LT) can significantly improve outcomes in some patients with PoPH, but is associated with significant operative and postoperative risks.
- The best management strategy in PoPH is uncertain, and the risk–benefit assessment of medical therapy alone or in combination with LT must account for a multitude of factors with limited evidence for guidance.

INTRODUCTION/HISTORY/DEFINITIONS/BACKGROUND

Portopulmonary hypertension (PoPH) is a type of pulmonary arterial hypertension (PAH) that exclusively affects those with underlying portal hypertension, typically in the context of chronic liver disease.[1–7] First formally recognized as a distinct disease entity in 1990 as part of the inaugural "lung–liver" meeting, the diagnostic criteria for PoPH have undergone several revisions since then.[8] Currently, PoPH is defined hemodynamically on right heart catheterization (RHC) by an elevated mean pulmonary arterial pressure (mPAP) greater than 20 mm Hg, a pulmonary capillary wedge pressure of 15 mm Hg or less, and a pulmonary vascular resistance (PVR) of 3 Wood Units or greater ($\geq$240 dyne•s•cm^{-5}), in the setting of portal hypertension.[1–3] Portal hypertension is determined clinically by the presence of classic sequelae (gastroesophageal varices, portal hypertensive gastropathy, abdominal ascites, hepatorenal syndrome, spontaneous bacterial peritonitis) or directly through measurement of an elevated hepatic venous pressure gradient greater than or equal to 6 mm Hg on venous catheterization.[9,10]

PREVALENCE/INCIDENCE/PATHOGENESIS

PoPH is estimated to afflict between 5% and 6% of all individuals with underlying portal hypertensive liver disease, with an incidence of approximately one to three per three million.[5,11] PoPH has been reported to be more common in female individuals and those with underlying autoimmune liver disease, although this association has not been validated in additional disease cohorts and remains unclear.[4] PoPH exhibits the same pulmonary vascular remodeling as other subtypes of PAH, characterized by smooth muscle hypertrophy, intimal fibrosis, and plexiform lesions, but the molecular pathogenesis

[a] Division of Pulmonary, Critical Care, and Sleep Medicine, University of Cincinnati, ML 0564, Medical Sciences Building, 231 Albert Sabin Way, Cincinnati, OH 45267, USA; [b] Department of Anesthesiology, University of Cincinnati, ML 3553, Medical Sciences Building, 231 Albert Sabin Way, Cincinnati, OH 45267, USA
* Corresponding author.
E-mail address: josean@ucmail.uc.edu

Heart Failure Clin 19 (2023) 55–65
https://doi.org/10.1016/j.hfc.2022.08.017
1551-7136/23/© 2022 Elsevier Inc. All rights reserved.

of PoPH is not well understood[12–14] (**Fig. 1**). Vasoactive peptides affecting vascular tone and remodeling pathways, such as endothelin-1 (ET1), are theorized to play a central role in disease pathogenesis.[4,12,15–18] ET1 is secreted by liver perivascular endothelial and stellate cells, has potent vasoconstrictive properties, and has been shown to be present in higher concentrations in the pulmonary vasculature of patients with PoPH as compared with those with non-PoPH liver cirrhosis. A deficiency of bone morphogenic protein 9 (BMP9), which is produced by hepatic stellate cells and promotes vascular quiescence through the vascular endothelial growth factor signaling pathway, may also play a role in PoPH disease pathogenesis.[19–21] BMP9 levels were significantly lower in patients with PoPH as compared with other types of PAH, and also predicted transplant-free survival in PoPH, suggesting BMP9 may have value as a disease-specific biomarker with diagnostic and prognostic utility. Unfortunately, evidence linking these vasoactive peptides to PoPH is limited, and our understanding of the mechanisms and corresponding biomarkers driving PoPH disease pathogenesis remains incomplete.

CLINICAL COURSE

PoPH exhibits among the worst survival of all PAH subtypes, with a 5-year survival of between 35% and 49%, as compared with a 5-year survival of 64% to 72% in patients with idiopathic PAH (IPAH).[5,22–25] Similar to other subtypes of PAH, survival is strongly linked to the degree of cardiac impairment and the extent of PVR elevation, but these prognostic factors do not fully explain the increased mortality observed in PoPH.[1,2,5,6,8] Patients with PoPH are estimated to have an approximately three-fold higher risk of mortality than comparable patients with IPAH, even after adjustment for demographic characteristics, RHC hemodynamics, and targeted pulmonary vascular therapy.[23] Interestingly, this increased mortality is despite patients with PoPH demonstrating less severe hemodynamic disease severity at diagnosis compared with patients with IPAH. It is believed that the excess mortality observed in patients with PoPH stems in part from the complex interplay between the liver and cardiovascular disease in these patients.[24–26]

Surprisingly, neither the severity of underlying liver disease (measured by the Model for End-stage Liver Disease [MELD] score) nor the extent of portal pressure elevation, has been shown to predict either the presence or severity of PoPH at diagnosis.[5,8,11] Stated another way, PoPH can occur in patients with any degree of liver dysfunction or portal pressure elevation, including those with relatively minor portal hypertension and no evidence of hepatic synthetic dysfunction. Despite the lack of association between liver disease severity and PoPH incidence, it is well established that liver disease severity (MELD score) strongly predicts survival in PoPH.[6,25–28] Other predictors, including hemodynamic disease severity (mPAP, PVR), demographics (age, race), and functional capacity, may also have prognostic utility in PoPH, but they have not consistently predicted outcomes across different disease cohorts. Registry studies also suggest patients with PoPH are also less likely to be college graduates, more likely to be unemployed, less likely to receive combination targeted PAH therapy, and more likely to be underinsured than patients with IPAH. In addition, patients with PoPH are also more likely to be hospitalized, more likely to visit the emergency department, and more likely to have higher health care resource usage when compared with portal hypertensive patients without pulmonary hypertension.[24–26,29] Precisely how socioeconomic determinants of health might predict survival in PoPH is not yet clear, and the optimal use of these metrics in risk stratification of patients with PoPH remains to be determined.

As alluded to earlier when discussing potential risk factors for developing PoPH, a sex disparity in PoPH outcomes has been observed.[30] Female

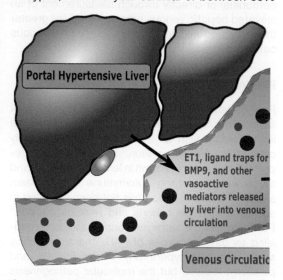

Fig. 1. Hypothesized mechanism of PoPH molecular pathogenesis. ET1, ligand traps that sequester BMP9, and other vasoactive peptides are released from the liver in response to portal hypertensive disease. These peptides enter the venous circulation, translocate to the pulmonary vasculature, and drive smooth muscle hypertrophy, intimal fibrosis, and plexiform lesion formation, the characteristic histopathological hallmarks of PoPH.

patients with PoPH have shown significantly higher PVR values than male patients at the time of diagnosis, yet demonstrate a significantly greater improvement in PVR with targeted therapy than their male counterparts. The reasons for this "sex paradox" in the development of PoPH and treatment response are unclear but may relate to abnormalities in both sex hormone levels (higher estrogen relative to dehydroepiandrosterone sulfate) and genetics (genetic variation in estrogen and aromatase enzyme genes) that have previously been associated with PoPH.[31–33]

THERAPEUTIC OPTIONS

Like other subtypes of PAH, treatment in PoPH is aimed at improving cardiac function, reducing vascular resistance, optimizing functional capacity, and achieving a "low-risk" clinical profile.[1,2] Owing to a limited number of high-quality clinical studies focusing on medical management of PoPH, and the exclusion of PoPH from almost all randomized controlled treatment studies of PAH, most of the evidence supporting targeted medical therapy in PoPH is extrapolated from case reports, case series, and expert opinion.

The most robust evidence supporting targeted therapy in PoPH comes from the PORTICO randomized controlled trial, which achieved its primary endpoint of a significant improvement in PVR more than 12 weeks of treatment with the endothelin receptor antagonist macitentan.[34] Secondary endpoints, including other metrics of PoPH hemodynamic disease severity, also improved in this study. Other cohort studies of endothelin receptor antagonist therapy in PoPH, using either ambrisentan or bosentan, reinforce the beneficial effect of endothelin receptor antagonist therapy in PoPH, with significant improvement in hemodynamic measures of PoPH disease severity (mPAP, PVR) in treated patients.[35–39]

The evidence for using other targeted pulmonary hypertension therapeutics in PoPH is primarily extrapolated from randomized controlled trials showing benefit in other PAH subtypes, supplemented with case series and observational data suggesting a comparable benefit in PoPH with these medications. Treatment with phosphodiesterase-5 inhibitor medications (sildenafil, tadalafil) has shown improved RHC hemodynamics and functional capacity in PoPH.[40–42] The soluble guanylate cyclase activator riociguat improved PoPH hemodynamics and functional status in a subgroup analysis of the larger PATENT randomized controlled trial.[43] Parenteral prostacyclin therapy, such as epoprostenol or treprostinil, is generally considered to be the most potent medication available to treat pulmonary vascular disease, and case series suggest comparable efficacy and clinical benefit when applied to the PoPH subtype of PAH.[44,45]

SURGICAL TECHNIQUES

Despite the use of targeted therapy to improve hemodynamics and functional status in PoPH, survival in PoPH is consistently inferior to that observed for other subtypes of PAH, even in the modern treatment era. Liver transplantation (LT) offers the tantalizing possibility of durable resolution of both pulmonary vascular and hepatic disease with a single procedure, but the unfortunate reality is considerably more complex. PoPH can fully resolve, improve to some degree, worsen considerably, or develop de novo following LT. Owing to significant perioperative and postoperative risks, as well as variable outcomes following LT, PoPH is not itself an indication for LT.[5,8]

As outcomes in PoPH are predicted by hemodynamic disease severity and cardiovascular dysfunction, as well as the extent of liver synthetic dysfunction (MELD score), it comes as no surprise that these variables also predict perioperative mortality during LT. There is a high risk of perioperative and postoperative mortality in patients with PoPH undergoing LT with an uncontrolled disease, but the precise hemodynamic thresholds at which LT is considered safe have shifted over time. In the early 2000s, it was appreciated that LT was associated with almost 100% mortality if performed in patients with PoPH with mPAP greater than 50 mm Hg, and 50% mortality for those patients with PoPH with mPAP values between 35 mm Hg and 50 mm Hg and a PVR greater than 3.1 Wood Units before LT.[3,5,46] Attempting to balance the increased risks of LT in uncontrolled PoPH with the potential cardiovascular, hepatic, and survival benefits in transplant recipients, the MELD exception study group and conference (MESSAGE) met in 2006 to update guidelines for LT in PoPH.[5,22,47] This group reached a consensus that patients with PoPH who were able to achieve and maintain control of their hemodynamic disease, defined as mPAP less than 35 mm Hg and a PVR less than 5 Wood Units on RHC testing, were eligible to be granted MELD exception points to expedite LT. Admittedly, this recommendation was based on limited data regarding the magnitude of increased LT risk relative to RHC hemodynamics. Quantification of risk based on mPAP was somewhat arbitrary, which was a limitation acknowledged by the MESSAGE investigators at the time. A recent update in 2020 expanded MELD exception point eligibility to patients with

PoPH and with mPAP values between 35 mm Hg and 45 mm Hg able to achieve and maintain a PVR less than 3 Wood Units.[22,48]

Despite this limitation in the MELD exception points for PoPH, it is well established that survival following LT in PoPH patients with adequate control of their hemodynamic disease is comparable with patients without PoPH and significantly better than in patients with PoPH who did not undergo LT. Those undergoing LT with MELD exception points experience 1 year and 3 year survival rates post-LT of approximately 85% to 95% and 75% to 80%, respectively, the same survival rates as those transplanted without exception points, and considerably higher than the estimated treated PoPH 3 year survival of approximately 50% in the modern era.[6,11,24,25,27,49–51] Although hemodynamic disease severity is established as a strong predictor of perioperative mortality during LT, the precise relationship between pre-LT hemodynamics and post-LT outcomes in PoPH remains unclear. Although previous studies have not identified a relationship between pre-LT hemodynamics and post-LT survival in PoPH, more recent evidence suggests a PVR threshold between 1.6 and 3.1 Wood Units and a mPAP threshold greater than 35 mm Hg may predict increased post-LT mortality in PoPH.[6,51–54] The evidence supporting these predictive thresholds comes primarily from retrospective evidence, and confirmatory prospective studies will be necessary before changes to the perioperative risk stratification and management of PoPH can be considered. Currently, it is unclear whether PoPH increases the risk of post-LT graft failure, and there is no evidence to suggest targeted therapy itself influences the risk of post-LT mortality or graft failure beyond its effects on pre-LT pulmonary vascular hemodynamics.[28,49,53]

Although PoPH can improve or resolve fully following LT, there is also considerable heterogeneity in the postoperative course experienced by these patients. There is ample evidence from the literature describing significant improvement or full resolution of PoPH following LT, with a considerable minority of patients with PoPH (estimated at up to 30%–50%) able to achieve and maintain normal pulmonary vascular hemodynamics in the absence of all targeted PoPH therapy.[5,22,54–60] However, case reports have also detailed significant worsening of PoPH after LT, as well as de novo precapillary PAH occurring following LT in patients without any pretransplant history of pulmonary vascular disease.[61–63] Adding to this uncertainty, there are no established predictors for the resolution of PoPH following LT, and no clear association between type, strength, and route of targeted pulmonary vascular therapy and the risk of persistent PoPH following LT. Reflecting the clinical equipoise that exists regarding the use of LT in PoPH, a survey of PoPH specialists indicated less than half (42%) believe that PoPH always improves following LT, and only a third (31%) consider treated PoPH to be a sole indication for LT (ie, in the absence of decompensated cirrhosis).[64] Current guidelines attempt to account for this variable response to LT in PoPH, suggesting serial Doppler echocardiographic monitoring of pulmonary vascular disease post-LT and judicious titration of targeted PoPH therapy.[5] Unfortunately, it remains unclear what factors predict hemodynamic response following LT in PoPH, which patients with PoPH are at greatest risk of decompensation after LT, and for how long after transplant this elevated risk is present, highlighting the need for additional research in this poorly understood area of post-LT management.

Further complicating the decision to undergo LT, patients with PoPH are also exposed to unique perioperative risks during the actual LT procedure, and pulmonary arterial catheter monitoring is considered the standard of care during these operations.[5,65] In a simplified manner, LT occurs in sequential "phases" based on the presence or absence of the liver: the preanhepatic, the anhepatic, the reperfusion, and the neohepatic phases[65–67] (**Fig. 2**). The preanhepatic phase occurs when the native liver is exposed and mobilized, the anhepatic phase occurs following native liver removal (with associated vascular clamping and bypass), the reperfusion phase is defined by the release of vascular clamps and reperfusion of the graft, and the neohepatic phase is defined by the situation of the graft organ and anastomosis of arterial and biliary trees. Relevant to LT in PoPH, the preanhepatic phase can be associated with volume shifts and decreased preload due to bleeding during dissection and liver mobilization, but these are generally managed successfully with volume resuscitation and vasopressor support.[65] The anhepatic phase, with associated vascular clamping and loss of all native liver function, poses a great intraoperative risk to the PoPH patients undergoing an LT procedure.[65,68,69] Vascular clamping results in a sudden drop in cardiac output and decreases in systemic and pulmonary vascular pressures, with a corresponding increase in PVR. Metabolic derangements including acidosis and hypocalcemia can be prominent. Although detrimental to cardiovascular homeostasis in the patients with pulmonary vascular disease, these effects are ultimately transient, and corrective measures must be approached cautiously. Vasopressor

Pre-anhepatic

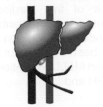

Bleeding

Decreased ventricular preload

Anhepatic

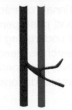

Decreased CO

Decreased SVR

Increased PVR

Decreased Preload

Acidosis

Hypocalcemia

Neohepatic

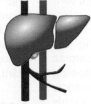

Cytokine release

Elevated risk of vascular thromboembolism

Reperfusion

Cytokine release

Acidosis

Hyperkalemia

Increased Ventricular Preload

Increased CO

Hypothermia

Hypotension

Elevated risk of arrhythmias

Frequent bleeding

Fig. 2. Unique risks confronted by patients with PoPH across phases of LT. Risks to patients with PoPH across phases of LT, from preanhepatic, anhepatic, reperfusion, and neohepatic phases.

medications can be helpful, but excess volume administration is typically avoided, as vascular unclamping that occurs later in the operation can result in a considerable increase in pulmonary arterial pressures, and excess resuscitation can precipitate right ventricular failure and cardiovascular collapse. Vascular unclamping signals the start of the reperfusion phase, arguably the most challenging part of the operation. Release of previously clamped "stagnant" blood and reperfusion of a grafted organ not only increases cardiac output and venous return, but can also stimulate significant cytokine release and hemodynamic instability due to the cold, acidotic, potassium-rich, inflammatory nature of the reperfused blood itself.[5,65,68–71] Hypotension, elevated pulmonary arterial pressures, increased right ventricular preload, hypothermia, increased bleeding, and an increased risk of cardiac arrhythmias are all possible manifestations. The neohepatic phase, where the graft is situated and anastomosed, is

also the phase in which venous thromboembolism risk (which can result in pulmonary embolism and cardiac arrest in patients with underlying pulmonary vascular disease) is at its highest. Postreperfusion syndrome is a particularly feared complication following the reperfusion phase, occurring in up to one-third of all cases. This syndrome, defined by a sustained drop in mean arterial pressure of 30% or greater in the first few minutes of reperfusion, can markedly increase pulmonary arterial pressures, diminish cardiac contractility, and precipitate right ventricular failure and asystole.[5,65,69–71] The morbidity and mortality of postreperfusion syndrome and reperfusion-associated right heart failure in PoPH LT are considerable. Adequate control of PoPH hemodynamic disease severity before LT may help protect against reperfusion-associated hemodynamic instability and postreperfusion syndrome, and administration of short-acting pulmonary vasodilators such as inhaled nitric oxide and support of the right ventricle with inotropic agents or extracorporeal life support may be helpful to rescue the patient from right ventricular failure when it does occur.

One final operative consideration in PoPH is the immediate postoperative period following LT. There are unpredictable increases in both cardiac function and PVR that occur in the days following LT, and therefore the health of the right ventricle is believed to be of paramount importance in this critical postoperative period.[5,22,65,70] Downtitration of targeted pulmonary vascular therapy is avoided during this period due to the uncertain trajectory of right ventricular recovery following LT, and serial cardiac visualization (typically via transthoracic echocardiogram, although some authorities suggest transesophageal echocardiography for superior visualization of posterior cardiac structures) is advised for monitoring.[5,65] Careful volume management, consultation with a pulmonary vascular disease specialist, and consideration for use of a pulmonary artery catheter for real-time hemodynamic monitoring are all recommended in the postoperative period to promote recovery. The health of the right ventricle in the postoperative period strongly determines outcomes following LT, as right ventricular dysfunction can result in left ventricular failure due to interventricular interdependence, graft congestion, graft loss, and place the patient at risk of postoperative ventilatory support, escalation of care, and increased length of stay.

Despite the importance of the right ventricle in tolerating the immediate postoperative period following LT, much is unknown about the role of the right ventricle in predicting overall post-LT outcomes. Case series and cohort studies both suggest that targeted PoPH therapy and LT improve right ventricular structure and function in PoPH, but whether these improvements translate into favorable post-LT outcomes in PoPH remains to be established.[8,40,51,59] Heterogeneity in the precise echocardiographic metrics best used to identify right ventricular dysfunction, and even disagreement on what thresholds constitute right ventricular dysfunction in PoPH, have limited the routine use of right ventricular morphometry in determining LT candidacy in PoPH, and currently, considerations on the health of the right ventricle do not factor into MELD exception point determinations.[8,22,48] Recognizing the importance of this cardiac chamber in PoPH, however, current expert opinion and guidelines do endorse both echocardiographic monitoring of the right ventricle intraoperatively to assess patient status, and the use of echocardiography to guide adjustment of targeted therapy following LT.[5,65,70] Although the health of

the right ventricle is critically important to recovery following LT, the relationship between structural and functional characteristics of this cardiac chamber and postoperative outcomes in patients with PoPH undergoing LT is undefined, and additional research is needed to best inform future perioperative, postoperative, and MELD exception point recommendations in PoPH and LT.

DISCUSSION

PoPH is a progressive, ultimately fatal disease of the pulmonary vasculature, occurring in patients with underlying portal hypertensive liver disease, with poor response to targeted medical therapy, and among the worst long-term survival rates of any PAH subtype. LT, although potentially beneficial (or even curative) in a subset of patients with PoPH, is associated with considerable perioperative and postoperative risks (including morbidity and mortality) and has an unpredictable effect on the clinical course of PoPH. Consequently, although LT may be appropriate in carefully selected patients, PoPH itself is not an indication for transplantation, and there is a constant struggle to identify the optimal management strategy (medical or surgical) for these extremely complex patients. Although targeted therapy for PAH is associated with improvements in pulmonary vascular hemodynamics, cardiac function, PVR, and risk metrics, evidence for these therapeutics in PoPH is backed by mostly small case series and observational data, and survival for treated patients with PoPH remains unsatisfactory. LT can offer substantial improvements to mortality for selected patients with PoPH, and MELD exception points are granted to these patients to expedite LT and take full advantage of this benefit. However, considerable uncertainty exists surrounding PoPH and LT, including the predictors of perioperative and postoperative survival and graft failure, the hemodynamic and clinical characteristics that predict optimal response to LT, and preoperative, intraoperative, and postoperative strategies to optimize favorable outcomes following LT in these patients.

When considering LT in PoPH, an appraisal of the risks and benefits of medical therapy versus transplantation should be personalized to reflect individual patient factors, and there is no strategy that can be applied to all patients with PoPH (Fig 3). However, the authors believe certain global recommendations can be made regarding PoPH care. The first step in managing PoPH should be optimization of hemodynamic disease severity and achievement of low-risk status, as these are treatment goals for all subtypes of PAH and are

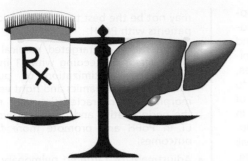

Fig. 3. Balance between medical therapy and liver transplant in portopulmonary hypertension. In patients with PoPH, there are both risks and benefits to medical therapy and surgical transplantation, and the overall balance does not favor one treatment strategy over the other. Thus, the optimal approach is best decided on an individual basis, with careful assessment of the risk–benefit ratio personalized for each patient.

5-year survival 35–49%	Post-LT survival in PoPH is comparable other populations
Targeted therapy improves pulmonary vascular hemodynamics	
Evidence for targeted therapy is primarily observational and case-series, few RCT's	Most patients experience improvement in PoPH disease severity, some are cured, but response to LT is variable
Does not reverse pulmonary arterial disease pathology	Control of PoPH is required to receive MELD exception points for LT listing
	LT has considerable perioperative and post-operative risk of morbidity and mortality
	PoPH alone is not an indication for LT

prerequisites for consideration of LT. Careful attention should be paid to the correction of both the PVR *and* the morphologic characteristics of the right ventricle such as dilation and dyskinesis. Only after the patient has achieved a truly low-risk profile, with both hemodynamic and cardiac structural optimization, should consideration of LT be entertained. In patients who achieve this low-risk state and have the necessary social and emotional support to successfully undergo a solid organ transplantation procedure, the authors believe LT offers significant benefits if it can be realized in the context of minimizing potential perioperative and postoperative risks. Successful LT has the potential to improve pulmonary vascular disease severity, and potentially confer a survival benefit when compared with patients with PoPH who did not undergo LT. Consequently, in appropriately optimized patients with PoPH, the authors would suggest pursuing LT as this currently offers the best chance of long-term survival. Finally, given the considerable uncertainty that currently exists,

the authors would take this opportunity to call for additional research into risk-stratification, predicting treatment response, and optimizing patient selection, operative course, and postoperative management of PoPH patients undergoing LT.

SUMMARY

PoPH is a devastating pulmonary vascular disease due to liver disease, with poor treatment response and dismal long-term survival, occurring in 5% to 6% of all patients with portal hypertensive liver disease. Pathogenic mechanisms are unknown, and outcomes are driven by both the underlying severity of liver disease and the cardiac adaptation to pulmonary vascular disease. Medical therapy for PoPH is comparable to other PAH subtypes, targeting pulmonary arterial vasodilation to improve cardiac function and lower PVR. Selected patients with PoPH are able to undergo LT, which can sometimes dramatically improve both their hepatic and cardiovascular diseases, but outcomes are variable, and perioperative and postoperative risks must be considered. Optimization of pulmonary vascular and right ventricular disease in PoPH may help minimize those risks and enhance post-LT outcomes, but currently, there are limited data available to help guide risk-stratification and prediction of perioperative and postoperative LT outcomes in PoPH, and further research is required. Ultimately, the struggle between LT and PoPH will need to be adjudicated on a case-by-case basis, with careful attention paid to hemodynamic and morphologic metrics of PAH disease severity, consideration of individual patient social, emotional, and cultural factors, and integration of input from colleagues in hepatology, anesthesiology, pulmonology, cardiology, and transplant surgery all necessary to optimize outcomes in these challenging clinical cases.

CLINICS CARE POINTS

- Portopulmonary hypertension (PoPH) affects between 5% and 6% of all individuals with underlying portal hypertensive liver disease. There is no association between the severity of portal hypertension or liver synthetic dysfunction and either presence or severity of PoPH.

- Outcomes in PoPH are driven by the severity of underlying liver disease and cardiac adaptation to elevated pulmonary vascular pressures.

- Treatment in PoPH is similar to other pulmonary arterial hypertension subtypes, centering around targeted pulmonary vasodilator therapy to reduce pulmonary pressures and pulmonary vascular resistance (PVR), improve cardiac function, and reach a "low-risk" clinical profile.

- Patients with PoPH who optimize their pulmonary vascular hemodynamics (mean pulmonary arterial pressure [mPAP] < 35 mm Hg and PVR < 5 Wood Units [WU], or mPAP 35–45 mm Hg with PVR < 3 WU) are eligible to receive Model for End-stage Liver Disease exception points to expedite liver transplantation (LT).

- LT is often beneficial in most patients with PoPH and can be curative in some patients, but is associated with a variable response, can be detrimental to some patients with PoPH, and predictors of PoPH cure following LT are unknown. In addition, LT is associated with considerable perioperative and postoperative risks of morbidity and mortality. It may not be the best treatment option for all patients with PoPH.

- Consideration of targeted medical therapy alone versus proceeding with LT in PoPH is challenging. Optimization of pulmonary vascular hemodynamics and right ventricular morphologic characteristics may minimize the perioperative and postoperative risks of LT in PoPH and promote more favorable outcomes.

- Adjustment of targeted pulmonary vascular therapy in PoPH is not recommended immediately following LT, due to variable trajectories of right ventricular healing. Serial echocardiography and careful adjustment of targeted therapy are suggested post-LT, but the optimal strategy for post-LT weaning of targeted therapy is undefined.

DISCLOSURE

The authors have no commercial or financial conflicts of interest pertaining to the contents of this article. A. Jose receives funding from the National Institutes of Health (2UL1RT00424, 2KL2TR001426), the Parker B. Francis Foundation, and the United Therapeutics Corporation through an investigator-sponsored grant. C.R. Jones has no funding disclosures. J.M. Elwing receives funding from United Therapeutics, Altavant, Aerovate, Bayer, and Gossamer Bio and serves as a consultant for Janssen, United Therapeutics, Liquidia, Phase Bio, Gossamer Bio, Bayer, Acceleron, and Altavant.

REFERENCES

1. Galie N, McLaughlin VV, Rubin LJ, et al. An overview of the 6th world symposium on pulmonary hypertension. Eur Respir J 2019;53(1):1802148.

2. Simonneau G, Montani D, Celermajer DS, et al. Haemodynamic definitions and updated clinical classification of pulmonary hypertension. Eur Respir J 2019;53:1801913.

3. Krowka MJ, Mandell MS, Ramsay MA, et al. Hepatopulmonary syndrome and portopulmonary hypertension: a report of the multicenter liver transplant database. Liver Transpl 2004;10(2):174–82.

4. Kawut S, Krowka MJ, Trotter JF, et al. Clinical risk factors for portopulmonary hypertension. Hepatology 2008;48(1):196–203.

5. Krowka MJ, Fallon MB, Kawut SM, et al. International liver transplant society practice guidelines: diagnosis and management of hepatopulmonary syndrome and portopulmonary hypertension.

Transplantation 2016;100(7):1440–52. https://doi.org/10.1097/TP.0000000000001229.

6. DuBrock HM, Goldberg DS, Sussman NL, et al. Predictors of waitlist mortality in portopulmonary hypertension. Transplantation 2017;101(7):1609–15.

7. Li J, Zhang Q, Zhang X, et al. Prevalence and prognosis of portopulmonary hypertension in 223 liver transplant recipients. Can Respir J 2018;2018:9629570.

8. Krowka MJ. Hepatopulmonary syndrome and portopulmonary hypertension: the pulmonary vascular enigmas of liver disease. Clin Liver Dis 2020;15(Suppl 1):S13–24.

9. Berzigotti A, Seijo S, Reverter E, et al. Assessing portal hypertension in liver diseases. Expert Rev Gastroenterol Hepatol 2013;7(2):141–55.

10. Bai W, Al-Karaghouli M, Stach J, et al. Test-retest reliability and consistency of HVPG and impact on trial design: a study in 289 patients from 20 randomized controlled trials. Hepatology 2021;74(6):3301–15.

11. Sithamparanathan S, Nair A, Thirugnanasothy L, et al. Survival in portopulmonary hypertension: outcomes of the United Kingdom National Pulmonary Arterial Hypertension registry. J Heart Lung Transpl 2017;36(7):770–9.

12. Porres-Aguilar M, Altamirano JT, Torre-Delgadillo A, et al. Portopulmonary hypertension and hepatopulmonary syndrome: a clinician-oriented overview. Eur Respir Rev 2012;21:223–33.

13. Saleemi S. Portopulmonary hypertension. Ann Thorac Med 2010;5(1):5–9.

14. Bartolome SD. Portopulmonary hypertension: diagnosis, clinical features, and medical therapy. Clin Liver Dis 2014;4(2):42–5.

15. Benjaminov FS, Prentice M, Sniderman KW, et al. Portopulmonary hypertension in decompensated cirrhosis with refractory ascites. Gut 2003;52(9):1355–62.

16. Pellicelli AM, Barbaro G, Puoti C, et al. Plasma cytokines and portopulmonary hypertension in patients with cirrhosis waiting for orthotopic liver transplantation. Angiology 2010;61(8):802–6.

17. Reynaert H, Thompson MG, Thomas T, et al. Hepatic stellate cells: role in microcirculation and pathophysiology of portal hypertension. Gut 2002;50(4):571–81.

18. Gandi CR. Hepatic stellate cell activation and profibrogenic signals. J Hepatol 2017;67(5):1104–5.

19. Nikolic I, Yung LM, Yang P, et al. Bone morphogenic protein 9 is a mechanistic biomarker of portopulmonary hypertension. Am J Respir Crit Care Med 2019;199(7):891–902.

20. Rochon ER, Krowka MJ, Bartolome S, et al. BMP 9/10 in pulmonary vascular complications of liver disease. Am J Respir Crit Care Med 2020;201(12):1575–8.

21. Breitkopf-Heinlein K, Meyer C, Konig C, et al. BMP-9 interferes with liver regeneration and promotes liver fibrosis. Gut 2017;66(5):939–54.

22. DuBrock HM, del Valle KT, Krowka MJ. Mending the MELD: an in-depth review of the past, present, and future of portopulmonary hypertension MELD exception. Liver Transplant 2022. https://doi.org/10.1002/lt.26422.

23. Kawut SM, Taichman DB, Ahya VN, et al. Hemodynamics and survival of patients with portopulmonary hypertension. Liver Transpl 2005;11(9):1107–11.

24. Krowka MJ, Miller DP, Barst RJ, et al. Portopulmonary hypertension: a report from the US-based REVEAL registry. Chest 2012;141(4):906–15.

25. Salvador ML, Loaiza CAQ, Padial LR, et al. Portopulmonary hypertension: prognosis and management in the current treatment era- results from the REHAP registry. Intern Med J 2021;51(3):355–65.

26. DuBrock HM, Burger CD, Bartolome S, et al. Health disparities and treatment approaches in portopulmonary hypertension and idiopathic pulmonary arterial hypertension: an analysis of the pulmonary hypertension association registry. Pulm Circ 2021;11(3). 20458940211020913.

27. Goldberg DS, Batra S, Sahay S, et al. MELD exceptions for portopulmonary hypertension: current policy and future implementation. Am J Transpl 2014;14:2081–7.

28. Aggarwal M, Li M, Bhardwaj A, et al. Predictors of survival in portopulmonary hypertension: a 20-year experience. Eur J Gastroenterol Hepatol 2022;34(4):449–56.

29. Sahay S, Tsang Y, Flynn M, et al. Burden of pulmonary hypertension in patients with portal hypertension in the United States: a retrospective database study. Pulm Circ 2020;10(4). https://doi.org/10.1177/2045894020962917. 2045894020962917.

30. DuBrock HM, Cartin-Ceba R, Channick RN, et al. Sex differences in portopulmonary hypertension. Chest 2021;159(1):328–36.

31. Al-Naamani N, Krowka MJ, Forde KA. Estrogen signaling and portopulmonary hypertension: the pulmonary vascular complications of liver disease study (PVCLD2). Hepatology 2021;73(2):726–37.

32. Roberts KE, Fallon MB, Krowka MJ, et al. Genetic risk factors for portopulmonary hypertension in patients with advanced liver disease. Am J Respir Crit Care Med 2009;179(9):835–42.

33. Shao Y, Yin X, Qin T, et al. Prevalence and associated factors of portopulmonary hypertension in patients with portal hypertension: a case-control study. Biomed Res Int 2021;5595614. https://doi.org/10.1155/2021/5595614.

34. Sitbon O, Bosch J, Cottreel E, et al. Macitentan for the treatment of portopulmonary hypertension (PORTICO): a multicenter, randomized, double-blind,

placebo-controlled, phase 4 trial. Lancet Respir Med 2019;7(7):594–604.

35. Preston IR, Burger CD, Bartolome S, et al. Ambrisentan in portopulmonary hypertension: a multicenter, open-label trial. J Heart Lung Transpl 2020;39(5):464–72.

36. Cartin-Ceba R, Swanson K, Iyer V, et al. Safety and efficacy of ambrisentan for the treatment of portopulmonary hypertension. Chest 2011;139(1):109–14.

37. Hoeper MM, Seyfarth HJ, Hoeffken G, et al. Experience with inhaled iloprost and bosentan in portopulmonary hypertension. Eur Respir J 2007;30(6):1096–102.

38. Hoeper MM, Halank M, Marx C, et al. Bosentan therapy for portopulmonary hypertension. Eur Respir J 2005;25(3):502–8.

39. Savale L, Magnier R, Le Pavec J, et al. Efficacy, safety and pharmacokinetics of bosentan in portopulmonary hypertension. Eur Respir J 2013;41(1):96–103.

40. Rossi R, Talarico M, Schepis F, et al. Effects of sildenafil on right ventricular remodeling in portopulmonary hypertension. Pulm Pharmacol Ther 2021;70:102071. https://doi.org/10.1016/j.pupt.2021.102071.

41. Reichenberger F, Vonswinckel R, Steveling E, et al. Sildenafil treatment for portopulmonary hypertension. Eur Respir J 2006;28:563–7.

42. Fisher JH, Johnson SR, Chau C, et al. Effectiveness of phosphodiesterase-5 inhibitor therapy for portopulmonary hypertension. Can Respir J 2015;22(1):42–6.

43. Cartin-Ceba R, Halank M, Ghofrani H, et al. Riociguat treatment for portopulmonary hypertension: a subgroup analysis from the PATENT-1/-2 studies. Pulm Circ 2018;8(2). https://doi.org/10.1177/2045894018769305. 2045894018769305.

44. Kuo PC, Johnson LB, Plotkin JS, et al. Continuous intravenous infusion of epoprostenol for the treatment of portopulmonary hypertension. Transplantation 1997;63(4):604–6.

45. Krowka MJ, Frantz RP, McGoon MD, et al. Improvement in pulmonary hemodynamics during intravenous epoprostenol (prostacyclin): A study of 15 patients with moderate to severe portopulmonary hypertension. Hepatology 1999;30(3):641–8.

46. Krowka MJ, Plevak DJ, Findlay JY, et al. Pulmonary hemodynamics and perioperative cardiopulmonary-related mortality in patients with portopulmonary hypertension undergoing liver transplantation. Liver Transpl 2000;6(4):443–50.

47. Freeman RB, Gish RG, Harper A, et al. Model for end-stage liver disease (MELD) exception guidelines: results and recommendations from the MELD exception study group and conference (MESSAGE) for the approval of patients who need liver transplantation with diseases not considered by the standard MELD formula. Liver Transpl 2006;12(S3):S128–36.

48. Enhancements to the National liver review board, OPTN liver and intestinal organ transplantation committee. 2020. Available at: https://optn.transplant.hrsa.gov/. Accessed March 1 2022.

49. Salgia RJ, Goodrich NP, Simpson H, et al. Outcomes of liver transplantation for portopulmonary hypertension in model for end-stage liver disease era. Dig Dis Sci 2014;59(8):1976–82.

50. Verma S, Hand F, Armstrong MJ, et al. Portopulmonary hypertension: still an appropriate consideration for liver transplantation. Liver Transpl 2016;22(12):1637–42.

51. Cartin-Ceba R, Burger C, Swanson K, et al. Clinical outcomes after liver transplantation in patients with portopulmonary hypertension. Transplantation 2020;105(10):2283–90.

52. DuBrock HM, Runo JR, Sadd CJ, et al. Outcomes of liver transplantation in treated portopulmonary hypertension patients with a mean pulmonary arterial pressure ≥ 35mmHg. Transpl Direct 2020;6:e630. https://doi.org/10.1097/TXD.0000000000001085.

53. Jose A, Shah SA, Anwar N, et al. Pulmonary vascular resistance predicts mortality and graft failure in transplantation patients with portopulmonary hypertension. Liver Transpl 2021;27(12):1811–23.

54. Cheng C, Wang Y, Wu T, et al. Sildenafil monotherapy to treat portopulmonary hypertension before liver transplant. Transpl Proc 2019;51(5):1435–8.

55. Sussman N, Kaza V, Barshes N, et al. Successful liver transplantation following medical management of portopulmonary hypertension: a single-center series. Am J Transpl 2006;6(9):2177–82.

56. Ramsay MA, Simpson BR, Nguyen AT, et al. Severe pulmonary hypertension in liver transplant candidates. Liver Transpl Surg 1997;3(5):494–500.

57. Plotkin JS, Kuo PC, Rubin J, et al. Successful use of chronic epoprostenol as a bridge to liver transplantation in severe portopulmonary hypertension. Transplantation 1998;65(4):457–9.

58. Koneru B, Ahmed S, Weisse AB, et al. Resolution of pulmonary hypertension of cirrhosis after liver transplantation. Transplantation 1994;58(10):1133–5.

59. Hollatz TJ, Musat A, Westphal S, et al. Treatment with sildenafil and treprostinil allows successful liver transplantation of patients with moderate to severe portopulmonary hypertension. Liver Transpl 2002;18(6):686–95.

60. Savale L, Sattler C, Coilly A, et al. Long-term outcome in liver transplantation candidates with portopulmonary hypertension. Hepatology 2017;65(5):1683–92.

61. Koch DG, Caplan M, Reuben A. Pulmonary hypertension after liver transplantation: case presentation and review of the literature. Liver Transpl 2009;15(4):407–12.

62. Rafanan AL, Maurer J, Mehta AC, et al. Progressive portopulmonary hypertension after liver

transplantation treated with epoprostenol. Chest 2000;118(5):1497–500.

63. Hemnes AR, Robbins IM. Sildenafil monotherapy in portopulmonary hypertension can facilitate liver transplantation. Liver Transpl 2009;15(1):15–9.

64. DuBrock HM, Salgia RJ, Sussman NL, et al. Porto-pulmonary hypertension: a survey of practice patterns and provider attitudes. Transpl Direct 2019; 5(6):e456.

65. Kandil S. Intraoperative anesthetic management of the liver transplant recipient with portopulmonary hypertension. Curr Opin Organ Transpl 2019;24(2): 121–30.

66. Reddy K, Mallett S, Peachy T. Venovenous bypass in orthotopic liver transplantation: time for a rethink? Liver Transpl 2005;11(7):741–9.

67. Steadman RH. Anesthesia for liver transplant surgery. Anesthesiol Clin North Am 2004;22(4):687–711.

68. Paulsen AW, Whitten CW, Ramsay MA, et al. Considerations for anesthetic management during veno-venous bypass in adult hepatic transplantation. Anesth Analg 1989;68(4):489–96.

69. Rudnick MR, De Marchi L, Plotkin JS. Hemodynamic monitoring during liver transplantation: a state of the art review. World J Hepatol 2015;7(10):1302–11.

70. Ramsay M. Portopulmonary hypertension and right heart failure in patients with cirrhosis. Curr Opin Anaesthesiol 2010;23(2):145–50.

71. Ramsay MA, Spikes C, East CA, et al. The perioperative management of portopulmonary hypertension with nitric oxide and epoprostenol. Anesthesiology 1999;90(1):299–301.

Microscopic Examination of Clots from Percutaneous Mechanical Embolectomies in Pulmonary Embolism

Vruksha Upadhyay, MD[a],*, Shameek Gayen, MD[b], Amandeep Aneja, MD[c],
Maruti Kumaran, MD[d], Riyaz Bashir, MD[e], Vladimir Lakhter, DO[e],
Joseph Panaro, MD[e], Gary Cohen, MD[e], Eduardo Bossone, MD[f],
Gerard Criner, MD[b], Parth Rali, MD[b]

KEYWORDS

- Histology • Pulmonary emboli • Thrombectomy • Thrombus dating • Age of a clot

KEY POINTS

- Pulmonary embolism (PE) is a prevalent disease with varying symptoms and mortality.
- There is little evidence to explain the varying severity and mortality in patients all diagnosed with "acute" PE as noted on computed tomography.
- By analyzing histology of thrombectomy clots, clots were aged and correlated to PE clinical presentation.

INTRODUCTION

Pulmonary embolism (PE) and deep vein thrombosis (DVT) have an estimated mortality of 100,000 people every year.[1] Computed tomography pulmonary angiogram (CTPA) is the diagnostic modality of choice for PE.[2,3] CTPA characteristics help identify acute from chronic PE. Patients presenting with acute PE and similar-appearing clot burden on CTPA may have varied clinical presentation in terms of severity. Baseline cardiovascular reserve is thought to be a potential contributor to differences in clinical presentation and outcomes.[3,4] Patients with high cardiovascular reserve with significant clot burden can have minimal hemodynamic instability, whereas patients with low cardiovascular reserve but a much lower clot burden PE may present in a state of shock.

However, other factors may influence the clinical presentation of PEs, including the true age of the PE. Patients come to an acute care setting with either acute (within 24–48 hours) or delayed (>48 hours) presentation depending on symptoms and overall health status. CTPA may not be able to determine the age of the clot (except classic chronic clot). Silver and colleagues[5] performed the first study to look at the histology of DVTs and PEs to qualitatively understand the age of a clot. In their study of 7 lower-extremity DVTs and 10 PE aspirates, they determined PEs to have earlier stage of thrombus than DVTs based on histology. However, there are very few studies that have attempted to estimate a clot age. It is important to define clot age, as it can impact the efficacy of treatment and type of treatment selection,

[a] Department of Internal Medicine, Temple University Hospital, 3401 North Broad Street, Philadelphia, PA, USA; [b] Department of Thoracic Medicine and Surgery, Temple University Hospital, 3401 North Broad Street, Philadelphia, PA, USA; [c] Department of Pathology, Temple University Hospital, 3401 North Broad Street, Philadelphia, PA, USA; [d] Department of Radiology, Temple University Hospital, 3401 North Broad Street, Philadelphia, PA, USA; [e] Department of Interventional Cardiology, Temple University Hospital, 3401 North Broad Street, Philadelphia, PA, USA; [f] Division of Cardiology, Cardarelli Hospital, Via Antonio Cardarelli, 9, Napoli, Naples 80131, Italy
* Corresponding author.
E-mail address: vruksha.upadhyay@tuhs.temple.edu

Heart Failure Clin 19 (2023) 67–73
https://doi.org/10.1016/j.hfc.2022.08.014
1551-7136/23/© 2022 Elsevier Inc. All rights reserved.

particularly in focus to reperfusion therapies. Older clots are more wall-adherent and may require longer infusion times of thrombolytic therapy or mechanical thrombectomy.[5] There are few to no data currently that help quantify in days how long an "acute" clot has been forming. There are also few data to further correlate the true age of the PE with the clinical course of patients. The authors aimed to quantify an estimate age of pulmonary artery thrombus aspirates and correlate clot age to radiologic features and clinical symptoms.

METHODS
Design and Study Population

The authors performed a retrospective analysis of patients with an intermediate- to high-risk PE who underwent mechanical thrombectomy. Intermediate- to high-risk PE was defined by right ventricle (RV) strain on imaging in addition to positive cardiac biomarkers per European Society of Cardiology risk-stratification guidelines. The decision to pursue a mechanical thrombectomy versus anticoagulation alone was made by a multidisciplinary pulmonary embolism response team (PERT) consisting of pulmonology, surgery, cardiology, and radiology. Factors that determined percutaneous mechanical intervention include clinical worsening, location of clot, and significance of right ventricular strain. Each patient was started on therapeutic anticoagulation as first line of therapy. Around 10% to 15% of patients with intermediate-risk PE at the authors' institution are deemed appropriate for advance reperfusion therapies beyond anticoagulation. The authors identified patients for whom pulmonary artery thrombus aspirate from percutaneous mechanical thrombectomy was sent for histopathologic examination. Patients were identified from the PERT database collected from the electronic medical record of the authors' institution. All patients' data were collected through retrospective chart review. The authors obtained Western Institutional Review Board approval (TEMP-9448). Only deidentified patients in the data set were combined for the purpose of data collection and analysis. The authors' institution granted waiver of consent owing to the retrospective nature of the study and the associated minimal risk. Patients ≥18 years of age who underwent percutaneous mechanical thrombectomy for intermediate-risk PE and for whom thrombus aspirate was sent for histopathologic examination were included.

Study Definitions

All patients were deemed to have acute PE and were treated under guidance of the authors'

center's PERT. All PEs were classified as acute, subacute, or chronic on CTPA by a blinded radiologist who had no information of the clinical context of the patient. Baseline variables of age, gender, and comorbid conditions, including malignancy, diabetes, chronic obstructive pulmonary disease (COPD), renal failure, and prior venous thromboembolism (VTE), were collected. Clinical characteristics and outcomes, including presence of DVT, onset of symptoms, oxygen requirement, and initial and follow-up transthoracic echocardiogram (TTE) findings, and mortality were collected. The age of thromboembolism based on histologic findings, was estimated and compared with patient clinical presentation and outcomes.

Thrombectomy Tissue Specimens

The thrombectomy tissue specimens after gross examination including measurements were transferred to an appropriately labeled tissue cassette and submitted for processing. Only cases whereby PE was thought to be unprovoked, and undiagnosed malignancy was in differential were sent for histopathologic examinations. Slides from each sample were stained with hematoxylin and eosin (H&E) stain. All sections were examined by light microscopy for the presence of thrombus components, including unusual findings, such as tumor, microorganisms, foreign body, and so forth. An attempt to estimate the age of thromboembolism based on histologic findings was performed (**Table 1**).[6]

RESULTS
Demographics and Baseline Characteristics

The authors collected PE aspirates from 13 patients with intermediate- to high-risk PE who underwent thrombectomy. Eight patients were men, and 5 patients were women. The average age was 58.2 years with a range of 31 to 79 years (SD ± 15.8 years). Two patients had a history of malignancy, and 5 patients had a history of prior VTE; one such patient also had history of malignancy. Further demographic information and comorbid conditions for each patient can be found in **Table 2**.

Thrombectomy Tissue Specimens

Histologically, of the 13 specimens evaluated, 6 (46.1%) specimens showed features of early/acute changes (<7 days), including lines of Zahn and neutrophilic pyknosis. One of these showed prominent eosinophils as the inflammatory component. Thrombi with features of acute organization (5–14 days), such as degeneration of

Table 1

Histology criteria used to estimate clot age

Patient No.	Estimated Time of Clot, d	Tumor	Lines of Zahn (0–3 d)	Neutrophil Pyknosis (2–7 d)	Macrophage Swelling (2–7 d)	Beginning of Endothelial Overgrowth at Edges (2–7 d)	Adherence to Vessel Wall (2–7 d)	Adventitial Hemorrhage (2–7 d)	Hemosiderin Macrophages (5–14 d)	Surface Endothelialization (5–14 d)	Degeneration of White Cells (5–14 d)	Degeneration and Homogenization of Fibrin Strands with Hyalinization of Thrombus (5–14 d)	Fibroblasts Ingrowth (5–14 d)	Collagenization with Granulation Tissue at Periphery of Thrombus at Junction of Thrombus with Vessel (2–5 wk)
1	2–7	Negative	Absent	Absent	Absent	Absent	Indeterminate	Indeterminate	Absent	Absent	Absent	Absent	Absent	Absent
2	0–3	Negative	Present	Present	Absent	Absent	Indeterminate	Indeterminate	Absent	Absent	Absent	Absent	Absent	Absent
2	0–3	Negative	Present	Present	Absent	Absent	Indeterminate	Indeterminate	Absent	Absent	Absent	Absent	Absent	Absent
3	2–7	Negative	Absent	Present	Absent	Absent	Indeterminate	Indeterminate	Absent	Absent	Present	Absent	Absent	Absent
4	5–14	Negative	Absent	Present	Absent	Present	Indeterminate	Indeterminate	Absent	Absent	Present	Present	Absent	Absent
5	5–14	Negative	Absent	Present	Absent	Present	Indeterminate	Indeterminate	Absent	Absent	Present	Present	Absent	Absent
6	5–14	Negative	Absent	Present	Present	Present	Indeterminate	Indeterminate	Present	Present	Present	Present	Present	Absent
6	5–14	Negative	Absent	Present	Present	Absent	Indeterminate	Indeterminate	Absent	Present	Present	Absent	Present	Absent
7	5–14	Negative	Absent	Present	Present	Present	Indeterminate	Indeterminate	Absent	Absent	Present	Present	Present	Absent
8	2–7	Negative	Present	Present	Present	Absent	Indeterminate	Indeterminate	Absent	Absent	Present	Present	Absent	Absent
9	5–14	Negative	Absent	Present	Present	Absent	Indeterminate	Indeterminate	Absent	Focal	Present	Absent	Absent	Absent
10	5–14	Negative	Absent	Present	Present	Present	Present	Absent	Absent	Present	Absent	Absent	Absent	Absent
11	2–7	Negative	Absent	Present	Present	Absent	Indeterminate	Indeterminate	Absent	Absent	Present	Absent	Absent	Absent
12	5–14	Negative	Absent	Present	Present	Present	Indeterminate	Indeterminate	Present	Present	Present	Present	Present	Absent
13	0–3	Negative	Present	Present	Present	Absent	Absent	Absent	Absent	Absent	Absent	Absent	Absent	Absent

Table 2
Baseline and comorbid characteristics

Patient	Age, y	Gender	Malignancy	Diabetes	COPD	CKD or ESRD	Prior VTE
1	62	Male	0	0	1	0	0
2	70	Male	0	0	0	0	1
3	61	Female	0	0	0	0	0
4	51	Male	0	0	0	0	0
5	36	Female	0	0	0	0	0
6	31	Male	0	0	0	0	0
7	38	Male	0	0	0	0	0
8	79	Male	1	0	0	1	0
9	67	Female	0	0	0	0	0
10	78	Female	0	0	0	0	0
11	63	Male	1	0	0	0	1
12	45	Male	0	0	0	1	1
13	75	Female	0	0	0	0	1

0 = N, 1 = Y.
Abbreviations: CKD, chronic kidney disease; ESRD, end stage renal disease.

white cells, homogenization of fibrin, and surface endothelialization, were noted in 7 out of 13 (53.9%) cases (**Fig. 1**). Overlapping features in the histopathology limited a precise day estimation. All 13 specimens were negative for tumor or microorganisms.

Clinical Characteristics

Symptom onset varied between the patients and did not seem to correspond with the age of clot on histology. On CTPA, all PEs were classified as acute with no features of chronic PE. CTPA images

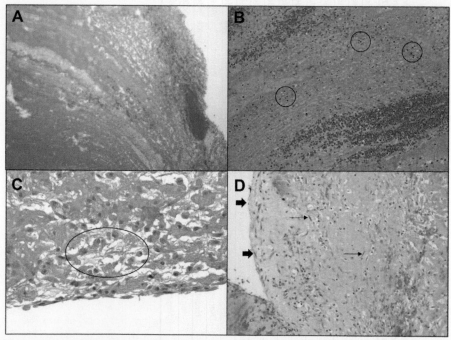

Fig. 1. Pulmonary artery thrombectomy specimens. (*A*) Lines of Zahn (0–3 days), ×200, H&E. (*B*) Thrombus with neutrophils pyknosis (*circles*) (2–4 days), ×200, H&E. (*C*) Thrombus with hemosiderin-laden macrophages with brown pigment (*highlighted*), macrophages showing swelling, degeneration of white blood cells (5–14 days), ×400, H&E. (*D*) Early fibroblast ingrowth (*arrows*) and surface endothelialization (*block arrows*) at the edge of an organizing thrombus (5–14 days), ×400, H&E.

Table 3
Clinical characteristics

Patient	Symptom Onset, d	Clot Age on CTPA	Clot Age via Histology, d	DVT Location	Initial Oxygen Requirement	Follow-Up Oxygen Requirement, L/min	Initial RV TTE Findings	Follow Upon RV TTE Findings	Survive to Discharge
1	3	Acute	2–7	3	50 L/min	5	Size: 5, function: 5	Size: 2, function: 2	1
2	1	Acute	0–3	0	100% Fio₂ via ventilator	n/a	Size: 2, function: 4	n/a	0
3	7	Acute	2–7	3	3 L/min	0	Size: 2, function: 2	Size: 2, function: 0	1
4	1	Acute	5–14	3	2 L/min	2	Size: 3, function: 4	n/a	1
5	7	Acute	5–14	3	3 L/min	0	Size: 4, function: 4	Size: 0, function: 0	1
6	7	Acute	>14	3	40% Fio₂ via ventilator	0	Size: 4, function: 6	n/a	1
7	6	Acute	>14	3	0 L/min	0	Size: 0, function: 3	Size: 0, function: 0	1
8	5	Acute	2–7	3	100% Fio₂ via CPAP	0	Size: 4, function: 5	Size: 0, function: 0	1
9	1	Acute	>14	0	5 L/min	2	Size: 2, function: 4	n/a	1
10	1	Acute	5–14	4	2 L/min	0	Size: 2, function: 2	Size: 0, function: 0	1
11	1	Acute	2–7	4	15 L/min	0	Size: 4, function: 4	n/a	1
12	7	Acute	5–14	3	4 L/min	0	Size: 5, function: 4	n/a	1
13	2	Acute	0–3	3	10 L/min	0	Size: 4, function: 4	Size: 0, function: 0	1

DVT: 0, negative; 1, unilateral above knee DVT; 2, unilateral below knee DVT; 3, unilateral entire leg; 4, B/L DVTs anywhere; RV size: 0, WNL; 1, ULN; 2, mildly dilated; 3, mildly to moderately dilated; 4, moderately dilated; 5, moderate to markedly dilated; 6, markedly dilated. n/a, not applicable; RV function: 0, WNL; 1, low normal; 2, mildly reduced; 3, mildly to moderately reduced; 4, moderately reduced; 5, moderately to markedly reduced; 6, markedly reduced.
Survive to Discharge: 0, N; 1, Y.

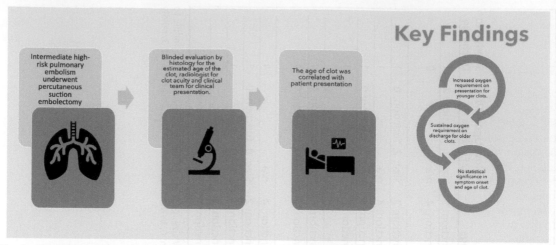

Fig. 2. Correlation of PE clinical presentation, radiology, and histology.

were reviewed independently by a chest radiologist who was not aware of histopathologic findings. Clot age via histology ranged from 0 to 3 days to greater than 14 days (**Table 3**). All 13 patients had evidence of RV strain TTE. Eleven of the 13 patients had concomitant DVT. The patients with the highest oxygen requirement (Fio$_2$ 100% via ventilator) on admission had PE less than 1 week based on histologic features compared with others. Patients with sustained oxygen requirement on discharge had PEs older than 1 week. One patient did not survive to discharge and had PE younger than 3 days on histopathology (see **Table 3**).

DISCUSSION

"Acute" PE presents with varying features, ranging from no symptoms at all to a complete hemodynamic collapse and death. If untreated, PE can have an overall mortality of up to 30%. With such variance in presentation and severity, it is important to better understand what "acute" PE consists of in order to better characterize disease course and potentially predict mortality. Review of literature shows that PE thrombectomies have previously been analyzed in autopsy studies in cases of PE fatalities, but never of survivors until most recently.[7–9] A study out of University of Rochester studied surgical thrombectomies (n = 16) from patients with PE in order to understand the morphology of a clot and correlate it to symptoms. All 16 aspirates had heterogenous morphology, and there was no correlation with symptom onset. Unlike the authors' study, they did not estimate the age of the clot. To the authors' knowledge, this is the first the study to correlate an estimated histologic age to disease presentation in cases of PE.

The authors' findings suggest that when aging PE via histology, there may be a correlation with differences in clinical presentation, outcomes, and potential treatment response (ie, need for oxygen support on discharge). In this cohort, treatment options focused predominately on thrombectomies. While awaiting thrombectomies, the patients were on anticoagulation, but for a mean of 50 hours. There may have been an effect of anticoagulation on the histology, but it would be minimal and would be uniform across all aspirates. Acute PEs, as categorized via CTPA, varied in their histologic age from 0 days to greater than 14 days. The authors' cohort demonstrated increased oxygen requirement on presentation for younger clots (<7 days). The only mortality in the case was also in a younger clot, specifically aged at less than 3 days. Right ventricular strain was seen in all 13 cases. Older clots were associated with sustained oxygen requirement despite treatment intervention. This may be related to vascularity changes, including tissue stiffness that occurs in older clots.[5] Onset of symptoms was not correlated to age of the clot; patients with clot age greater than >14 days based on histology often presented with 1 to 2 days of symptom onset, and these findings suggest the silent nature of the disease before symptoms onset. The authors' findings highlight a possible explanation for varying clinical presentations of "acute" PE. It also highlights the importance of recognizing that an "acute" PE can be as old as greater than 14 days in age or as young as less than 1 day old, which in turn could explain varying clinical presentations of similarly classified PEs.

Limitations of this study include its retrospective nature as well as its small sample size. As such, it is difficult to make strong connections between the histopathologic age of PE and the clinical severity of the PE (**Fig. 2**).

SUMMARY

"Acute" PEs, as determined via imaging, can have varying clinical presentations, despite similar classifications. The histopathologic age of thrombus can be a potential explanation for the varied presentation of acute PE, as seen in the authors' study. The authors found that patients with "younger" PE determined via histopathology tended to have more severe clinical presentations, whereas those with "older" PE determined via histopathology tended to require long-term oxygen therapy. This is most likely secondary to vascular stiffness that develops in older clots. Distinguishing young clots from older clots can change management as well. The authors' cohort showed minimal improvement on immediate need for oxygen requirement after percutaneous thrombectomies for older clots, but sharp improvement in the younger clots. Further studies are required to elucidate a potential correlation between thromboembolism histopathologic age and PE clinical presentation and severity.

CLINICS CARE POINTS

- It is important to note that different acute pulmonary emboli have different clinical presentations.
- An explanation for this may be found in the histopathology of clots, which can determine the true age of the clot.
- Although it is unclear if these findings can guide real-time management of patients with pulmonary embolism, they can serve to better understand the varying clinical presentation and severity of an "acute" pulmonary embolism.

DISCLOSURE

The authors have no conflicts of interest to disclose. This article has no relevant disclosures

in the form of grants, gifts, or other forms of financial support. The authors have no relationships with industry in relationship to any of the contents in the article.

REFERENCES

1. Beckman MG, Hooper WC, Critchley SE, et al. Venous thromboembolism: a public health concern. Am J Prev Med 2010;38(4 Suppl):S495–501. PMID: 20331949.

2. Konstantinides SV, Meyer G, Becattini C, et al. 2019 ESC Guidelines for the diagnosis and management of acute pulmonary embolism developed in collaboration with the European Respiratory Society (ERS). Eur Heart J 2020;41(4):543–603.

3. Demelo-Rodriguez P, Galeano-Valle F, Salzano A, et al. Pulmonary embolism: a practical guide for the busy clinician. Heart Fail Clin 2020;16(3):317–30.

4. Bělohlávek J, Dytrych V, Linhart A, et al. Pulmonary embolism, part I: Epidemiology, risk factors and risk stratification, pathophysiology, clinical presentation, diagnosis and nonthrombotic pulmonary embolism. Exp Clin Cardiol 2013;18(2):129–38.

5. Silver MJ, Kawakami R, Jolly MA, et al. Histopathologic analysis of extracted thrombi from deep venous thrombosis and pulmonary embolism: Mechanisms and timing. Catheter Cardiovasc Interv 2021;97(7): 1422–9. Epub 2021 Feb 1. PMID: 33522027.

6. Burke AP, Aubry M-C, Maleszewski JJ, et al. Pulmonary Embolism and Infarction. Practical Thoracic Pathology: Diseases of the Lung, Heart, and Thymus. 65; 300-309 Lippincott Williams & Wilkins.

7. Mansueto G, Costa D, Capasso E, et al. The dating of thrombus organization in cases of pulmonary embolism: an autopsy study. BMC Cardiovasc Disord 2019;19:250.

8. Ruppert ADP, de Matos Soeiro A, de Almeida MCF, et al. Clinical manifestations and pulmonary histopathological analysis related to different diseases in patients with fatal pulmonary thromboembolism: an autopsy study. Open Access Emergency Medicine: OAEM 2014;6:15–21.

9. Newcomb G, Wilson BL, White RJ, et al. An untapped resource: characteristics of thrombus recovered from intermediate or high risk pulmonary embolus patients. Cardiovasc Pathol 2022;57:107392.

Pregnancy and Pulmonary Hypertension
From Preconception and Risk Stratification Through Pregnancy and Postpartum

Jenny Y. Mei, MD[a], Richard N. Channick, MD[b],*, Yalda Afshar, MD, PhD[a],*

KEYWORDS

• Pregnancy • Pulmonary hypertension • Maternal co-morbidities • Heart failure

KEY POINTS

• Pulmonary hypertension carries significant morbidity and mortality in pregnancy.
• Patients in this high-risk cohort necessitate preconception risk-stratification, multidisciplinary care throughout their pregnancy and coordinated delivery planning.
• Optimal delivery planning and close postpartum monitoring are the key to minimize cardiopulmonary morbidity and mortality in pulmonary hypertension patients.

INTRODUCTION

Pulmonary hypertension (PH) is one of the highest risk medical conditions in pregnancy. Mortality due to PH has been increasing in the United States (5.5/100,000 in 2001 to 6.5/100,000 in 2010) and especially among women[1] (**Fig. 1**). The rate of hospitalizations for PH has also increased by 57% over this time period, with women accounting for 63% of hospitalizations.[2] PH can initially manifest as nonspecific symptoms such as dyspnea on exertion and fatigue.[1] Disease progression and increasing pulmonary pressures can lead to right ventricular (RV) failure, which leads to more pronounced symptoms such as chest pain, syncope on exertion, peripheral edema, and right upper quadrant pain and anorexia due to hepatic congestion.[1]

In pregnant people without a previous diagnosis, the diagnosis is commonly delayed due to the nonspecific nature of early symptoms; only 24% of PH due to congenital heart disease is diagnosed during pregnancy.[3] Further contributing to the delay or non-diagnosis of PH in pregnancy is that, even in healthy pregnant women, some degree of dyspnea, fatigue, and lower extremity edema are quite common. PH during pregnancy has high morbidity and mortality, with associated mortality rates as high as 25% to 56%.[3,4]

Pregnancy-related complications are due to cardiac inability to accommodate increased plasma volume and cardiac output, decreased systemic vascular resistance (SVR), and hypercoagulability in pregnancy.[1]

As a result, the World Health Organization (WHO) classifies pulmonary arterial hypertension (PAH) from any cause as class IV heart disease, wherein pregnancy is contraindicated.[5] However, the incidence of pregnancies complicated by PH is on the rise in the United States.[6] Apart from the associated maternal morbidity and mortality, the associated obstetric complications include fetal growth restriction, preterm birth, and fetal loss.[3,4]

PRECONCEPTION COUNSELING

Preconception care and counseling is primary prevention and an integral first step toward a healthy pregnancy. The goal of preconception counseling

[a] Division of Maternal-Fetal Medicine, Department of Obstetrics and Gynecology, University of California, Los Angeles, 200 Medical Plaza Suite 430, Los Angeles, CA, USA; [b] Division of Pulmonology, University of California, Los Angeles, 200 Medical Plaza Suite 365, Los Angeles, CA, USA
* Corresponding authors.
E-mail addresses: RChannick@mednet.ucla.edu (R.N.C.); YAfshar@mednet.ucla.edu (Y.A.)

Heart Failure Clin 19 (2023) 75–87
https://doi.org/10.1016/j.hfc.2022.08.019
1551-7136/23/© 2022 Elsevier Inc. All rights reserved.

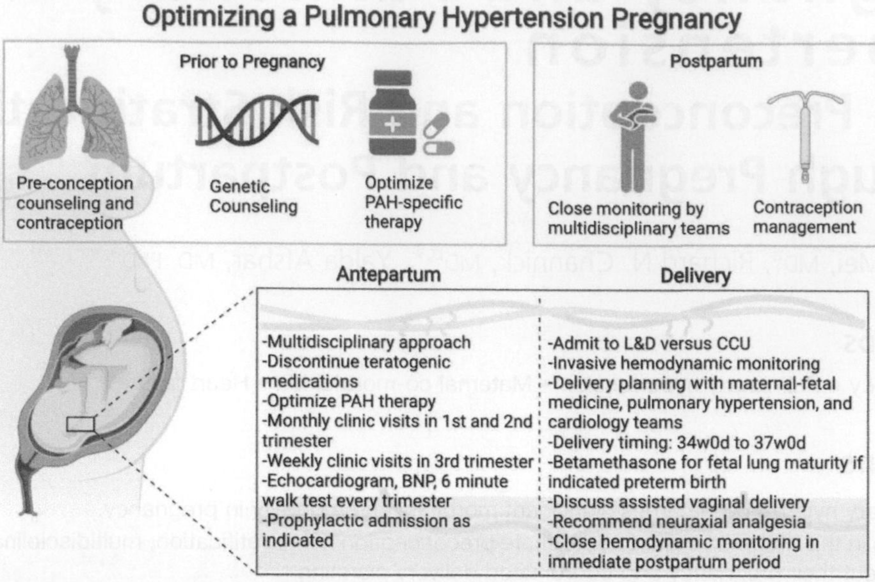

Fig. 1. Pulmonary hypertension in pregnancy. The optimal approach to having a successful pregnancy with pulmonary hypertension starts before to pregnancy, involves multidisciplinary management during the antepartum period, close monitoring and involved decision-making for delivery planning, and close outpatient follow-up in the postpartum period. PAH, pulmonary arterial hypertension; BNP, brain natriuretic peptide; L&D, labor and delivery; CCU, cardiac care unit.

is the reduction of potential harm and the recognition of modifiable risk factors related to pregnancy. More so, preconception counseling stratifies pregnancies on a continuum of low to high risk and women with PH qualify as high risk. The early initiation of care relies on counseling about potential pregnancy risks and preventative strategies that are provided before conception. Preconception care should be incorporated into any visit with a reproductive age woman, as nearly half of all pregnancies in the United States are unplanned.[7] The challenge of preconception care lies in addressing pregnancy planning for women who seek any medical care and to screen and educate all reproductively capable women on an ongoing basis to identify potential maternal and fetal risks and hazards to pregnancy before and between pregnancies. This counseling should be done concomitantly by PH and maternal fetal medicine (cardio-obstetrics) teams comfortable with PH.

Counseling about options for in vitro fertilization (IVF) and gestational carriers is a potential way for patients to avoid pregnancy, though the cost is prohibitive to many. Patients would also need to consider anesthesia risk for oocyte retrieval, though this risk is overall minimal. Overall, proper preconception counseling including risk stratification and optimization of medical illnesses is vital to a healthy and safe pregnancy in this high-risk population.

Pulmonary Hypertension Diagnosis

If symptoms and physical examination raise concern for PH, echocardiography is typically the next test performed.

Echocardiography can provide an estimate pulmonary artery systolic pressure indirectly by assessing velocity of the tricuspid regurgitant jet (which increases as pulmonary resistance increases) and estimating central venous pressure (CVP) as a surrogate for right atrial pressure (which increases in PH).[8] An estimation of the CVP involves assessing the size and compressibility of the inferior vena cava.

If the likelihood of PH is intermediate or high based on these measurements, confirmation with right heart catheterization is required.

The accepted hemodynamic definition of PH is a mean pulmonary arterial pressure, measured by right heart catheterization, of at least 20 mm Hg, as it represents 2 standard deviations above the normal mean pulmonary artery pressure of 14 ± 3.3 mm Hg.[9] In addition, a pulmonary capillary wedge pressure less than 16 mm Hg and a pulmonary vascular resistance of greater than 3 Wood units defines precapillary PH.

Owing to the physiologic changes of pregnancy, the accuracy of PH detection via transthoracic echocardiography in pregnancy is unclear. In pregnancy, despite the increase in blood volume, pulmonary vascular resistance decreases, and the mean pulmonary artery pressure should be less than 25 mm Hg.[10] However, pregnant patients have increased circulating volumes 40% to 50% above the nonpregnant state, and thus, their CVP and corresponding right atrial pressures may be overestimated on echocardiography.[8]

In the limited literature comparing echocardiographic assessments of PH with right heart catheterization in pregnant patients, case series have suggested overestimation of pulmonary artery pressure and RV systolic pressure on transthoracic echocardiography as compared with catheterization.[11,12] Thus, echocardiography can be considered a screening test, and confirmation with right heart catheterization should not be delayed in pregnancy.

A recent analysis of the US National Inpatient Sample and delivery records included 1,519 pregnant people with PH with birth hospitalizations.[6] Of this cohort, 59.6% had isolated PH, of whom 5.8% had idiopathic PH and 3% had coexisting Eisenmenger syndrome. The remaining 40.3% had underlying cardiac disease, most frequently valvular heart disease. Of note, chronic thromboembolic disease was identified in 87.9% of all patients and 85.1% of isolated PH patients (**Fig. 2**).

Physiologic Changes of Pregnancy

The cardiovascular system undergoes major hemodynamic and structural changes over the course of pregnancy to sustain a high-volume load.[13] Pregnancy is thus considered a natural stress test and can have profound impacts on patients with underlying cardiopulmonary disease.

Hemodynamic Changes

Antepartum

Throughout pregnancy, there is a continuous increase in cardiac output and plasma volume and decrease in maternal SVR.[14] Plasma volume increases to 150% normal levels, which can significantly impact patients with underlying cardiopulmonary disease, which starts as early as 6 weeks of gestation, even before most women realize they are pregnant. These levels peak at the onset of third trimester around 28 weeks of gestation. This is due to increases in estrogen and progesterone, along with activation of the renin–angiotensin–aldosterone system.

Blood pressure nadirs in the second trimester and then steadily increases over the third trimester.[15] Uterine mechanical compression of the inferior vena cava can reduce venous return to the right ventricle and portend postural hypotensive syndrome.[16]

Intrapartum and postpartum

Significant hemodynamic changes occur during labor and birth, with significant increases in cardiac output, heart rate, blood pressure, and plasma volume.[17] Immediately after the birth of the neonate and placenta, plasma volume increases by 500 mL quickly due to autotransfusion.[17] Cardiac output increases up to 80% immediately and then decreases within the first hour after delivery.

Patients with cardiovascular disease, including PH, are particularly susceptible to pulmonary edema with increased hydrostatic pressure and decreased colloid osmotic pressure during this time. Heart rate and blood pressure normally decrease in the first 48 hours postpartum, though they may rise between days 3 and 6 postpartum in the setting of fluid shifts, portending patients with hypertensive comorbidities to worsening disease and fluid overload.[18]

Natural postpartum diuresis occurs with increasing plasma atrial natriuretic peptide levels in the first week.[19] Overall hemodynamics return to a prepregnancy state 3 to 6 months postpartum. Of note, even an early miscarriage or termination still undergoes the hemodynamic shifts for the pregnant person.

Structural changes

The heart structurally adapts to the plasma volume increase during pregnancy as well.

The left ventricular mass increases by 50%, and RV mass by 40%.[20] Ejection fractions can vary among patients, although up to 20% of women have diastolic dysfunction at term, manifesting as dyspnea on exertion.[21] Structural cardiac changes should return to baseline by 1 year postpartum.

It can be difficult to distinguish cardiopulmonary complications from physiologic dyspnea in pregnancy. A recent algorithm established by the California Maternal Quality Care Collaborative (CMQCC) Cardiovascular Disease in Pregnancy and Postpartum Task Force identified certain severe symptoms and vital sign abnormalities labeled as "Red Flags" concerning for cardiovascular disease.[22] These included shortness of breath at rest, severe orthopnea necessitating four or more pillows, resting heart rate ≥120 beats per minute, resting systolic blood pressure ≥160 mm Hg, resting respiratory rate of ≥30 breaths per minute, and an oxygen saturation ≤94%. The presence of any of these "Red Flags" especially in the setting of known cardiovascular or pulmonary disease should prompt further workup and evaluation by maternal fetal medicine and medical subspecialties.

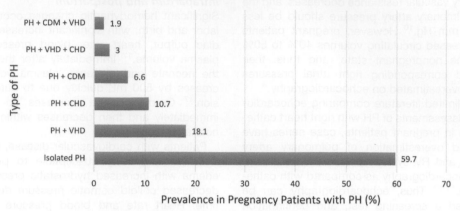

Fig. 2. Distribution of pulmonary hypertension subclasses in pregnancy. Breakdown of subclasses among the total 1519 patients with pulmonary hypertension as published by Thomas and colleagues. Most of the cases are isolated PH, followed by PH in the setting of valvular heart disease and congenital heart disease, respectively. Less commonly, patients have PH in the setting of cardiomyopathy or a combination of multiple cardiac comorbidities. CDM, cardiomyopathy; CHD, congenital heart disease; PH, pulmonary hypertension; VHD, valvular heart disease. (*Adapted from* Thomas E, Yang J, Xu J, Lima FV, Stergiopoulos K. Pulmonary Hypertension and Pregnancy Outcomes: Insights From the National Inpatient Sample. J Am Heart Assoc. 2017;6(10):e006144. Published 2017 Oct 24.)

Hematologic and coagulation changes

Although there is an increase in red blood cell mass by 20% to 30% in pregnancy, this change is proportionally lower than the notable 40% to 50% increase in plasma volume, creating a physiologic anemia due to hemodilution **Fig. 3**.

The risk of thromboembolism is also significantly increased in pregnancy as a result of physiologic and structural changes, including hypercoagulability, venous stasis, decreased venous outflow, and compression of the inferior vena cava and pelvic veins from the gravid uterus.[23] Altered levels of coagulation factors amplify the thrombogenic state, further increasing risk of thromboembolism.[23]

Prognosis

The majority of knowledge on morbidity and mortality in pregnant patients with PH is derived from case series or registries. Recent data from the US National Inpatient Sample reported PH affected 0.02% of pregnancy admissions, out of 6,759,101 patients.[6]

Not surprisingly, compared with women without heart disease or PH, women with PH experienced significantly higher cardiopulmonary morbidity (24.8 vs 0.4%). Up to 62% of PH patients had one or more major adverse cardiac events during pregnancy, primary heart failure and arrhythmias in women with combined PH, cardiomyopathy, and valvular heart disease. Women with PH also had significantly higher risk for preterm delivery and intrauterine fetal demise.

A recent retrospective review of 49 women with PH across four academic institutions found a mortality rate of 16% (8/49), with all deaths occurring postpartum.[24] Seven of eight deaths occurred in women with WHO group 1 PH, with an overall mortality rate of 23% (7/30) in this cohort. Of note, more than 50% of the women required advanced therapies including inotropic support, pulmonary vasodilators, nitric oxide, or extracorporeal membrane oxygenation (ECMO). Those with severe or group 1 PH or Eisenmenger syndrome carried the highest risk of mortality and preterm birth.

More recent data, including a systematic review of pregnancy cohorts between 2008 and 2018, showed a slightly low mortality rate of 12% overall, though higher for idiopathic PAH (20%).[25] Most of the patients (74%) had good functional class (NYHA I/II), and the majority (68%) had underlying congenital heart disease as the etiology. Causes of death included right heart failure, cardiac arrest, PH crisis, preeclampsia, and sepsis; 61% of maternal deaths occurred within 4 days postpartum.

Given these substantial risks for major morbidity and mortality, patients should be strongly advised against pregnancy, or even consider pregnancy termination in certain circumstances. Contraception and family planning are important topics that do not consistently occur.[26] A multidisciplinary team consisting of maternal–fetal medicine, pulmonology, cardiology, and obstetrician gynecologists is vital to taking care of these tenuous patients.

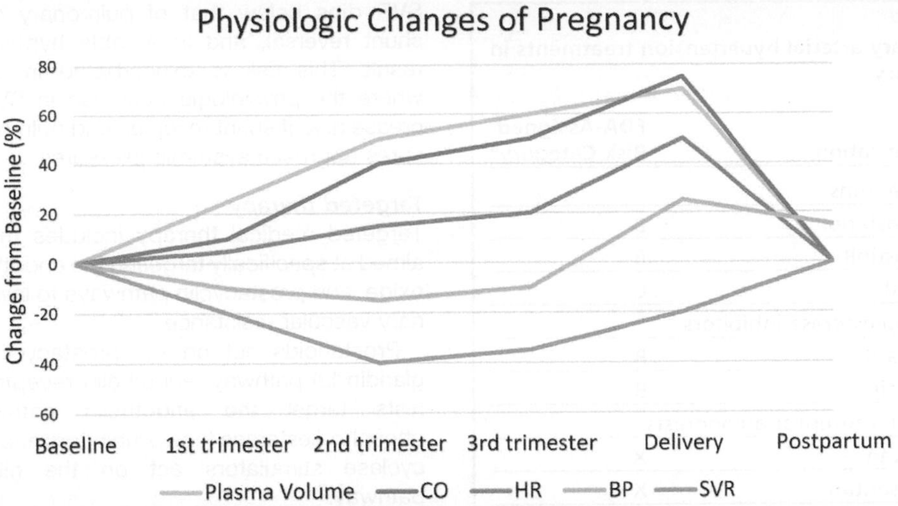

Fig. 3. Physiologic changes of pregnancy. Physiologic hemodynamic and cardiovascular changes over the course of pregnancy. Cardiac output steadily increases over the course of pregnancy, peaks at delivery, and slowly returns to baseline 3 to 6 weeks postpartum. Heart rate slowly increases over pregnancy and also peaks at delivery. Blood pressure nadirs in the second trimester peaks at delivery and returns to baseline 3 to 6 weeks postpartum. Plasma volume increases 150% over the course of pregnancy and can result in anemia due to hemodilution. Systemic vascular resistance nadirs in the second trimester and slowly returns to baseline postpartum. CO, cardiac output; HR, heart rate; BP, blood pressure; SVR, systemic vascular resistance. (*Data from* American College of Obstetricians and Gynecologists' Presidential Task Force on Pregnancy and Heart Disease and Committee on Practice Bulletins—Obstetrics. ACOG Practice Bulletin No. 212: Pregnancy and Heart Disease. Obstet Gynecol. 2019;133(5):e320-e356.)

Pulmonary Hypertension Management

Treatment overview

Treatment of PAH is based on clinical presentation, etiology, severity, and disease response to therapy (**Table 1**).

PH treatment consists of supportive measures and medical therapy.[27] Supportive measures include supervised exercise guidance, preventive care (including immunizations against influenza and pneumococcus), social support, and counseling on avoiding excessive physical activity that can exacerbate symptoms.

For patients with PH due to left heart or lung disease, treatment is aimed at targeting the underlying cause.

For patients with PAH (Group 1), in addition to supportive therapies such as oxygen, if needed, and diuretics, treatment is directly targeted. These patients are managed in centers of expertise for PH.

Medical Therapies: Considerations in Pregnancy

Anticoagulation

Endothelial cell activation in idiopathic PAH increases thrombosis risk, specifically microscopic thrombotic lesions in the pulmonary vasculature.[28] Thromboembolic events in the pulmonary vasculature leads to increased pulmonary pressure, which can worsen right heart function and precipitate cardiac morbidity and mortality. The European Society of Cardiology Guidelines recommend anticoagulation for patients with idiopathic PAH.[8]

In pregnancy, anticoagulation should be continued for patients who have a preexisting indication for anticoagulation. Prophylactic anticoagulation can be considered for those not previously on anticoagulation. Warfarin should be avoided if possible given teratogenicity, and low-molecular-weight heparin should be used in its place.[29]

Direct oral anticoagulants (DOACs), including direct thrombin inhibitors and factor Xa inhibitors, are also considered contraindicated in pregnancy.

Supplemental oxygen

Hypoxemia can lead to pulmonary vascular vasoconstriction, and thus supplemental oxygen should be administered to maintain oxygen saturation above 90% in nonpregnant patient.[1] There is limited data on goal oxygen saturation in pregnancy. Higher altitude can also worsen vasoconstriction related to hypoxemia and thus should also be avoided.

Diuretics

Diuretics are a mainstay of therapy in PAH to decrease RV preload and improve renal function.

Table 1
Pulmonary arterial hypertension treatments in pregnancy

PAH Medication	FDA-Assigned Risk Category[a]
Prostaglandins	
Epoprostenol	B
Treprostinil	B
Iloprost	C
Phosphodiesterase inhibitors	
Sildenafil	B
Tadalafil	B
Endothelin receptor antagonists	
Bosentan	X
Ambrisentan	X
Macitentan	X
Soluble guanylate cyclase stimulators	
Riociguat	X
Others	
Nitric oxide	C
Enoxaparin	B
Heparin	C
Calcium channel blockers	C
Furosemide	C

Table of most commonly used PAH treatments and their respective FDA-assigned risk categories.

Abbreviations: FDA, US Food and Drug Administration; PAH, pulmonary arterial hypertension.

[a] FDA pregnancy categories. B: no well-controlled studies have been conducted in humans; animal studies show no risk to the fetus; C: no well-controlled studies have been conducted in humans; animal studies have demonstrated an adverse effect on the fetus; X: controlled studies in animals or humans demonstrate fetal abnormalities; the risk in pregnant women outweighs possible benefit.

Maintaining euvolemia is especially important in the pregnant PAH patient, given the volume expansion that occurs in the second and third trimesters.

Calcium channel blockers

A small percentage of patients with PAH, in response to acute vasodilator testing, will demonstrate significant pulmonary vasoreactivity. These patients have been shown to benefit from calcium channel blockers.

However, in the vast majority of patients who are not vasoreactive, calcium blockers should be avoided. These agents are nonselective vasodilators and thus will also lower SVR, which may lead to severe hypotension.

In addition, in patients with intracardiac shunts (such as ventricular or atrial septal defects), if the SVR dips below that of pulmonary circulation, shunt reversal, and intractable hypoxemia may result. This risk is exacerbated in pregnancy, where the physiologic decrease in SVR can increase risk of shunt reversal, and pulmonary pressures approach systemic pressures.

Targeted therapy

Targeted medical therapy includes medications aimed at specifically targeting the endothelin, nitric oxide, and prostacyclin pathways to lower pulmonary vascular resistance.

Prostanoids act on the prostacyclin (prostaglandin I2) pathway, endothelin receptor antagonists target the endothelin pathway, and phosphodiesterase type 5 inhibitors and guanylate cyclase stimulators act on the nitric oxide pathway.[30]

There are no current guidelines for standard targeted therapy in pregnancy, though cases have been described.[24,31,32] Prostaglandins have no known teratogenic effect, however, have not been extensively studied in humans. When its use is necessary, its benefits to the mother are deemed to outweigh any potential risk to the fetus.[33]

Phosphodiesterase type-5 inhibitors have been used in pregnancies either alone or in combination with prostaglandins.[29]

Endothelin receptor antagonists and soluble guanylate cyclase stimulators should be avoided due to teratogenicity concerns.

A case series of six postpartum women with severe PH also unfortunately ended with maternal mortality for all six within several months.[24]

Ultimately, decompensating patients should be evaluated for lung transplant, especially if they are New York Heart Association class III to IV on maximal medical therapy, declining exercise scores, failing epoprostenol, have heart failure with cardiac index less than 2 L/min/m^2, and have elevated right atrial pressure 15 mm Hg or above.[8]

PREGNANCY OUTCOMES
Individualized Counseling

Pregnant patients with PAH require individualized counseling and multidisciplinary collaboration at the centers of expertise in PH, ideally with access to ECMO and transplant teams.[5,34,35]

Following a pregnancy, planned or unplanned, rediscussion of pregnancy intention and risk stratification must be initiated, including consideration of termination for maternal benefit.[5,8] If termination of pregnancy occurs, it should occur in a center with advanced cardiopulmonary support measures including ECMO and transplant as consideration for obstetric and cardiac anesthesia is important.

Antenatal Management

Physiologic changes of pregnancy can worsen cardiac and pulmonary status and predispose morbidity and mortality for patients with PH. These changes begin in the first trimester but markedly increase in the second and third trimester. The overall goals during pregnancy and postpartum are maintaining circulatory volume and avoiding systemic hypotension, hypoxemia, and acidosis.[5]

Over half of the pregnant patients with PH in the Registry of Pregnancy and Cardiac Disease were admitted to the hospital at some point in their pregnancy, with cardiac indications (specifically heart failure) being the most common indication for admission.[36] Over one-third of the patients required more than one admission, with the mean gestational age at admission being 27 weeks (1st–3rd quartile 19.6–35.1 weeks).

In the first trimester, the patient's baseline cardiopulmonary status should be evaluated carefully. The patient should be extensively counseled on consideration of termination of pregnancy as an option in light of high associated morbidity and mortality.

Targeted medication therapy should be generally continued, aside from ones that are potentially teratogenic, such as endothelin antagonists and soluble guanylate cyclase stimulators. Calcium channel blockers should be continued if the patient had a positive vasoreactivity test response. A multinational, prospective registry examining contemporary outcomes of pregnancies with PAH found improved pregnancy outcomes in long-term responders to calcium channel blockers.[37]

In the second trimester, increased volume expansion and cardiac output occur simultaneously with systemic and pulmonary vasodilation. These physiologic changes can lead to RV overload and predispose patients to heart failure or decompensation.

The beginning of the third trimester marks the point of maximal physiologic change until labor and delivery, thus necessitating frequent assessments throughout. It is recommended that patients have frequent assessments with maternal-fetal medicine and PH specialists throughout pregnancy, up to every 1 to 2 weeks in the second and third trimester.[1] Patients will need regular echocardiograms, B-type natriuretic peptide testing, and 6-min walk testing to monitor cardiopulmonary status.[37]

Inpatient admission is recommended if heart failure develops, with consideration for right heart catheterization. Some patients may warrant elective inpatient hospitalization for closer monitoring before symptom develops in more severe cases.[38]

Intrapartum Management

PH patients are especially at risk for RV decompensation during labor and delivery. In the setting of pain, anxiety, and catecholamine increase, there is a significant increase in cardiac output and oxygen consumption.

Furthermore, significant Valsalva can decrease venous return, which can precipitate hypotension and prevent the necessary right heart filling to overcome increased pulmonary resistance. In the immediate postpartum period, a significant increase in venous return can precipitate ventricular overload, heart failure, and even death.

On admission, IV prostacyclins should be initiated as appropriate. In addition to noninvasive cardiac and pulmonary monitoring in the form of telemetry and pulse oximetry, invasive monitoring should be considered, such as a central venous catheter to monitor RV preload. This may necessitate intensive care unit admission or labor and delivery depending on hospital policy and resources. This may be particularly important for patients with severe PH, group 1 PAH, or Eisenmenger syndrome.

Arterial lines should be considered for blood pressure monitoring for waveform contour assessment to monitor cardiac output.[39] While less commonly used, pulmonary artery catheters can play a role in assessing pulmonary artery pressure and pulmonary vascular resistance.[24,37,40]

Of note, the immediate postpartum period portends the greatest risk for decompensation, morbidity, and mortality, and thus any intensive monitoring should be continued through that period.

Anesthesia

Adequate intrapartum analgesia is essential in minimizing fluctuations in cardiac output for patients with PH as the goal of sympathetic blockade. Although the use of general anesthesia has successfully described in pregnant patients with PAH, some studies have found an increased risk for maternal mortality in women receiving general anesthesia compared with neuraxial.[3,24,37,40]

Endotracheal intubation and mechanical ventilation should be avoided, if possible, given that positive pressure ventilation increases intrathoracic and pulmonary artery pressure, subsequently decreasing venous return.

Table 2
Considerations in a delivery plan for pulmonary hypertension patients

Timing	Intervention
Antepartum	Indicate WHO, CARPREG, ZAHARA risk stratification as appropriate
	Indicate potential cardiopulmonary risks for the patient: atrial arrhythmia, ventricular arrhythmia, heart failure, volume overload
Admission	Notify appropriate subspecialty teams
	Establish continuous telemetry and pulse oximetry
	Evaluate need for cardiac or ICU nurse
	Establish invasive hemodynamic monitoring: pulmonary artery catheter, CVP line, arterial line
	Place compression socks or sequential compression devices
	Place bubble or particle filters as appropriate
	Obtain baseline EKG
	Obtain baseline laboratories: CBC, CMP, magnesium, BNP, PT/INR
	Set electrolyte repletion goals
	Recommend epidural placement from cardiopulmonary perspective
	Establish contingency plans in case of cardiopulmonary complications
Peripartum Management	Maintain strict ins and outs and make sure that they are recorded
	Start IV prostacyclin and inhaled vasodilators
	Avoid IV fluids if possible:
	If needed for fetal resuscitation, use 0.5 mL/kg/h maintenance fluids after NPO > 6 h
	Limit IVF boluses to 250 cc except if resuscitating for significant blood loss
	Use diuretics as needed to maintain CVP <10 mm Hg
	Avoid:
	Ergometrine and sulprostone—contraindicated in cardiac disease
	Carboprost—Contra-indicated in pulmonary edema, cyanotic heart disease, and pulmonary hypertension
	Use with caution:
	Pitocin—caution with fluid retention over long period of infusion
	Terbutaline—caution with cardiac arrhythmia risk
	Methylergonovine—caution in patients with hypertensive or cardiac disease
	If need for infective endocarditis prophylaxis:
	Ampicillin 2 g IV OR Cefazolin or ceftriaxone 1 g IV, 30–60 min before anticipated delivery
	If PCN allergy: clindamycin 600 mg IV, 30–60 min before anticipated delivery
	ECMO team on standby with the consideration of ECMO sheaths placed at start of induction
Delivery Management	Establish if any obstetric or cardiac indications for cesarean birth
	Establish if patient may push without any limitations (outside of obstetric indications) during second stage of labor
	Establish if patient should minimize pushing during second stage of labor; if so, consider laboring down, offering operative delivery
	Notify anesthesia, nursing, multidisciplinary teams if patient is going for cesarean birth
	Recognize 500 mL autotransfusion in the immediate postpartum setting

(continued on next page)

Table 2 (continued)	
Timing	**Intervention**
Recovery/Postpartum	Continue strict fluid management Establish if postpartum recovery vs CCU for monitoring Establish if echocardiogram is needed before discharge Obtain postpartum laboratories: CBC, BMP, magnesium with appropriate repletion; repeat BNP
Discharge Planning	Coordinate outpatient follow-up with subspecialty teams Finalize contraception plan

Abbreviations: BNP, brain natriuretic peptide; CBC, complete blood count; CCU, cardiac care unit; CMP, comprehensive metabolic panel; EKG, electrocardiogram; ICU, intensive care unit; NPO, nothing by mouth; PCN, penicillin; PT/INR, prothrombin time/international normalized ratio.
Consider making final delivery planning recommendations with multidisciplinary team of maternal–fetal medicine, pulmonary hypertension, and cardiology.

Neuraxial anesthesia, on the other hand, can adequately provide pain control without increasing intrathoracic pressure. Epidural or combined low-dose spinal–epidural anesthesia is preferred over spinal to help maintain venous return and avoid hypotension.[24,31,32]

Patients with Eisenmenger's physiology are particularly sensitive to changes in SVR, as decrease in SVR below pulmonary circulation can worsen right-to-left shunting, leading to worsening hypoxia and death. Although both general and neuraxial anesthesia can decrease SVR and increase mortality risks, neuraxial analgesia administered in a controlled fashion can minimize such fluctuations.[41]

Timing and Mode of Delivery

Planned delivery timing should be considered for pregnant patients with PH to use appropriate resource and personnel availability, controlling location of delivery, and timing of birth before maternal decompensation (**Table 2**).

Some studies have advocated for scheduled deliveries in the late preterm period, between 34 and 36 weeks of gestation.[29,42] Indeed prematurity rates, both spontaneous and indicated, range from 22% to 78% in the setting of maternal PH.[6,24,36,37,42]

The ECMO team should be consulted and on standby in all deliveries and timing and location should be optimized as appropriate, even if the birthing person must labor and deliver in the ICU, as appropriate.

The recommended mode of birth is controversial, as there are notable risks with both physiologic stress of labor and surgical procedures. Nevertheless, in our opinion, no strong evidence to date demonstrates that a cesarean birth is more beneficial than an assisted vaginal birth

(forceps or vacuum-assisted vaginal birth). As such, we routinely offer assisted vaginal birth for our pregnant patients with PH, outside of the routine obstetric indications for cesarean birth.

The second stage of labor (after the women's cervix is completed dilated and "pushing" begins) elicits Valsalva maneuver, which increases intrathoracic and abdominal pressure, thereby decreasing venous return. PH patients rely on adequate preload to maintain cardiac output; thus, Valsalva can quickly drop preload and lead to cardiopulmonary collapse.

The physiologic stress of labor also increases the level of catecholamines and sympathetic tone, increases heart rate and oxygen consumption, and can constrict the pulmonary vasculature.

Adequate neuraxial analgesia is imperative to minimize these effects, and in our center, we discuss neuraxial analgesia as a prerequisite to a vaginal birth. Operative vaginal birth, namely forceps-assisted or vacuum-assisted vaginal birth, can be used to avoid or minimize Valsalva and also shorten the second stage of labor.

In the Registry of Pregnancy and Cardiac Disease, 63% of patients with PH underwent a cesarean birth, with 90% of those cases planned for cardiac indications, but what is unclear is what the true cardiac indication, other than PH was in these cases.[36]

In a recent series of patients with PH who delivered, mortality rates were higher in the cesarean birth group (18%) compared with the vaginal birth group (5%).[24] In this cohort, 61% of patients underwent a trial of labor, of whom 75% had a successful vaginal birth. Of note, the greatest risk for mortality was in group 1 PH patients who underwent an intrapartum cesarean birth.

Although some historical management trends have favored planned cesarean birth, the latest

Table 3
Contraceptive options in pulmonary hypertension patients

Contraceptive Method	Hormonal Component	Typical Effectiveness	How to Use	Limitations
Sterilization	None	Failure rate <1%	Bilateral tubal ligation or salpingectomy surgery is permanent	Requires surgery
Copper IUD	None	Failure rate <1%	Placed by provider, effective up to 11 y Can also be used as emergency contraception if placed within 5 d	Increased menstrual cramping and bleeding
Hormonal IUD	Progestin	Failure rate <1%	Placed by provider, effective up to 3–7 y	Irregular bleeding common
Subdermal implant	Progestin	Failure rate <1%	Placed by provider, effective up to 3–5 y	Irregular bleeding common
DMPA injection	Progestin	Failure rate 6–10%	Repeat injection every 13–15 wk	Irregular bleeding common, can decrease bone density
Progestogen-only pill	Progestin	Failure rate 6–10%	Take 1 pill daily	Requires strict daily timing (30–60 min window)
Barrier (condoms, diaphragm, spermicides)	None	Failure rate 13–21%	Use consistently with each episode of intercourse	Requires consistent use, user dependent
Behavioral (fertility awareness, withdrawal)	None	Failure rate up to 22%	Fertility awareness requires recognition and monitoring of ovulatory cycle with periodic abstinence	Requires close monitoring, user dependent
Emergency contraception (ulipristal acetate or levonorgestrel)	Progestin	Depends on timing after intercourse	Use as soon as possible after unprotected intercourse, up to 3 d for levonorgestrel, and up to 5 d for ulipristal	Effectiveness depends on timing May be less effective if over 165 pounds for levonorgestrel and over 195 pounds for ulipristal

Abbreviations: IUD, intrauterine device; DMPA, medroxyprogesterone acetate.

guidelines from the European Society of Cardiology overall state that both planned cesarean or vaginal birth carry lower risk than an intrapartum or emergent cesarean delivery.[5]

Cesarean births overall carry higher rates of maternal morbidity and mortality, including hemorrhage, shock, cardiac arrest, renal failure, venous thromboembolic event, and infection.[43] Cardiac output in the immediate postpartum period increases significantly, as previously noted, regardless of delivery route.

Factors that should be considered when deciding include the patient's obstetric history, likelihood of successful vaginal birth, characteristics of their PH, WHO functional class, and specific hemodynamic indices.[44] At our center, we maintain cesarean birth for women with PH only for routine obstetric indications and recommend planned induction of labor in the late preterm or early term period with an early epidural and a forceps-assisted vaginal birth.

Postpartum Care and Contraception

Most of the maternal mortality with PH occurs in the first week postpartum.[3,4,24,36]

Major hemodynamic changes occur during this time, and patients' volume status should be monitored vigilantly. Rising CVP is a sign of rising right heart pressure that should be used to guide diuresis therapy and prevent RV overload.[35] On discharge, patients should be followed closely especially with routine assessment of right heart function.

As discussed during preconception care, contraception and planned pregnancy is an essential topic to discuss and ideally have a reliable option chosen. Combined oral contraceptives should be ideally avoided in this patient cohort due to increased thromboembolism risk.

Long-acting reversible contraceptives, namely an intrauterine device or hormonal implant, should be strongly considered given efficacy and ideal side effect profile. Sterilization should be discussed and offered as appropriate as well **Table 3**.

SUMMARY

PH carries significant morbidity and mortality in pregnancy. Patients in this high risk cohort necessitate preconception counseling and risk stratification as well multidisciplinary care throughout their pregnancy and delivery planning. Optimal delivery planning and close postpartum monitoring are the key to minimize cardiopulmonary morbidity and mortality in PH patients.

CLINICS CARE POINTS

- Pulmonary hypertension carries significant morbidity and mortality in pregnancy, with mortality rates as high as 25% to 56% in the setting of right ventricular failure.

- Pregnancy-related complications arise from cardiac inability to accommodate increased plasma volume and cardiac output, decreased systemic vascular resistance, and hypercoagulability.

- Patients with pulmonary hypertension, especially pulmonary arterial hypertension, should be strongly counseled to avoid pregnancy, and termination should be offered.

- Patients in this high-risk cohort necessitate multidisciplinary care throughout their pregnancy and delivery planning.

- Prostaglandins, phosphodiesterase inhibitors, calcium channel blockers, and anticoagulation should be considered as appropriate. Endothelin receptor blockers and soluble guanylate cyclase stimulators should be avoided due to teratogenicity.

- The highest risk for maternal morbidity and mortality is in the peripartum and immediate postpartum period.

- Deliberate delivery planning and close monitoring are the key to minimize cardiopulmonary morbidity and mortality.

- Close hemodynamic monitoring is recommended during delivery, including consideration of central venous catheter, arterial lines, and careful attention to volume status.

- Timing and mode of delivery should consider multiple factors and should be tailored to the individual. We recommend late preterm birth.

- Neuraxial anesthesia is recommended over general or spinal anesthesia whenever possible.

- Operative vaginal birth (namely forceps) should be considered to minimize physiologic cardiovascular stress in the second stage of labor.

- Contraception counseling is essential in the postpartum setting, with avoidance of estrogen-containing methods given increased venous thromboembolism risk.

DISCLOSURE

The authors have nothing to disclose.

REFERENCE

1. Martin SR, Edwards A. Pulmonary Hypertension and Pregnancy. Obstet Gynecol 2019;134:974–87.

2. George MG, Schieb LJ, Ayala C, et al. Pulmonary hypertension surveillance. United States, 2001 to 2010. Chest 2014;146:476–95.

3. Bedard E, Dimopoulos K, Gatzoulis MA. Has there been any progress made on pregnancy outcomes among women with pulmonary arterial hypertension? Eur Heart J 2009;30:256–65.

4. Weiss BM, Zemp L, Seifert B, et al. Outcome of pulmonary vascular disease in pregnancy: a systematic overview from 1978 through 1996. J Am Coll Cardiol 1998;31:1650–7.

5. Regitz-Zagrosek V, Blomstrom Lundqvist C, Borghi C, et al. ESC guidelines on the management of cardiovascular diseases during pregnancy: the Task Force on the Management of Cardiovascular Diseases during Pregnancy of the European Society of Cardiology (ESC). Eur Heart J 2011;32:3147–97.

6. Thomas E, Yang J, Xu J, et al. Pulmonary hypertension and pregnancy outcomes: insights from the national inpatient sample. J Am Heart Assoc 2017;6: 1–12.

7. Henshaw SK. Unintended pregnancy in the United States. Fam Plann Perspect 1998;30:24–9, 46.

8. Galiè N, Humbert M, Vachiery JL, et al. 2015 ESC/ERS guidelines for the diagnosis and treatment of pulmonary hypertension: the Joint Task Force for the Diagnosis and Treatment of Pulmonary Hypertension of the European Society of Cardiology (ESC) and the European Respiratory Society (ERS): endorsed by: Association for European Paediatric and Congenital Cardiology (AEPC), International Society for Heart and Lung Transplantation (ISHLT). Eur Heart J 2016;37:67–119.

9. Simonneau G, Montani D, Celermajer DS, et al. Haemodynamic definitions and updated clinical classification of pulmonary hypertension. Eur Respir J 2019;53:1–13.

10. Liu S, Elkayam U, Naqvi TZ. Echocardiography in pregnancy: part 1. Curr Cardiol Rep 2016;18:92.

11. Penning S, Robinson KD, Major CA, et al. A comparison of echocardiography and pulmonary artery catheterization for evaluation of pulmonary artery pressures in pregnant patients with suspected pulmonary hypertension. Am J Obstet Gynecol 2001;184:1568–70.

12. Wylie BJ, Epps KC, Gaddipati S, et al. Correlation of transthoracic echocardiography and right heart catheterization in pregnancy. J Perinat Med 2007; 35:497–502.

13. American College of Obstetricians and Gynecologists' Presidential Task Force on Pregnancy and Heart Disease and Committee on Practice Bulletins—Obstetrics. ACOG Practice Bulletin No. 212: Pregnancy and Heart Disease. Obstet Gynecol 2019;133:e320–56.

14. Sanghavi M, Rutherford JD. Cardiovascular physiology of pregnancy. Circulation 2014;130:1003–8.

15. Nama V, Antonios TF, Onwude J, et al. Mid-trimester blood pressure drop in normal pregnancy: myth or reality? J Hypertens 2011;29:763–8.

16. Kinsella SM, Lohmann G. Supine hypotensive syndrome. Obstet Gynecol 1994;83:774–88.

17. Kuhn JC, Falk RS, Langesaeter E. Haemodynamic changes during labour: continuous minimally invasive monitoring in 20 healthy parturients. Int J Obstet Anesth 2017;31:74–83.

18. Sibai BM. Etiology and management of postpartum hypertension-preeclampsia. Am J Obstet Gynecol 2012;206:470–5.

19. Castro LC, Hobel CJ, Gornbein J. Plasma levels of atrial natriuretic peptide in normal and hypertensive pregnancies: a meta-analysis. Am J Obstet Gynecol 1994;171:1642–51.

20. Ducas RA, Elliott JE, Melnyk SF, et al. Cardiovascular magnetic resonance in pregnancy: insights from the cardiac hemodynamic imaging and remodeling in pregnancy (CHIRP) study. J Cardiovasc Magn Reson 2014;16:1.

21. Melchiorre K, Sharma R, Khalil A, et al. Maternal cardiovascular function in normal pregnancy: evidence of maladaptation to chronic volume overload. Hypertension 2016;67:754–62.

22. Hameed A, Foster E, Main E, et al. Cardiovascular disease assessment in pregnant and postpartum women, a California maternal quality care collaborative quality Improvement Toolkit, 2017.

23. Thromboembolism in pregnancy. ACOG Practice Bulletin No. 196. American College of Obstetricians and Gynecologists. Obstet Gynecol 2018;132: e1–17.

24. Meng ML, Landau R, Viktorsdottir O, et al. Pulmonary hypertension in pregnancy: a report of 49 cases at four tertiary North American sites. Obstet Gynecol 2017;129:511–20.

25. Low TT, Guron N, Ducas R, et al. Pulmonary arterial hypertension in pregnancy-a systematic review of outcomes in the modern era. Pulm Circ 2021;11(2). 20458940211013671.

26. Kovacs AH, Harrison JL, Colman JM, et al. Pregnancy and contraception in congenital heart disease: what women are not told. J Am Coll Cardiol 2008;52:577–8.

27. Galiè N, Channick RN, Frantz RP, et al. Risk stratification and medical therapy of pulmonary arterial hypertension. Eur Respir J 2019;53:1–11.

28. Chin KM, Channick RN. Pulmonary hypertension. In: Broaddus VC, Mason RJ, Ernst JD, et al, editors. Murray and Nadel's textbook of respiratory medicine. 6th ed. Philadelphia, PA: Elsevier; 2016. p. 1031–49.

29. Hemnes AR, Kiely DG, Cockrill BA, et al. Statement on pregnancy in pulmonary hypertension from the pulmonary vascular research institute. Pulm Circ 2015;5:435–65.

30. Del Pozo R, Hernandez Gonzalez I, Escribano-Subias P. The prostacyclin pathway in pulmonary arterial hypertension: a clinical review. Expert Rev Respir Med 2017;11:491–503.

31. Bonnin M, Mercier FJ, Sitbon O, et al. Severe pulmonary hypertension during pregnancy: mode of delivery and anesthetic management of 15 consecutive cases. Anesthesiology 2005;102:1133–7.

32. Bendayan D, Hod M, Oron G, et al. Pregnancy outcome in patients with pulmonary arterial hypertension receiving prostacyclin therapy. Obstet Gynecol 2005;106:1206–10.

33. Briggs GG, Freeman RK, Towers CVT, et al. Drugs in pregnancy and lactation, a reference guide to fetal and neonatal risk. 11th edition. Philadelphia, PA: Wolters Kluwer; 2017.

34. Stout KK, Daniels CJ, Aboulhosn JA, et al. 2018 AHA/ACC guideline for the management of adults with congenital heart disease: a report of the American College of Cardiology/American Heart Association Task Force on Clinical Practice Guidelines. Circulation 2018;139(14):e698–800. [Epub ahead of print].

35. Kiely DG, Condliffe R, Webster V, et al. Improved survival in pregnancy and pulmonary hypertension using a multiprofessional approach. BJOG 2010;117:565–74.

36. Sliwa K, van Hagen IM, Budts W, et al. ROPAC investigators. Pulmonary hypertension and pregnancy outcomes: data from the Registry of Pregnancy and Cardiac Disease (ROPAC) of the European Society of Cardiology. Eur J Heart Fail 2016;18:1119–28.

37. Jais X, Olsson KM, Barbera JA, et al. Pregnancy outcomes in pulmonary arterial hypertension in the modern management era. Eur Respire J 2012;40:881–5.

38. Sahni S, Palkar AV, Rochelson BL, et al. Pregnancy and pulmonary arterial hypertension: a clinical conundrum. Pregnancy Hypertens 2015;5:157–64.

39. Sangkum L, Liu GL, Yu L, et al. Minimally invasive or noninvasive cardiac output measurement: an update. J Anesth 2016;30:461–80.

40. O'Hare R, McLoughlin C, Milligan K, et al. Anaesthesia for caesarean section in the presence of severe primary pulmonary hypertension. Br J Anaesth 1998;81:790–2.

41. Yuan S. Eisenmenger syndrome in pregnancy. Braz J Cardiovasc Surg 2016;31:325–9.

42. Konstantinides SV. Trends in pregnancy outcomes in patients with pulmonary hypertension: still a long way to go. Eur J Heart Fail 2016;18:1129–30.

43. American College of Obstetricians and Gynecologists (College); Society for Maternal-Fetal Medicine, Caughey AB, Cahill AG, et al. Safe prevention of the primary cesarean delivery. J Obstet Gynecol 2014;210:179–93.

44. Sharma K, Afshar YR, Bairey-Merz CN, et al. Guidelines and consensus: statement on pregnancy in pulmonary hypertension from the Pulmonary Vascular Research Institute. Pulm Circ 2016;6:143.

Genetics of High-Altitude Pulmonary Edema

Christina A. Eichstaedt, PhD[a,b,c,*], Nicola Benjamin, MSc[a,c], Ding Cao, MD[a,b], Eglė Palevičiūtė, MD[d], Ekkehard Grünig, MD[a,c]

KEYWORDS

- Pulmonary artery pressure • Pulmonary hypertension • Hypoxia • High-altitude pulmonary edema
- Polymorphisms • Mutations

KEY POINTS

- Pulmonary hypertension and high-altitude pulmonary edema are characterized by increased pulmonary artery pressures.
- Genetic studies highlighted genes involved in hypoxia response in particular related to the hypoxia-inducible factor.
- Case-control studies and families with several HAPE-susceptible members may inform about contributing genetic factors.

INTRODUCTION

High-altitude pulmonary edema (HAPE) is noncardiogenic lung edema characterized by elevated pulmonary artery pressures, dyspnea, cough, and reduced exercise capacity. In advanced stages body temperature can rise up to 38.5°C, frothy pink sputum, cyanosis and tachycardia may occur.[1] Its occurrence rate depends on the speed and mode of ascent, exhaustion, personal susceptibility to HAPE and the final altitude reached. The edema mainly results from exaggerated pulmonary vasoconstriction in response to hypoxia and exercise leading to elevated pulmonary artery pressures[2] and an alveolar-capillary leakage.[3] Impaired fluid uptake in the lungs also contributes to edema formation.[4] Diagnosis of HAPE is suspected when respective symptoms and current or preceding altitude exposure are present, oxygen saturation is reduced and rales are audible at auscultation. The diagnosis is confirmed by x-ray and supported by alveolar hemorrhage in bronchoalveolar lavage and "comet-trails" or "B-lines" seen by echocardiography.[5,6]

HAPE can occur in 7%-15% of mountaineers who ascent within the same day to extreme elevations above 4000 m.[7–9] In contrast, slow ascending mountaineers reaching an altitude of 2000 m only have an average HAPE risk of 0.01%.[10] If left untreated HAPE is the main cause of nontraumatic death at altitude. Treatment includes immediate descent in person or by air evacuation, supplemental oxygen, a hyperbaric Gamow bag or, if these options are not possible or available, medical intervention such as the calcium channel blocker nifedipine, and phosphodiesterase 5 inhibitors (PDE5i) can be given.[11] In mountaineers the best prevention of HAPE is a slow ascent with multiple acclimatization nights at increasing altitude and days of rest. If susceptibility to HAPE is known, preventive medication such as nifedipine or the PDE5i tadalafil or sildenafil may be taken.[11]

a Centre for Pulmonary Hypertension, Thoraxklinik Heidelberg gGmbH at Heidelberg University Hospital, Röntgenstraße 1, Heidelberg 69126, Germany; b Laboratory for Molecular Genetic Diagnostics, Institute of Human Genetics, Heidelberg University, Im Neuenheimer Feld 366, Heidelberg 69120, Germany; c Translational Lung Research Center Heidelberg (TLRC), Member of the German Center for Lung Research (DZL), Heidelberg, Germany; d Clinic of Cardiac and Vascular Diseases, Institute of Clinical Medicine, Vilnius University, Santariskiu-2, Vilnius 08661, Lithuania
* Corresponding author. Centre for Pulmonary Hypertension, Thoraxklinik Heidelberg gGmbH at Heidelberg University Hospital, Röntgenstraße 1, Heidelberg 69126, Germany.
E-mail address: christina.eichstaedt@med.uni-heidelberg.de

Heart Failure Clin 19 (2023) 89–96
https://doi.org/10.1016/j.hfc.2022.07.002

Abbreviations

HAPE   High-altitude pulmonary
                        edema
PAH   Pulmonary arterial
                        hypertension

The most well-known form of HAPE occurs in lowland residents performing treks or climbs at high altitude. Another type of HAPE has been described in highland residents who spent a few days or weeks at lower altitudes and develop HAPE despite the previous acclimatization upon return to high altitude.[12] This phenomenon is called "re-entry HAPE."[13,14] Only very few cases have been described of the third form of HAPE referred to as "resident HAPE," which may occur in individuals who live permanently at high altitude who have not undergone a change in altitude.[15–17]

CLUES TO GENETIC SUSCEPTIBILITY

The earliest clue toward a possible genetic susceptibility emerged from studies demonstrating an inherent exaggerated pulmonary arterial pressure response of HAPE susceptibles (HAPE-S) to normoxic exercise and hypoxia exposure compared to controls.[2,18] These findings were confirmed in a subsequent larger study.[19] While an exaggerated pressure response is characteristic for HAPE-S, not all individuals presenting with this response are, however, prone to develop HAPE.[20] The mechanism behind HAPE development and the exaggerated pressure response could be partly due to reduced pulmonary nitric oxide (NO) production in HAPE-S compared to HAPE resistant mountaineers.[21]

Reduced NO and elevated pulmonary arterial pressure are also underlying factors in the development of pulmonary arterial hypertension (PAH). For PAH a genetic predisposition is known and has been discovered primarily in familial PAH but also in around 20% of patients with sporadic PAH.[22,23] A significantly greater elevated pulmonary arterial systolic pressure during exercise and hypoxia was identified in healthy family members of PAH patients with a genetic predisposition for PAH vs. those family members without a genetic predisposition.[24] These results were confirmed in a large, European, multicentre study showing the exaggerated pulmonary pressure response to exercise and hypoxia to be more prevalent in healthy variant carriers than in those family members without a genetic variant for PAH.[9] Finally, patients have been described, who suffered from pulmonary hypertension and HAPE,

further illustrating the connection between the two diseases and possibly a shared or similar genetic predisposition.[14,25–27]

Further evidence pointing at a genetic background of HAPE is the recurrence rate in HAPE-S mountaineers. HAPE-S who have suffered from one HAPE episode have a 60% chance to develop a second episode when re-exposed to altitude.[28]

Rarely, also families have been reported with several HAPE cases.[14,29] These families were characterized by re-entry HAPE. Interestingly, the incidence of re-entry HAPE is very low in indigenous high-altitude populations whose ancestors have adapted over millennia to counteract the adverse environment of high altitude such as lower oxygen levels, aridity, cold, and increased solar radiation. There are only a few case reports of HAPE-S Tibetan or Nepali individuals.[30,31] Similarly, only a limited number of HAPE reports exist from the native populations of the South American Andes.[32]

In summary, it has been assumed, that HAPE susceptibility is at least in some cases genetically determined. This hypothesis has been supported by several findings: (a) the observation of an exaggerated pulmonary pressure response during exercise and hypoxia, which has been seen in HAPE-S[2] and in gene carriers of familial PAH,[9,33] (b) the high recurrence rate of HAPE in the same individual,[28] (c) familial aggregation of HAPE in some families,[14,29] (d) protection from HAPE in long-term altitude populations, (e) the finding of genetic abnormalities mainly in PAH genes detected in HAPE susceptibles.[14] The hypothesis has been evaluated by different forms of studies (**Fig. 1**).

SEQUENCING OF SINGLE-NUCLEOTIDE POLYMORPHISMS IN PATIENTS WITH HIGH-ALTITUDE PULMONARY EDEMA

Before the current genome-wide sequencing techniques such as high throughput next-generation sequencing or genotyping were available, the main focus of analyses was the frequency of specific variants in single candidate genes. These variants are assumed to be associated with HAPE susceptibility and their frequency is compared between HAPE-S and ideally HAPE resistant controls. Variants which are analyzed in these studies are often present at rather high

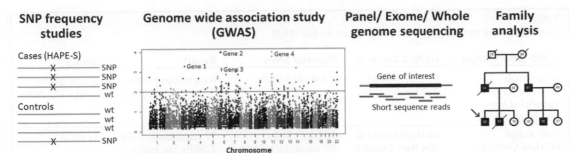

Fig. 1. Types of genetic studies to identify genetic HAPE susceptibility. Predefined single-nucleotide polymorphisms (SNPs) may be overrepresented in comparison to the wildtype (wt) variant in patients vs. controls. Genome-wide association studies (GWAS) focus on genome-wide SNPs and compare frequencies of cases and controls. High throughput techniques can sequence a number (panel) or all genes in the genome (whole-exome / -genome sequencing). Family studies look at the cosegregation of specific gene variants with HAPE susceptibility.

frequencies (>5%) in the general population. These variants would be considered to be benign polymorphisms without a directly disease-causing effect following the strict rules of variant characterization guidelines by the American Medical College of Genetics and Genomics.[34] Nevertheless, these variants may have some influence on a specific part of the disease phenotype, or be in linkage, i.e. linked by physical proximity on the genome to a disease-modifying variant.

Previously, researchers focused on genes with physiologically relevant functions in HAPE pathogenesis such as the enzyme endothelial NO synthase (NOS3) producing the vasodilator NO,[35,36] genes from the renin–angiotensin system[37–40] or genes in general involved in or known from lung diseases such as the microRNA host gene MIR17HG[41] known from asthma, or the telomer helicase gene RTEL1 known from pulmonary fibrosis.[42] Similarly, genes were investigated which encode altered biomarkers in patients with HAPE such the gene encoding IL6, which is upregulated in bronchoalveolar lavage of patients with HAPE.[43] Since all of these studies have only focused on known polymorphisms, which are considered to be prevalent in the general population they will most likely, even if significantly overrepresented in HAPE susceptibles, pose only a small overall risk for HAPE development.

GENOME-WIDE ASSOCIATION STUDIES IN PATIENTS WITH HIGH-ALTITUDE PULMONARY EDEMA

Genome-wide association studies (GWAS) are based on the same principle of higher SNP frequencies in cases vs. controls. However, instead of only analyzing selected known variants, hundreds of thousand of variants are sequenced in cases vs. controls. The GWAS studies conducted

for HAPE-S vs. HAPE resistant controls are summarised in **Table 1**. Some strengthened already previously assumed gene-disease associations e.g. with the endothelial NO synthase gene NOS3. Other studies highlighted genes located around the identified variants with significantly different allele frequencies. Overall, a clear functional contribution to HAPE development from these studies still remains limited.

LARGER SCALE SEQUENCING APPROACHES

A recent study employed a new approach and performed *whole mitochondrial genome sequencing* of HAPE resistant and HAPE-S Han Chinese.[48] This study identified two noncoding variants in the mitochondrial genome at different frequencies in the two groups, however, without providing any explanation for a possible mechanism of disease contribution.

Another study took a different approach and investigated *30 SNPs selected for possible functional consequence* in two relevant hypoxia genes in HAPE susceptible and HAPE protected Indians. EGLN1 the proly hydroxlase 2 and the HIF1AN hydroxylase were analyzed. Both enzymes are responsible for the hydroxylation of the hypoxia-inducible factor 1 alpha (HIF1α) under normoxic conditions leading either to its degradation or inhibition of HIF1α to bind complex proteins required for full functionality.[49] The study revealed three SNPs in the gene EGLN1 which led to an increased gene expression in a functional analysis of the variants in a cell culture reporter gene expression model (luciferase assay). The plasma protein levels were also measured in HAPE-S and HAPE resistant groups and revealed higher protein levels of the hydroxylase PHD2 (encoded by EGLN1) in HAPE susceptible Indo-Aryan subjects. A higher level of PHD2 should lead to reduced activity of

Table 1
Genome-wide association studies conducted for HAPE

HAPE-S Population	HAPE-R Controls	Number SNPs	Result	Study
First stage 96 Indo-Aryan Second stage 201 Indo-Aryan	96 Indo-Aryan 200 Indo-Aryan	1,140,419 SNPs	4 candidate SNPs in eNOS (NOS3)	Kanipakam et al,[44] 2021
First stage 68 Han Chinese Second stage 199 Han Chinese	84 HapMap CHB 304 Han Chinese	906,600 SNPs 68 candidate SNPs	77 candidate SNPs 7 SNPs, no coding variant	Li et al,[45] 2017
First stage 96 Indo-Aryan Second stage 104 Indo-Aryan	96 Indo-Aryan 104 Indo-Aryan	1,140,419 SNPs 138 candidate SNPs in 10 genes	138 candidate SNPs 3 SNPs in apelin (APLN), 2 SNPs in its receptor (APLNR), 3 in eNOS (NOS3)	Mishra et al,[36] 2015
23 Han Chinese	17 Han Chinese	1,140,419 SNPs	39 candidate SNPs	Duan et al,[46] 2014
40 Han Chinese	22 Han Chinese	1,140,419 SNPs	57 candidate SNPs	Yang et al,[47] 2013

Abbreviations: eNOS, endothelial nitric oxide synthase; HAPE-R / S, high altitude pulmonary edema resistant / susceptible; SNP, single-nucleotide polymorphism.

the HIF and subsequent downstream genes. Interestingly, the *EGLN1* has been shown to be strongly reduced in well-adapted native high-altitude populations in the Himalayas preventing erythrocytosis and subsequent chronic mountain sickness.[50,51] In Andean highlanders alterations in the same signaling cascade may also lead to a better adaptation to high altitude.[52] Thus, it remains unclear how in the one population the same gene can have an adaptive advantage (native highlanders) leading to a blunted hypoxia response, while in HAPE-S its overexpression is associated with increased pulmonary artery pressures and HAPE development.

We have investigated a set of 42 genes in HAPE-S mountaineers[14] using a *PAH-specific gene panel.*[22,53] The genes were either genes known to be able to cause pulmonary arterial hypertension (PAH) or were associated with PAH. This approach was chosen due to the aforementioned overlap and similarities between HAPE and PAH concerning the elevated pulmonary artery pressure, reduced NO, patients with, both conditions, pulmonary hypertension and HAPE and the increased pulmonary artery pressure during normobaric hypoxia and moderate exercise in HAPE-S and in family members of PAH patients with a predisposing pathogenic variant in the *BMPR2* gene.[2,9,33] This gene panel approach revealed two likely pathogenic variants in two out of 64 Caucasian HAPE-S mountaineers.[14] The first

variant was located in the monooxygenase genes cytochrome P1B1 (*CYP1B1*) and the second variant in the histidine-rich glycoprotein (*HRG*). Both genes were candidate genes for PAH and their functional disruption could have led to increased endothelial permeability (*HRG*) and an inhibited vasodilatory response (*CYP1B1*) in the HAPE-S mountaineers. However, they await further validation for their role in HAPE susceptibility.

Yet another approach was taken by Yuhong and colleagues[54] who focused on changes in *gene transcription* instead of gene variants. The authors measured transcriptional changes on RNA level in whole blood from 12 male HAPE-S Han Chinese and compared them to 9 male controls.[54] In this study the gene expression was measured of 84 candidate genes involved in hypoxia signaling. Expression was measured in blood either during acute HAPE and after symptoms resolved (HAPE-S) or during altitude exposure without any HAPE symptoms (controls). All subjects arrived at altitude with a similar ascent profile. Of the investigated genes, 9 genes were significantly up- or down-regulated in patients with HAPE during the acute HAPE phase compared to expression at recovery and compared to controls at the same altitude. While this approach highlighted important genes involved in the acute phase of HAPE the preselection of hypoxia genes and the fact that the oxygen saturation of patients with acute HAPE was very low (56% at 3780 m compared to 90% in controls) somewhat limits the explanatory power for HAPE development or physiology by the highlighted genes. It should have been expected that any genes regulated by HIF1α were to demonstrate stronger differences in acutely hypoxic individuals.

FAMILIES WITH MULTIGENERATIONAL HIGH-ALTITUDE PULMONARY EDEMA

Two families have been investigated so far on a genetic level who show multigenerational HAPE.[14,29] In both cases the respective family members suffered from re-entry HAPE after residing a short period of time at lower altitude. Lorenzo and colleagues performed genotyping for 500,658 SNPs in a family with 6 HAPE-S family members. The study identified a haplotype, which is a block of physically neighboring SNPs in affected individuals. The haplotype was assigned to HIF2α (EPAS1 gene). However, on closer inspection, only 4 out of the 7 SNPs within the haplotype showed statistical significance. Moreover, the haplotype block itself was around 8 Mb up-stream of the EPAS1 gene location.[29] Thus, this family may offer a hint on where to focus but does not provide conclusive evidence for EPAS1 leading to HAPE susceptibility.

The second so far described HAPE family was analyzed by us with our PAH-specific gene panel.[14] This family included two HAPE susceptible children and their aunt whose HAPE episode was only ascertained by clinical history. One of the children developed PAH during adulthood at 23 years of age after she had several HAPE episodes. We could identify a likely pathogenic missense variant in the gene Janus Kinase 2 (JAK2) in both HAPE susceptible children. The same variant was also present in another HAPE-resistant sibling and their HAPE-resistant father. Interestingly, the HAPE-S children were born at low altitude and moved back to >3000 m a few weeks after birth. The two other variant carriers were born and raised at high altitude. These results could point to another layer for HAPE susceptibility, namely environmental influences or epigenetic changes. The altitude of birth and subsequent lung development may have influenced HAPE susceptibility in this family.

ANIMAL MODELS FOR HIGH-ALTITUDE PULMONARY EDEMA

Various researchers have tried to develop animal models to resemble HAPE. Interesting molecular candidates were aquaporins, which encode water channel proteins and may play a part in disturbed lung water clearance during HAPE. Previously, homozygous aquaporin 5 knockout mice were shown to have an impaired water permeability between airspace and capillaries.[55] Thus, a Chinese team of researchers anticipated an increased occurrence of capillary leakage due to hypoxia-induced pulmonary pressure increase in these knockout mice.[56] They compared mice at rest and at exercise on a treadmill in a hypobaric hypoxic chamber, which simulated an altitude of 5000 m.[56] In these animals HAPE or HAPE-like lung injury was demonstrated by an elevated number of proteins in the bronchoalveolar lavage and a higher ratio of the wet lung to dry lung was identified compared to control mice. While lung edema was apparent in particular in the mice exercising at hypoxia, no difference in the wildtype vs. aquaporin 5 knockout mice could be detected. The same model of exercise plus hypoxia also led to lung edema in wildtype Sprague-Dawley rats, which had to walk on a treadmill for 48 h with only short feeding breaks at a simulated altitude of 4800 m.[57] Hypoxia-exposed rats that exercised had higher levels of red blood cells and albumin in the bronchoalveolar lavage compared to those, who were allowed to rest at the same environmental conditions.[57] In addition, the wet/dry lung ratio of the studied rats was significantly increased with synergistic effects of hypoxia and exercise. While this model resembled HAPE pathophysiology it is a complex animal model for other researchers to establish.

Another animal model for HAPE was generated recently by inducing a conditional, cell-specific homozygous knockout of the Von-Hippel-Lindau (VHL) gene in mice.[58] The gene encodes ubiquitin ligase, which is required for the degradation of HIF1α during normoxic conditions. The disturbance of the VHL ligase leads to a constant gene activation of HIF downstream genes as it is physiologically seen during hypoxia. Gojkovic and colleagues generated mice that only carry the homozygous VHL gene disruption in myeloid cells. The mice developed pulmonary edema without hypoxia exposure at rest, which could simplify further experiments investigating HAPE physiology as no hypobaric hypoxia chamber and treadmill training were required. However, the mice lacked a cardinal symptom of HAPE, i.e. the elevated pulmonary artery pressure. Thus, this model may be used only for specific questions after edema formation as it does not resemble the same mechanism leading the capillary stress failure as seen in HAPE patients with pulmonary hypertension.

FUTURE DIRECTIONS

HAPE susceptibility is a large burden and danger for affected individuals in alpine sports and trekking. Thus, it would be of high importance to have diagnostic procedures to identify susceptible individuals. One option may be the screening of individuals using echocardiography during exercise or a simulated exposure for 120 minutes at high altitude in a hypoxic chamber. An exaggerated pulmonary pressure response may point toward an underlying genetic predisposition or at least an increased susceptibility to HAPE. Overall, only few possibly contributing genetic factors have been identified for HAPE development. Future studies should advance the genetic analyses in clinically well characterized HAPE-S including in particular families with several HAPE cases. The genetic characterization employing next-generation sequencing such as whole exome and whole-genome sequencing of re-entry families could assist to discover underlying factors contributing to HAPE susceptibility. To identify the complex triggers of HAPE in one individual compared to a HAPE-free individual with the same ascent profile various aspects including genetic differences, transcriptional changes, and epigenetic differences should be considered and investigated. The molecular and clinical findings from HAPE-S families and individuals may then, in turn, be also informative for pulmonary hypertension, characterized by the same elevated pulmonary artery pressure.

SUMMARY

Different types of studies have identified interesting candidate genes associated with HAPE development in mountaineers or in high-altitude residents who developed HAPE after a short time at lower altitudes. So far there is no specific gene, which has crystallised to be the single most important HAPE susceptibility gene. The acute disease appears to be influenced not only by external factors such as mode of ascent, speed of ascent, and maximum altitude reached but also by individual genetic and possibly epigenetic factors.

CLINICS CARE POINTS

- HAPE diagnosis is confirmed by x-ray
- Patients with HAPE should immediately descent or be air evacuated

---

- Medical treatment includes nifedipine and phosphodiesterase 5 inhibitors
- Preventive treatment includes sildenafil, tadalafil, and nifedipine
- If an individual previously had HAPE, there is a 60% chance of HAPE recurrence

DISCLOSURE

CAE, NB: report no conflicts of interest. EG: has received grants and personal fees from Actelion, Bayer AG, and MSD; grants from GSK, Novartis, and United Therapeutics and personal fees from SCOPE, OrPha Swiss GmbH, and Zurich Heart House, outside the submitted work. EP: has received speaker honoraria fees from Johnson and Johnson and Medis Pharma, outside the submitted work.

REFERENCES

1. Bärtsch P, Mairbäurl H, Swenson ER, et al. High altitude pulmonary oedema. Swiss Med Wkly 2003; 133(27–28):377–84.
2. Grünig E, Mereles D, Hildebrandt W, et al. Stress Doppler echocardiography for identification of susceptibility to high altitude pulmonary edema. J Am Coll Cardiol 2000;35(4):980–7.
3. Bärtsch P, Swenson ER. Clinical practice: acute high-altitude illnesses. N Engl J Med 2013;368(24): 2294–302.
4. Höschele S, Mairbäurl H. Alveolar flooding at high altitude: failure of reabsorption? News Physiol Sci 2003;18:55–9.
5. Lichtblau M, Bader PR, Carta AF, et al. Extravascular lung water and cardiac function assessed by echocardiography in healthy lowlanders during repeated very high-altitude exposure. Int J Cardiol 2021;332: 166–74.
6. Swenson ER, Maggiorini M, Mongovin S, et al. Pathogenesis of high-altitude pulmonary edema: inflammation is not an etiologic factor. JAMA 2002; 287(17):2228–35.
7. Luks AM, Swenson ER, Bärtsch P. Acute high-altitude sickness. Eur Respir Rev 2017;26(143).
8. Singh I, Kapila CC, Kahanna PK, et al. High-altitude pulmonary oedema. Lancet 1965;1(7379):229–34.
9. Grünig E, Weissmann S, Ehlken N, et al. Stress Doppler echocardiography in relatives of patients with idiopathic and familial pulmonary arterial hypertension: results of a multicenter European analysis of pulmonary artery pressure response to exercise and hypoxia. Circulation 2009;119(13):1747–57.
10. Roach JM, Schoene RB. High-altitude pulmonary edema. In: Pandoff KB, Burr RE, editors. Medical

aspects of harsh environments. 1st edition. Ft. Belvoir: Defense Technical Information Center; 2002. p. 789–814.

11. Luks AM, Auerbach PS, Freer L, et al. Wilderness medical society clinical practice guidelines for the prevention and treatment of acute altitude illness: 2019 update. Wilderness Environ Med 2019;30(4S):S3–18.

12. Houston CS, Harris DE, Zeman EJ. Going higher: oxygen, man and mountains. 5th edition. Seattle: The Mountaineers Books; 2005. p. 318.

13. Gray GW. High altitude pulmonary edema. Semin Respir Med 1983;5(2):141–50.

14. Eichstaedt CA, Mairbäurl H, Song J, et al. Genetic predisposition to high-altitude pulmonary edema. High Alt Med Biol 2020;21(1):28–36.

15. Ebert-Santos C. High-altitude pulmonary edema in mountain community residents. High Alt Med Biol 2017;18(3):278–84.

16. Giesenhagen AM, Ivy DD, Brinton JT, et al. High altitude pulmonary edema in children: a single referral center evaluation. J Pediatr 2019;210:106–11.

17. Kelly TD, Meier M, Weinman JP, et al. High-altitude pulmonary edema in colorado children: a cross-sectional survey and retrospective review. High Alt Med Biol 2022;23(2):119–24.

18. Bärtsch P, Grünig E, Hohenhaus E, et al. Assessment of high altitude tolerance in healthy individuals. High Alt Med Biol 2001;2(2):287–96.

19. Dehnert C, Grünig E, Mereles D, et al. Identification of individuals susceptible to high-altitude pulmonary oedema at low altitude. Eur Respir J 2005;25(3):545–51.

20. Dehnert C, Mereles D, Greiner S, et al. Exaggerated hypoxic pulmonary vasoconstriction without susceptibility to high altitude pulmonary edema. High Alt Med Biol 2015;16(1):11–7.

21. Busch T, Bärtsch P, Pappert D, et al. Hypoxia decreases exhaled nitric oxide in mountaineers susceptible to high-altitude pulmonary edema. Am J Respir Crit Care Med 2001;163(2):368–73.

22. Eichstaedt CA, Sassmannshausen Z, Shaukat M, et al. Gene panel diagnostics reveals new pathogenic variants in pulmonary arterial hypertension. Respir Res 2022;23(1):74.

23. Pfarr N, Szamalek-Hoegel J, Fischer C, et al. Hemodynamic and clinical onset in patients with hereditary pulmonary arterial hypertension and BMPR2 mutations. Respir Res 2011;12:99.

24. Grünig E, Dehnert C, Mereles D, et al. Enhanced hypoxic pulmonary vasoconstriction in families of adults or children with idiopathic pulmonary arterial hypertension. Chest 2005;128(6 Suppl):630S–3S.

25. Brill AK, Kunz A, Ott SR, et al. When "high" is not very high: high altitude pulmonary edema as first manifestation of sarcoidosis-related pulmonary hypertension. High Alt Med Biol 2012;13(4):285–7.

26. Corvinus C, Bärtsch P, Dehnert C, et al. Pulmonary hypertension in a patient with Abt-Letterer-Siwe syndrome and episodes of HAPE. Eur Respir J 2010;36(5):1212–4.

27. Naeije R, De Backer D, Vachiery JL, et al. High-altitude pulmonary edema with primary pulmonary hypertension. Chest 1996;110(1):286–9.

28. Bärtsch P, Maggiorini M, Mairbäurl H, et al. Pulmonary extravascular fluid accumulation in climbers. Lancet 2002;360(9332):571 [author reply: 571-2].

29. Lorenzo VF, Yang Y, Simonson TS, et al. Genetic adaptation to extreme hypoxia: study of high-altitude pulmonary edema in a three-generation Han Chinese family. Blood Cells Mol Dis 2009;43(3):221–5.

30. Baniya S, Holden C, Basnyat B. Reentry High Altitude Pulmonary Edema in the Himalayas. High Alt Med Biol 2017;18(4):425–7.

31. Wu T. A Tibetan with chronic mountain sickness followed by high altitude pulmonary edema on reentry. High Alt Med Biol 2004;5(2):190–4.

32. Hultgren HN, Marticorena EA. High altitude pulmonary edema. Epidemiologic observations in Peru. Chest 1978;74(4):372–6.

33. Grünig E, Janssen B, Mereles D, et al. Abnormal pulmonary artery pressure response in asymptomatic carriers of primary pulmonary hypertension gene. Circulation 2000;102(10):1145–50.

34. Richards S, Aziz N, Bale S, et al. Standards and guidelines for the interpretation of sequence variants: a joint consensus recommendation of the American College of Medical Genetics and Genomics and the Association for Molecular Pathology. Genet Med 2015;17(5):405–24.

35. Ahsan A, Mohd G, Norboo T, et al. Heterozygotes of NOS3 polymorphisms contribute to reduced nitrogen oxides in high-altitude pulmonary edema. Chest 2006;130(5):1511–9.

36. Mishra A, Kohli S, Dua S, et al. Genetic differences and aberrant methylation in the apelin system predict the risk of high-altitude pulmonary edema. Proc Natl Acad Sci U S A 2015;112(19):6134–9.

37. Stobdan T, Ali Z, Khan AP, et al. Polymorphisms of renin-angiotensin system genes as a risk factor for high-altitude pulmonary oedema. J Renin Angiotensin Aldosterone Syst 2011;12(2):93–101.

38. Bhagi S, Srivastava S, Tomar A, et al. Positive Association of D Allele of ACE Gene With High Altitude Pulmonary Edema in Indian Population. Wilderness Environ Med 2015;26(2):124–32.

39. Dehnert C, Weymann J, Montgomery HE, et al. No association between high-altitude tolerance and the ACE I/D gene polymorphism. Med Sci Sports Exerc 2002;34(12):1928–33.

40. Hotta J, Hanaoka M, Droma Y, et al. Polymorphisms of renin-angiotensin system genes with high-altitude

pulmonary edema in Japanese subjects. Chest 2004;126(3):825–30.

41. Si L, Wang H, Jiang Y, et al. MIR17HG polymorphisms contribute to high-altitude pulmonary edema susceptibility in the Chinese population. Sci Rep 2022;12(1):4346.

42. Rong H, He X, Zhu L, et al. Association between regulator of telomere elongation helicase1 (RTEL1) gene and HAPE risk: a case-control study. Medicine (Baltimore) 2017;96(39):e8222.

43. He X, Wang L, Zhu L, et al. A case-control study of the genetic polymorphism of IL6 and HAPE risk in a Chinese Han population. Clin Respir J 2018; 12(9):2419–25.

44. Kanipakam H, Sharma K, Thinlas T, et al. Structural and functional alterations of nitric oxide synthase 3 due to missense variants associate with high-altitude pulmonary edema through dynamic study. J Biomol Struct Dyn 2021;39(1):294–309.

45. Li X, Jin T, Zhang M, et al. Genome-wide association study of high-altitude pulmonary edema in a Han Chinese population. Oncotarget 2017;8(19): 31568–80.

46. Duan RF, Liu W, Long CL, et al. [Genome-wide association study of high altitude pulmonary edema]. Zhongguo Ying Yong Sheng Li Xue Za Zhi 2014; 30(2):101–5.

47. Yang J, Li X, Al-Lamki RS, et al. Sildenafil potentiates bone morphogenetic protein signaling in pulmonary arterial smooth muscle cells and in experimental pulmonary hypertension. Arterioscler Thromb Vasc Biol 2013;33(1):34–42.

48. Wang Y, Huang X, Peng F, et al. Association of variants m.T16172C and m.T16519C in whole mtDNA sequences with high altitude pulmonary edema in Han Chinese lowlanders. BMC Pulm Med 2022; 22(1):72.

49. Sharma K, Mishra A, Singh HN, et al. High-altitude pulmonary edema is aggravated by risk loci and associated transcription factors in HIF-prolyl hydroxylases. Hum Mol Genet 2021;30(18):1734–49.

50. Simonson TS, Yang Y, Huff CD, et al. Genetic evidence for high-altitude adaptation in Tibet. Science 2010;329(5987):72–5.

51. Lorenzo FR, Huff C, Myllymaki M, et al. A genetic mechanism for Tibetan high-altitude adaptation. Nat Genet 2014;46(9):951–6.

52. Eichstaedt CA, Pagani L, Antao T, et al. Evidence of Early-Stage Selection on EPAS1 and GPR126 Genes in Andean High Altitude Populations. Scientific Rep 2017;7(1):13042.

53. Song J, Eichstaedt CA, Rodríguez Viales R, et al. Identification of genetic defects in pulmonary arterial hypertension by a new gene panel diagnostic tool. Clin Sci (London, Engl : 1979) 2016;130(22):2043–52.

54. Yuhong L, Tana W, Zhengzhong B, et al. Transcriptomic profiling reveals gene expression kinetics in patients with hypoxia and high altitude pulmonary edema. Gene 2018;651:200–5.

55. Ma T, Fukuda N, Song Y, et al. Lung fluid transport in aquaporin-5 knockout mice. J Clin Invest 2000; 105(1):93–100.

56. She J, Bi J, Tong L, et al. New insights of aquaporin 5 in the pathogenesis of high altitude pulmonary edema. Diagn Pathol 2013;8:193.

57. Bai C, She J, Goolaerts A, et al. Stress failure plays a major role in the development of high-altitude pulmonary oedema in rats. Eur Respir J 2010;35(3): 584–91.

58. Gojkovic M, Darmasaputra GS, Velica P, et al. Deregulated hypoxic response in myeloid cells: A model for high-altitude pulmonary oedema (HAPE). Acta Physiol (Oxf) 2020;229(2):e13461.

Use of Oral Anticoagulant Drugs in Patients with Pulmonary Hypertension

Pablo Demelo-Rodriguez, MD, PhD[a,b,c,1], Francisco Galeano-Valle, MD[a,b,c,1], Marco Proietti, MD, PhD[d,e,f,1,*]

KEYWORDS

- Pulmonary hypertension • Oral anticoagulant drugs • VKAs • DOACs

KEY POINTS

- In patients with pulmonary hypertension, there is a significant burden of adverse outcomes and mortality.
- Pathophysiological and clinical data support the use of oral anticoagulants (OACs) in pulmonary arterial hypertension (PAH) and chronic thromboembolic pulmonary hypertension (CTEPH).
- The use of OAC seems to be able to mitigate this risk, even though supported mainly by observational data.
- Most studies so far used vitamin K antagonists, whereas data on direct oral anticoagulants (DOACs) still seem limited.
- If the use of OAC seems to be a mainstay in treatment of PAH and CTEPH, more data are still needed to support more solidly guidelines and evaluate use of DOACs.

INTRODUCTION

Pulmonary embolism (PE) and deep vein thrombosis are the main clinical manifestations of venous thromboembolism (VTE). Acute PE is the third most common acute cardiovascular condition. Acute PE is burdened by remarkable mortality, ranging from 7% (when correctly diagnosed and promptly treated) to 34% (in patients presenting with hemodynamic instability).[1] Annual incidence rates for PE range from 39 to 115 per 100,000 population and are increasing over time. Incomplete thrombus resolution occurs in 25% to 50% of patients after acute PE despite adequate anticoagulation but bears no clinical significance in most cases; therefore, no routine follow-up computed tomography pulmonary angiogram (CTPA) imaging is needed in such patients treated for PE.[2]

The post-PE syndrome (PPES) occurs in up to 50% of PE survivors[3] and is defined as new or progressive dyspnea, exercise intolerance, and/or impaired functional or mental status after at least 3 months of adequate anticoagulation following acute PE, which cannot be explained by other (preexisting) comorbidities.[4] Chronic thromboembolic pulmonary hypertension (CTEPH) is the most severe clinical presentation of PPES.

[a] Venous Thromboembolism Unit, Internal Medicine, Hospital General Universitario Gregorio, Marañón, Calle Doctor Esquerdo 46, Madrid 28007, Spain; [b] Department of Medicine, School of Medicine, Universidad Complutense de Madrid, Madrid, Spain; [c] Sanitary Research Institute Gregorio Marañón, Calle Doctor Esquerdo 46, Madrid 28007, Spain; [d] Department of Clinical Sciences and Community Health, University of Milan, Via Francesco Sforza 35, Milan 20122, Italy; [e] Geriatric Unit, IRCCS Istituti Clinici Scientifici Maugeri, Via Camaldoli 64, Milan 20138, Italy; [f] Liverpool Centre for Cardiovascular Science, University of Liverpool and Liverpool Heart & Chest Hospital, West Derby Street, Liverpool 6 8TX, UK
[1] All the authors contributed equally to the article.
* Corresponding author. Geriatric Unit, IRCCS Istituti Clinici Scientifici Maugeri, Via Camaldoli 64, Milan 20138, Italy.
E-mail address: marco.proietti@unimi.it
Twitter: @MProiettiMD (M.P.)

Heart Failure Clin 19 (2023) 97–106
https://doi.org/10.1016/j.hfc.2022.08.018
1551-7136/23/© 2022 Elsevier Inc. All rights reserved.

On the other hand, pulmonary arterial hypertension (PAH) is a clinical condition characterized by the presence of precapillary PH and pulmonary vascular resistance (PVR) greater than 3 Wood units, in the absence of other causes of precapillary PH.

In this review, the authors disclose the role of oral anticoagulant (OAC) drugs for the main clinical presentations of pulmonary hypertension (PH), PAH, and CTEPH as well as the main guideline recommendations.

DEFINITIONS
Classification of Pulmonary Hypertension

PH is a hemodynamic and pathophysiological condition defined as an increase in mean pulmonary artery pressure (PAP) $\geq$25 mm Hg at rest as assessed by right heart catheterization. PH can be found in multiple clinical conditions.[5] The clinical classification of PH includes five groups according to their similar clinical presentation, pathological findings, hemodynamic characteristics, and treatment strategy[6,7]:

- PAH, group 1, is a clinical condition characterized by the presence of precapillary PH and PVR greater than 3 Wood units, in the absence of other causes of precapillary PH such as PH due to lung diseases, CTEPH, or other rare diseases. PAH includes different forms that share a similar clinical picture and virtually identical pathological changes of the lung microcirculation (ie, idiopathic, heritable, drug induced, associated with connective tissue disease, and so forth).
- PH due to left heart disease (group 2).
- PH due to lung diseases and/or hypoxia (group 3).
- CTEPH and other pulmonary artery obstructions (group 4), includes CTEPH and other pulmonary artery obstructions (angiosarcoma, arteritis, congenital pulmonary arteries stenoses, and hydatidosis).
- PH with unclear and/or multifactorial mechanisms (group 5).

Pulmonary Artery Hypertension

PAH is a proliferative vasculopathy characterized by vasoconstriction, cell proliferation, fibrosis, and thrombosis. Pathologic findings include intimal hyperplasia and fibrosis, medial hypertrophy, and in situ thrombi of the small pulmonary arteries and arterioles.[8,9] The small pulmonary arteries and arterioles seem qualitatively similar in the pathologic studies in all patients with PAH. It is unclear whether these mechanisms are shared

with most other types of PH. A previous pathophysiologic review suggested that abnormalities of both coagulation and the fibrinolytic system lead to a prothrombotic state in patients with idiopathic PAH.[10] Patients with PH are at increased risk for intrapulmonary thrombosis and thromboembolism due to sluggish pulmonary blood flow, dilated right heart chambers, venous stasis, and immobility. Even a small thrombus can produce hemodynamic deterioration in a patient with a compromised pulmonary vascular bed.[9] There is a high prevalence of vascular thrombotic lesions at postmortem examination in patients with PAH.[6]

Chronic Thromboembolic Pulmonary Hypertension

Approximately 40% of PE survivors have persistent perfusion defects. Despite that, the diagnosis of CTEPH is rare, presenting with a prevalence in PE survivors of 2% to 3%, and 5% to 8% in PE survivors with persistent dyspnea.[4,11]

CTEPH is a disease caused by the persistent obstruction of pulmonary arteries by fibrotic organized thrombi causing fixed mechanical obstruction that leads to overflow of the open pulmonary arteries and remodeling of the pulmonary microvascular bed, which leads to a progressive increase in PVR.[12] Interestingly, there is no clear correlation between the degree of mechanical obstruction found at imaging and hemodynamics. Most patients diagnosed with CTEPH are derived from cohorts with acute PE.[13]

Associated conditions include thrombophilia disorders, particularly antiphospholipid antibody syndrome and high coagulation factor VIII levels, cancer, a history of splenectomy, inflammatory bowel disease, ventricular-atrial shunts, and infection of chronic intravenous lines and devices such as implantable pacemakers. Median age at diagnosis of CTEPH is 63 years, and both sexes are equally affected. Clinical symptoms and signs are nonspecific or absent in early stages; thus, early diagnosis remains a challenge. When present, the clinical symptoms of CTEPH may resemble those of acute PE or of PAH. Scores for predicting or ruling out CTEPH are limited by a lack of specificity.[14,15]

The diagnosis of CTEPH requires a mean PAP of $\geq$25 mm Hg along with a pulmonary arterial wedge pressure of $\leq$15 mm Hg, documented at right heart catheterization in a patient with mismatched perfusion defects on ventilation/perfusion lung scan, performed after at least 3 months of adequate anticoagulation (to distinguish this condition from acute PE). Specific diagnostic signs for CTEPH on CTPA include ring-like stenoses, webs, slits, and chronic total occlusions.[6] Of note, a change to decrease mean PAP to ≥20 mm Hg to define PH has been proposed but is not yet incorporated into diagnostic criteria of CTEPH.[11]

CTEPH is defined as chronic pulmonary vascular obstruction with normal mean PAP pressure at rest, but with limited exercise tolerance, which is attributed, at least in part, to an increased slope of the PAP-flow relationship (>3 mm Hg/L/min) during exercise or dead space ventilation.[16] The dead-space fraction is decreased with exercise, whereas ventilatory efficiency, measured by the ventilatory equivalent for carbon dioxide slope, is decreased.[17,18] Currently, there is no sufficient data to support the definition of "PH on exercise."[6]

Based on the elements described above, both PAH and CTEPH receive a direct indication to be prescribed with OAC in the European Society of Cardiology (ESC) and other international guidelines.[6,19]

ADVERSE OUTCOMES IN PATIENTS WITH PULMONARY HYPERTENSION

Irrespective of its relatively low prevalence and incidence, the presence of PH is burdened by significant morbidity and mortality.[6,20] Indeed, PH and the consequential right heart failure can often lead to complications affecting every organ and system, from those more commonly known as consequences on left heart side function, kidney function, and cognitive function, to the less known as those affecting endocrine system, gut and liver function, immune system, and others.[20]

Despite the significant advances in the specific clinical and pharmacological management achieved in the last years,[6,21,22] the most concerning effect of PH is the increased medium- and long-term risk of mortality.[23] Even though several specific pharmacological treatments are currently available,[21,22] and despite the diffusion of pulmonary endarterectomy (PEA) as treatment of choice for CTEPH,[6] data coming from observational registries did not show significant improvement in the risk of death in long-term follow-up (**Table 1**).[13,23–27] Indeed, the data coming from a French nationwide registry including 674 patients with PH in 2006 documented an overall mortality rate of almost 12% in incident PH patients at 1 year of follow-up.[24] Ling and colleagues[25] reported an overall mortality rate of almost 27% over a 5-year follow-up time also in incident PH patients, and Kerr and colleagues[27] reported an overall mortality rate of 6.53%, which increases up to 11.5% in inoperable patients, in a registry of CTEPH only patients. Evidence coming from the observational registries also confirmed

that over time, PH patients report a significant clinical deterioration and worsening, both the general PH cohorts[26] and those with CTEPH only.[27]

Significant evidence of an important burden of adverse outcomes comes also from other clinical scenarios. In a large systematic review and meta-analysis including more than 16,000 patients, Kolte and colleagues[28] reported that even patients with mild PH (defined as PAP <25 mm Hg) show a significant increase in the risk of all-cause death (risk ratio [R + R 1.52, 95% confidence interval [CI] 1.32–1.74), over a long-term follow-up observation. Similar data were also reported in specific clinical populations. Indeed, Brinza and colleagues[29] reported a twofold increased risk of death in PH patients receiving a kidney transplant, and Xiong and colleagues[30] reported a more than threefold increased risk of death in systemic sclerosis-associated PH.

IMPACT OF ORAL ANTICOAGULANT ON ADVERSE OUTCOMES IN PULMONARY HYPERTENSION PATIENTS

As reported above, both PAH and CTEPH recognize a specific indication for treatment with OAC.[6] The importance of OAC in both patients with PAH and CTEPH has been clear since the earlier article studying the various forms of PH, underlining the role of thrombotic mechanisms in the developing of both conditions.[31] Although nowadays the advances of specific pharmacological therapy for PAH reduced the importance of OAC in those patients, it remains a mainstay for treatment of patients with CTEPH.[31] Since the earlier studies reporting specific data about the use of vitamin K antagonists (VKAs) in PH patients, it became clear how the use of OAC would have been useful to reduce the risk of death on long-term follow-up.[32]

In a systemic review and meta-analysis published in 2018, Khan and colleagues[33] aimed to summarize the evidence available about the effectiveness of OAC in PAH. In this study, which included data about more than 2,500 patients, OAC was associated with a significant reduction in risk of death (hazard ratio [HR] 0.72, 95% CI 0.57–0.93), particularly in patients with idiopathic PAH.[33] Importantly, in the 12 studies included in the meta-analysis, in almost all of them VKAs were the only OAC used. Furthermore, modeling data seem to confirm the beneficial effect of OAC in idiopathic PAH patients, with a significant improvement in risk of outcomes and gain in terms of quality of life.[34]

Table 1
Main outcome data coming from observational registries in patients with pulmonary hypertension

Study, Year	Geographic Location	Patients	FU	Outcomes
Humbert et al,[24] 2006	France	674 *Prevalent: 553* *Incident: 121*	1 year	Mortality in Incident Group: 11.6%
Pepke-Zaba et al,[13] 2011	Europe/Canada	679	NR	Overall Mortality: 9.9%
Ling et al,[25] 2012	UK/Ireland	482	5 years	Overall Mortality: 26.8% 1-year Survival: 92.7% 2-year Survival: 84% 3-year Survival: 73.3% 5-year Survival: 61.1%
Frost et al,[26] 2013	US	3001	2 years	Overall Survival: 80.2% ± 0.7% Overall Survival-Free from Major Events: 78.9% ± 0.8% Clinically Worsened: 1340 (44.6%) Overall Mortality: 6.53%
Kerr et al,[27] 2021	US	750 *Operated: 566* *Operable/No Surgery: 88* *Inoperable: 96*	1 year	*WHO Functional Classes:* *Operated: III 82.9%* *Operable/No Surgery: III 56%* *Inoperable: III 48.2%*
Chang et al,[23] 2022	US	935	496 days[a]	Overall Mortality: 12.9% 1-year Mortality: 8% 2-year Mortality: 16% 3-year Mortality: 21%

Abbreviations: FU, Follow-Up; NR, Not Reported; US, United States; UK, United Kingdom; WHO, World Health Organization.
[a] Median follow-up.

The use of OAC in CTEPH is pivotally indicated by its thromboembolic origin, even though this indication has not been supported by specific studies and the specific evidence is substantially scarce.[2] Since their introduction, the direct oral anticoagulants (DOACs) have become an attracting treatment option for patients with CTEPH and generally for PH patients.[31] Notwithstanding, so far only very few observational studies have addressed this issue.[35] Recently, two systematic reviews emerged from the literature.[36,37] In the article by Sedhom and colleagues, six cohorts were included in the systematic review, for a total of 2145 patients. In this study, the investigators underlined a trend in lower risk of major bleeding in patients treated with DOACs, with a still contradictory impact in terms of thrombotic event recurrence.[37] In another systematic review and meta-analysis, presented during the latest American College of Cardiology meeting, the investigators included four observational studies with a total of 1750 patients with CTEPH, showing a safety advantage of DOACs treatment.[36] Indeed, although there was no significant difference in terms thrombotic event recurrence (odds ratio [OR] 2.07, 95% CI 0.65–6.65), the risk of major bleeding was significantly lower with DOACs than VKAs (OR 0.51, 95% CI 0.28–0.93),[36] also with no relevant heterogeneity regarding this pooled outcome data (I^2 0%). Interestingly, the investigators also reported a strong trend in reduction of risk of death (OR 0.45, 95% CI 0.20–1.01, $P = 0.05$), despite a moderate-to-high heterogeneity (I^2 66%). Clearly, these data need to be further confirmed in larger cohorts, hopefully in a randomized controlled trial.

CHOICE OF ORAL ANTICOAGULANT DRUGS

VKAs are a group of OACs that act by antagonizing the effect of vitamin K and thus decreasing the levels of vitamin K-dependent coagulation factors (II, VII, IX, and X). VKAs are drugs with a large body of clinical experience, low cost and widely available. The main disadvantages of VKA are the requirement for frequent monitoring and the several food and drug interactions. VKAs have been for decades the treatment of choice in patients with atrial fibrillation and VTE.[38,39]

On the other hand, DOACs are OACs introduced more than a decade ago, indicated as first option in patients with atrial fibrillation and VTE.[39,40] Their mechanism of action consists in inhibiting factor Xa (rivaroxaban, apixaban, and edoxaban) or thrombin (dabigatran). They do not require regular monitoring of levels and have less drug-to-drug interactions than VKAs.[38–41]

Choice of Oral Anticoagulant in Patients with Pulmonary Arterial Hypertension

Interruption and consequent modulation of the coagulation cascade should theoretically improve survival in patients with PAH. This presents a plausible rationale for the use of OAC in PAH. However, because of the nonexistence of randomized controlled trials on anticoagulation versus placebo for the treatment of PH, effectiveness, and benefits of OAC therapy in these patients is confined to observational data.[6,9]

Hence, the evidence regarding the use of anticoagulation in patients with idiopathic PAH is mostly based in small series and retrospective studies.[32,42,43] As already reported, Khan and colleagues[33] performed a systematic review, which reported a moderate risk of bias, to examine the impact of adjunctive OAC in patients with PAH. In 11 of the 12 studies included, patients received warfarin as anticoagulant therapy. In the remaining study, 93% patients received warfarin, 6% heparins, and only 1% were treated with DOACs.[42] Thus, warfarin has been the treatment of choice when anticoagulation is considered in patients with PAH, based on the available experience. Interestingly, international normalized ratio (INR) is targeted at 1.5 to 2.5 in many centers in the United States and Japan,[19,44] whereas many European centers target INR at 2 to 3. Based on the aforementioned studies, guidelines recommend the use of warfarin in patients with PAH when anticoagulation is considered.[6,19,45]

Currently, there is no evidence to support the use of DOACs in patients with PAH. There is no published study regarding the use of DOAC in these patients.[29] Several factors may limit the use of DOACs in patients with PAH. Renal and hepatic failure is frequent in patients with PAH, and this may limit the use of DOACs and might increase the risk of bleeding and decrease the efficacy of the drug.[46] Also, DOACs may present drug–drug interactions with PH-targeted therapies. DOACs bioavailability might be increased by P-glycoprotein (P-gp) or CYP3A4 inhibition, thus increasing the risk of bleeding. Type 5 phosphodiesterase inhibitors (sildenafil, tadalafil, and vardenafil) are P-gp inhibitors, whereas other therapies such as prostanoid receptor agonist (selexipag), guanylate cyclase stimulator (riociguat), or endothelin antagonist (ambrisentan) are P-gp substrates.[47]

Choice of Oral Anticoagulant in Patients with Chronic Thromboembolic Pulmonary Hypertension

The use of OAC is considered the first step and the cornerstone in the management of CTEPH. In fact, the diagnosis of CTEPH is based on findings obtained after at least 3 months of effective anticoagulation.[6] There is a general agreement that therapeutic OAC should be continued indefinitely, regardless of the surgical or medical treatment of CTEPH, although as already reported this recommendation has not been validated in a clinical trial.[7] Guidelines recommend the use of VKAs as the treatment of choice, given the scarce evidence of DOACs in this setting.[2,6]

As addressed above, the currently available evidence comes exclusively from observational studies, also with conflicting results. A recent study compared consecutive CTEPH patients undergoing PEA between 2007 and 2018 (794 treated with VKAs and 206 with DOACs). Hemodynamic outcomes, bleeding events and mortality were similar in both groups, but VTE recurrence was higher with DOACs (0.76% vs 4.62% person-year, $P = 0.008$).[48] However, another study including 501 CTEPH patients between 2011 and 2018 (312 treated with warfarin and 134 with rivaroxaban) found that major bleeding was significantly higher with warfarin (HR 1.94, 95% CI 1.05–3.62), with no difference in the rates of VTE recurrence (HR 1.21, 95% CI 0.64–2.23).[49] Hayashi and colleagues[50] compared 120 CTEPH patients (70 treated with VKA and 50 treated with DOACs), and they found no significant differences in the risk of bleeding or VTE recurrence.

Results coming from single studies, as well as the pooled data coming from the recent systematic reviews and meta-analyses,[36,37] suggest that DOACs represent a safe alternative to VKAs and also underline the need for more solid and well-conducted studies to elucidate the actual impact of DOACs versus VKAs in patients with CTEPH and PAH, also taking proper account of issues regarding bioaccumulation and drug–drug interactions.[51]

GUIDELINES RECOMMENDATIONS

The ESC and the European Respiratory Society (ERS) published their last guidelines on the diagnosis and treatment of PH back in 2015[6] (**Table 2**). The experts recommended the use of OAC in patients with idiopathic PAH, hereditary PAH and PAH due to anorexigens (Recommendation Class IIb, Level of Evidence C). This recommendation was based on single-center experience and retrospective studies. However, ESC/ERS guidelines did not give recommendations regarding the type of OAC to be used, indicating that the role of DOACs was still unclear.[6] There is less evidence regarding the use of oral anticoagulation in patients with Eisenmenger syndrome due to the

high risk of thrombosis and bleeding. In these patients, oral anticoagulation should only be considered in cases of PA thrombosis, signs of heart failure, and absent or mild hemoptysis (Recommendation Class IIb, Level of Evidence C). In patients with PAH associated with connective tissue disease, OAC may be considered on an individual basis and in the presence of thrombophilia predisposition (Recommendation Class IIb, Level of Evidence C) according to ESC/ERS guidelines. In patients with PAH associated with portal hypertension, OAC is not recommended due to high risk of bleeding (Recommendation Class III, Level of Evidence C).[6] In patients with PAH associated with Human Immunodeficiency Virus (HIV) infection, OAC is also not recommended due to high bleeding risk and the lack of data on the efficacy/risk ratio (Recommendation Class III, Level of Evidence C). In patients with CTEPH, lifelong anticoagulation is recommended (Recommendation Class I, Level of Evidence C), even after PEA. Again, experts indicated the absence of data on the efficacy and safety of DOACs in these patients.

The Spanish Society of Pulmonology and Thoracic Surgery Guidelines, published in 2018, give similar recommendations, including OAC for patients with idiopathic PAH, heritable PAH, and PAH caused by anorexigens. OAC is also recommended for patients with CTEPH, and the experts recommend the use of VKAs, as there is no evidence with sufficient strength to support the use of DOACs.[45]

Interestingly, the CHEST Guideline and Expert Panel Report on Therapy for Pulmonary Hypertension in Adults, published in 2019, chose not to make any recommendations regarding the use of OAC in patients with PAH. The experts found that studies addressing anticoagulation in PAH patients could not be included in meta-analysis due to the small sample, different interventions, and different subpopulations.[52]

SUMMARY

In this narrative, the authors summarized the evidence regarding the use of OAC in patients with PH, specifically those with PAH and CTEPH. The presence of both conditions entails an increased risk for adverse outcomes, particularly an increased risk of all-cause death. Even though coming exclusively from observational studies, current evidence underlines a beneficial effect of OAC therapy in these patients, beyond the other pharmacological therapy. Despite appearing as a promising alternative to VKAs, the use of DOACs in these patients is still debated and demands more evidence (**Fig. 1**).

Table 2
ESC guidelines recommendations regarding OAC in patients with pulmonary hypertension

Type of PH	OAC Recommended	Choice of OAC	Class of Recommendation	Level of Evidence
Idiopathic PAH	Yes	VKAs	IIb	C
Hereditary PAH	Yes	VKAs	IIb	C
PAH due to Anorexigens	Yes	VKAs	IIb	C
PAH due to Congenital Heart Disease	No (consider if pulmonary artery thrombosis or signs of heart failure)	-	IIb	C
PAH with Connective Tissue Disease	No (consider if thrombophilia predisposition)	-	IIb	C
PAH Associated with Portal Hypertension	No	-	III	C
PAH associated with HIV	No	-	III	C
Chronic Thromboembolic Pulmonary Hypertension	Yes	VKA	I	C

Abbreviations: HIV, Human Immunodeficiency Virus; OAC, Oral Anticoagulant; PAH, Pulmonary Artery Hypertension; VKAs, Vitamin K Antagonists.

This article clearly underlines how, in the context of a currently advanced clinical management and pharmacotherapy,[16] patients with both PAH and CTEPH are still burdened by significant morbidity and mortality.[6,20] Thus, irrespective of the overall low prevalence and incidence of this condition, figures regarding the risk of adverse outcomes, in particular mortality, seem to be still unacceptably high. In this light, the use of OAC seems to remain an important and pivotal mainstay of the overall treatment of these patients. This is certainly true even when considering the general evidence about the effectiveness of OAC in reducing mortality also in other clinical scenarios.[53]

Standing on these premises seems important to obtain more solid and clear evidence about the impact of OAC in PH patients. Indeed, as underlined, if the international guidelines now

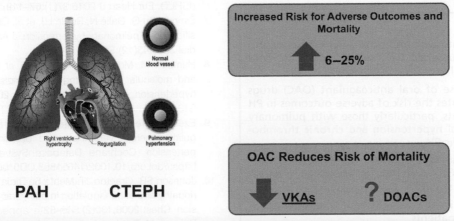

Increased Risk for Adverse Outcomes and Mortality

6–25%

OAC Reduces Risk of Mortality

VKAs   ? DOACs

PAH   CTEPH

Fig. 1. Impact and use of OAC in patients with pulmonary hypertension. CTEPH, chronic thromboembolic pulmonary hypertension; DOACs, direct oral anticoagulants; OAC, oral anticoagulant; PAH, pulmonary artery hypertension; VKAs, vitamin K antagonists.

recommend the use of OAC with substantially high degree of recommendation, this evidence is basically supported by a limited number of observational studies, weakening the strength of evidence.[6] Such lack of a strong scientific background could seem in some way unacceptable, considering the important clinical impact of this condition. Moreover, more studies are strongly needed to understand whether the use of DOACs could significantly reduce the risk of adverse outcomes without any relevant safety concern. Given the availability of these drugs, which surely made possible an important implementation of OAC therapy in other conditions, as atrial fibrillation, it seems pivotal to clarify their possible role in managing PH patients.[31]

Moreover, given the important impact of PH on patients' health, we can underline how the use of OAC and specific pharmacological therapy are important cornerstones of a clinical management that should be more comprehensive and holistic to address the many clinical consequences of PH presence.[20] This aligns with a more modern approach that is now suggested for several cardiovascular conditions.[40,54,55]

In conclusion, the use of OAC, particularly VKAs, is substantially recommended in patients with PAH and CTEPH, given the important risk of adverse outcomes they could experience and the positive impact of these drugs on this risk. Notwithstanding, given the substantial lack of solid evidence, more studies are needed to better substantiate guidelines recommendations. This is particularly needed to clarify the possible utility of DOACs in this clinical scenario, which still demands more evidence.

CLINICS CARE POINTS

- Patients with pulmonary hypertension (PH) are burdened with relevant morbidity and mortality.

- The use of oral anticoagulant (OAC) drugs mitigates the risk of adverse outcomes in PH patients, particularly those with pulmonary arterial hypertension and chronic thromboembolic PH.

- Data so far support the use of vitamin K antagonists, even though based on observational studies.

- So far is still unclear the role of direct OACs in these patients.

- More data are needed to better substantiate guidelines in the future

FUNDING

None.

DISCLOSURE

All the authors declare no significant disclosure to be declared.

REFERENCES

1. Demelo-Rodriguez P, Galeano-Valle F, Salzano A, et al. Pulmonary embolism: a practical guide for the busy clinician. Heart Failure Clin 2020;16(3):317–30.

2. Konstantinides Sv, Meyer G, Becattini C, et al. 2019 ESC Guidelines for the diagnosis and management of acute pulmonary embolism developed in collaboration with the European Respiratory Society (ERS). Eur Heart J 2020;41(4):543–603.

3. Boon GJAM, Huisman Mv, Klok FA. Determinants and management of the post–pulmonary embolism syndrome. Semin Respir Crit Care Med 2021;42(02):299–307.

4. Klok FA, van der Hulle T, den Exter PL, et al. The post-PE syndrome: a new concept for chronic complications of pulmonary embolism. Blood Rev 2014;28(6):221–6.

5. Hoeper MM, Bogaard HJ, Condliffe R, et al. Definitions and diagnosis of pulmonary hypertension. J Am Coll Cardiol 2013;62(25):D42–50.

6. Galiè N, Humbert M, Vachiery J-L, et al. 2015 ESC/ERS Guidelines for the diagnosis and treatment of pulmonary hypertension: The Joint Task Force for the Diagnosis and Treatment of Pulmonary Hypertension of the European Society of Cardiology (ESC) and the European Respiratory Society (ERS): Endorsed by: association for European Paediatric and Congenital Cardiology (AEPC), International Society for Heart and Lung Transplantation (ISHLT). Eur Heart J 2016;37(1):67–119.

7. Simonneau G, Galiè N, Rubin LJ, et al. Clinical classification of pulmonary hypertension. J Am Coll Cardiol 2004;43(12):S5–12.

8. Humbert M, Morrell NW, Archer SL, et al. Cellular and molecular pathobiology of pulmonary arterial hypertension. J Am Coll Cardiol 2004;43(12):S13–24.

9. Ezedunukwe IR, Enuh H, Nfonoyim J, et al. Anticoagulation therapy versus placebo for pulmonary hypertension. Cochrane Database Syst Rev 2014. https://doi.org/10.1002/14651858.CD010695.pub2.

10. Johnson SR, Granton JT, Mehta S. Thrombotic arteriopathy and anticoagulation in pulmonary hypertension. Chest 2006;130(2):545–52.

11. Delcroix M, Torbicki A, Gopalan D, et al. ERS statement on chronic thromboembolic pulmonary hypertension. Eur Respir J 2021;57(6):2002828.

12. Dorfmüller P, Günther S, Ghigna M-R, et al. Microvascular disease in chronic thromboembolic pulmonary hypertension: a role for pulmonary veins and systemic vasculature. Eur Respir J 2014;44(5):1275–88.

13. Pepke-Zaba J, Delcroix M, Lang I, et al. Chronic thromboembolic pulmonary hypertension (CTEPH): results from an international prospective registry. Circulation 2011;124(18):1973–81.

14. Klok FA, Dzikowska-Diduch O, Kostrubiec M, et al. Derivation of a clinical prediction score for chronic thromboembolic pulmonary hypertension after acute pulmonary embolism. J Thromb Haemost 2016;14(1):121–8.

15. Klok FA, Tesche C, Rappold L, et al. External validation of a simple non-invasive algorithm to rule out chronic thromboembolic pulmonary hypertension after acute pulmonary embolism. Thromb Res 2015;135(5):796–801.

16. Kim NH, Delcroix M, Jais X, et al. Chronic thromboembolic pulmonary hypertension. Eur Respir J 2019;53(1):1801915.

17. Claeys M, Claessen G, la Gerche A, et al. Impaired cardiac reserve and abnormal vascular load limit exercise capacity in chronic thromboembolic disease. JACC: Cardiovasc Imaging 2019;12(8):1444–56.

18. Klok FA, Ageno W, Ay C, et al. Optimal follow-up after acute pulmonary embolism: a position paper of the European Society of Cardiology Working Group on Pulmonary Circulation and Right Ventricular Function, in collaboration with the European Society of Cardiology Working Group on Atherosclerosis and Vascular Biology, endorsed by the European Respiratory Society. Eur Heart J 2022;43(3):183–9.

19. Fukuda K, Date H, Doi S, et al. Guidelines for the treatment of pulmonary hypertension (JCS 2017/JPCPHS 2017). Circ J 2019;83(4):842–945.

20. Rosenkranz S, Howard LS, Gomberg-Maitland M, et al. Systemic consequences of pulmonary hypertension and right-sided heart failure. Circulation 2020;141(8):678–93.

21. Yaghi S, Novikov A, Trandafirescu T. Clinical update on pulmonary hypertension. J Investig Med 2020;68(4):821–7.

22. Papamatheakis DG, Poch DS, Fernandes TM, et al. Chronic Thromboembolic Pulmonary Hypertension. J Am Coll Cardiol 2020;76(18):2155–69

23. Chang KY, Duval S, Badesch DB, et al. Mortality in pulmonary arterial hypertension in the modern era: early insights from the pulmonary hypertension association registry. J Am Heart Assoc 2022;11(9).

24. Humbert M, Sitbon O, Chaouat A, et al. Pulmonary arterial hypertension in france. Am J Respir Crit Care Med 2006;173(9):1023–30.

25. Ling Y, Johnson MK, Kiely DG, et al. Changing demographics, epidemiology, and survival of incident pulmonary arterial hypertension. Am J Respir Crit Care Med 2012;186(8):790–6.

26. Frost AE, Badesch DB, Miller DP, et al. Evaluation of the predictive value of a clinical worsening definition using 2-year outcomes in patients with pulmonary arterial hypertension. Chest 2013;144(5):1521–9.

27. Kerr KM, Elliott CG, Chin K, et al. Results from the United States chronic thromboembolic pulmonary hypertension registry. Chest 2021;160(5):1822–31.

28. Kolte D, Lakshmanan S, Jankowich MD, et al. Mild pulmonary hypertension is associated with increased mortality: a systematic review and meta-analysis. J Am Heart Assoc 2018;7(18). https://doi.org/10.1161/JAHA.118.009729.

29. Brinza C, Covic A, Stefan AE, et al. Pulmonary arterial hypertension and adverse outcomes after kidney transplantation: a systematic review and meta-analysis. J Clin Med 2022;11(7):1944.

30. Xiong A, Liu Q, Zhong J, et al. Increased risk of mortality in systemic sclerosis-associated pulmonary hypertension: a systemic review and meta-analysis. Adv Rheumatol 2022;62(1):10.

31. Bertoletti L, Mismetti V, Giannakoulas G. Use of anticoagulants in patients with pulmonary hypertension. Hämostaseologie 2020;40(03):348–55.

32. Rich S, Kaufmann E, Levy PS. The effect of high doses of calcium-channel blockers on survival in primary pulmonary hypertension. N Engl J Med 1992;327(2):76–81.

33. Khan MS, Usman MS, Siddiqi TJ, et al. Is Anticoagulation Beneficial in Pulmonary Arterial Hypertension? Circ Cardiovasc Qual Outcomes 2018;11(9). https://doi.org/10.1161/CIRCOUTCOMES.118.004757.

34. Jose A, Eckman MH, Elwing JM. Anticoagulation in pulmonary arterial hypertension: a decision analysis. Pulm Circ 2019;9(4):1–12.

35. Brokmeier H, Kido K. Off-label use for direct oral anticoagulants: valvular atrial fibrillation, heart failure, left ventricular thrombus, superficial vein thrombosis, pulmonary hypertension—a systematic review. Ann Pharmacother 2021;55(8):995–1009.

36. Burmeister C, Ghazaleh S, Patel N, et al. Direct Oral Anticoagulants Versus Vitamin K Antagonists for The Treatment of Chronic Thromboembolic Pulmonary Hypertension: A Systematic Review and Meta-Analysis. J Am Coll Cardiol 2022;79(9):1655.

37. Sedhom R, Megaly M, Gupta E, et al. Use of direct oral anticoagulants in chronic thromboembolic pulmonary hypertension: a systematic review. J Thromb Thrombolysis 2022;53(1):51–7.

38. Salzano A, Demelo-Rodriguez P, Marra AMAM, et al. A focused review of gender differences in antithrombotic therapy. Curr Med Chem 2017;24(24):2576–88.

39. Stevens SM, Woller SC, Baumann Kreuziger L, et al. Executive summary: antithrombotic therapy for VTE disease: second update of the CHEST guideline

and expert panel report. Chest 2021;160(6): 2247–59.

40. Hindricks G, Potpara T, Dagres N, et al. 2020 ESC Guidelines for the diagnosis and management of atrial fibrillation developed in collaboration with the European Association for Cardio-Thoracic Surgery (EACTS). Eur Heart J 2021;42(5):373–498.

41. Corsini A, Ferri N, Proietti M, et al. Edoxaban and the issue of drug-drug interactions: from pharmacology to clinical practice. Drugs 2020;80(11):1065–83.

42. Olsson KM, Delcroix M, Ghofrani HA, et al. Anticoagulation and survival in pulmonary arterial hypertension: results from the Comparative, Prospective Registry of Newly Initiated Therapies for Pulmonary Hypertension (COMPERA). Circulation 2014;129(1): 57–65.

43. Fuster V, Steele PM, Edwards WD, et al. Primary pulmonary hypertension: natural history and the importance of thrombosis. Circulation 1984;70(4):580–7.

44. McLaughlin Vv, Archer SL, Badesch DB, et al. ACCF/AHA 2009 Expert Consensus Document on Pulmonary Hypertension. J Am Coll Cardiol 2009; 53(17):1573–619.

45. Barberà JA, Román A, Gómez-Sánchez MÁ, et al. Guidelines on the diagnosis and treatment of pulmonary hypertension: summary of recommendations. Archivos de Bronconeumologia 2018;54(4):205–15.

46. Gabriel L, Delavenne X, Bedouch P, et al. Risk of direct oral anticoagulant bioaccumulation in patients with pulmonary hypertension. Respiration 2016; 91(4):307–15.

47. Margelidon-Cozzolino V, Delavenne X, Catella-Chatron J, et al. Indications and potential pitfalls of anticoagulants in pulmonary hypertension: Would DOACs become a better option than VKAs? Blood Rev 2019;37:100579.

48. Bunclark K, Newnham M, Chiu Y, et al. A multicenter study of anticoagulation in operable chronic thromboembolic pulmonary hypertension. J Thromb Haemost 2020;18(1):114–22.

49. Sena S, Bulent M, Derya K, et al. Real-life data of direct anticoagulant use, bleeding risk and venous thromboembolism recurrence in chronic thromboembolic pulmonary hypertension patients: an observational retrospective study. Pulm Circ 2020;10(1): 1–10.

50. Hayashi H, Tsuji A, Ueda J, et al. Comparison of efficacy and safety between direct oral anticoagulant and warfarin in patients with chronic thromboembolic pulmonary hypertension. Circulation 2018; 138:A15733.

51. Porres-Aguilar M, Hoeper MM, Rivera-Lebron BN, et al. Direct oral anticoagulants in chronic thromboembolic pulmonary hypertension. J Thromb Thrombolysis 2021;52(3):791–6.

52. Klinger JR, Elliott CG, Levine DJ, et al. Therapy for pulmonary arterial hypertension in adults: update of the chest guideline and expert panel report. Chest 2019;155(3):565–86.

53. Rivera-Caravaca JM, Roldán V, Esteve-Pastor MA, et al. Cessation of oral anticoagulation is an important risk factor for stroke and mortality in atrial fibrillation patients. Thromb Haemost 2017;117(6).

54. Romiti GF, Pastori D, Rivera-Caravaca JM, et al. Adherence to the "atrial fibrillation better care" pathway in patients with atrial fibrillation: impact on clinical outcomes-a systematic review and meta-analysis of 285,000 patients. Thromb Haemost 2022;122(3):406–14.

55. Lip GYH, Lane DA, Lenarczyk R, et al. Integrated care for optimizing the management of stroke and associated heart disease: a position paper of the European Society of Cardiology Council on Stroke. Eur Heart J 2022;43(26):2442–60.

Management of COVID-19 in Patients with Pulmonary Arterial Hypertension

Ioannis T. Farmakis, MD, MSc[a,b], George Giannakoulas, MD, PhD[a,*]

KEYWORDS

• COVID-19 • Pulmonary arterial hypertension • PAH-targeted therapies • Pulmonary hypertension

KEY POINTS

• PAH is significant comorbidity that can lead to unfavorable outcomes during COVID-19.
• PAH-targeted therapies should be continued during the course of COVID-19.
• The development of chronic pulmonary hypertension after COVID-19 remains to be investigated.

INTRODUCTION

The COVID-19 pandemic has caused more than 6 million deaths worldwide as of April 2022, while model data suggest that the toll of the pandemic on mortality could be at least three times greater.[1] Early in the course of the pandemic, observational studies from China indicated that patients with comorbidities were particularly vulnerable to complications from the SARS-CoV-2 infection and at high risk for severe disease and mortality.[2] Patients with a history of cardiovascular disease, diabetes, and cancer remain at increased risk for complications from COVID-19. In fact, nationwide inpatient data from Germany show that deceased hospitalized patients were more commonly elderly (≥70 years), with a higher Charlson comorbidity index compared with survivors, and were more likely to suffer from cardiovascular comorbidities (hypertension 52%, coronary artery disease 23%, and heart failure 31%).[3]

On the other hand, pulmonary arterial hypertension (PAH) is associated with significant morbidity and mortality. In PAH, elevated pulmonary vascular resistance and the development of decompensated right heart response are eventually the key mechanisms leading to death for most of the patients. PAH-related hospitalizations amount to ~30 per million population annually and are associated with 6% inpatient mortality.[4] A primary cardiac discharge diagnosis is recorded in almost half of the PAH-related hospitalizations, but primary cardiac hospitalizations show a decreasing trend from 2001 to 2014 falling from 52.9% to 41.4% of all hospitalizations.[5] Extra-cardiac reasons for hospitalization in patients with PAH are overall associated with greater inpatient mortality than a primary cardiac diagnosis (6.9% vs 5.3%). Remarkably, a sepsis diagnosis is associated with a 25% risk for inpatient mortality, while pneumonia with 9.4% and respiratory insufficiency or arrest with 21.4%.

The aforementioned evidence and rationale suggest that patients with PAH could be at increased risk for complications and, subsequently, worse outcomes following COVID-19. In this review, we discuss the evidence regarding the course and the management of COVID-19 in patients with PAH, the challenges in PAH management during the pandemic and, lastly, the long-term complications of COVID-19 in relation to pulmonary vascular disease (**Fig. 1**).

Type of submission: Review article.
[a] Department of Cardiology, AHEPA University Hospital, Stilp. Kiriakidi 1, Thessaloniki 54637, Greece; [b] Center for Thrombosis and Hemostasis, University Medical Center Mainz, Langebeckstr. 1, 55131, Mainz, Germany
* Corresponding author. Aristotle University of Thessaloniki, AHEPA Hospital, Cardiology Department, Stilp. Kiriakidi 1, Thessaloniki 54637, Greece.
E-mail address: ggiannakoulas@auth.gr

Heart Failure Clin 19 (2023) 107–114
https://doi.org/10.1016/j.hfc.2022.07.003
1551-7136/23/© 2022 Elsevier Inc. All rights reserved.

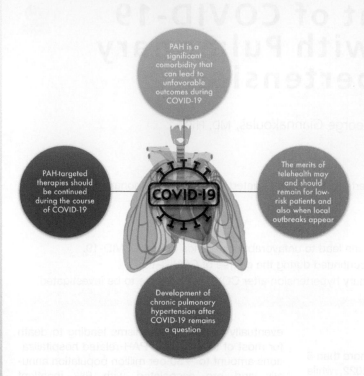

Fig. 1. The interplay between pulmonary hypertension and COVID-19

PAH is a significant comorbidity that can lead to unfavorable outcomes during COVID-19

PAH-targeted therapies should be continued during the course of COVID-19

The merits of telehealth may and should remain for low-risk patients and also when local outbreaks appear

COVID-19

Development of chronic pulmonary hypertension after COVID-19 remains a question

EARLY EVIDENCE: COULD PATIENTS WITH PULMONARY ARTERIAL HYPERTENSION HAVE FAVORABLE OUTCOMES DURING COVID-19 INFECTION?

Early studies in the course of the pandemic showed controversial results regarding the outcome of patients with PAH and suggested that the SARS-CoV-2 infection could have a favorable outcome in this population (**Table 1**). A case series of 13 patients from more than 32 US expert PH centers in late March 2020 showed that intubation was required only in 3 patients, while only one patient died.[6] Similarly, in a case series of 4 patients in the Lombardy region of Italy, none of the patients developed acute right heart failure and all survived the disease.[7] Lastly, a case series from Spain comprising 10 patients with PAH and COVID-19 (7 of them in a low-risk status) showed that 70% of patients required hospitalization, while none of them died, an unexpectedly favorable outcome.[8] These results led the investigators to form hypotheses that certain pathophysiological features of PAH, as well as benefits attributed to the targeted medical PAH therapies could lead to a protective effect in COVID-19. The suggested mechanisms included reduced viral entrance through decreased angiotensin-converting enzyme (ACE)-2 expression in PAH, an attenuated response to lung perfusion changes due to basal abnormal lung perfusion in PAH and chronic

vasodilator treatment, especially the protective effect of endothelin receptor antagonists against acute respiratory distress syndrome (ARDS).

FURTHER EVIDENCE

The largest study conducted comes from the French PH registry and included 211 patients with precapillary PH (among them 58.3% with a diagnosis of PAH) and a diagnosis of COVID-19 from February 2020 to April 2021.[9] In this prospective cohort, 32.2% of patients were hospitalized in a common ward, while an additional 27.5% of patients were hospitalized in an intensive care unit (ICU); the median length of stay was 9[5–15] days. High-flow nasal cannula and corticosteroids were increasingly used after September 2020, while the proportion of patients receiving mechanical ventilation (11.1%) was similar between the 2 first waves of the pandemic. One-fourth of patients (24.6%) died (23% among group 1 PH), the proportion was 41.3% of hospitalized patients. Half of the patients who died and nearly a quarter of the hospitalized ones had documented limitations to care escalation (incl. do-not-resuscitate orders). The study was powered for limited inferential analysis regarding mortality; however, significant predictors of mortality were male sex, older age, and comorbidities (including chronic renal failure and chronic lung disease), which were more significant than the PH group per se.

Table 1
Studies reporting COVID-19 infection among patients with pulmonary arterial hypertension

Study	Centers	Countries	Study Period	Population	N of patients	COVID-19 Incidence	Hospitalization Rate	Case Fatality Rate
Sulica et al,[39] 2021	1	US	March–May 2020	PAH + CTEPH	11	3.1%	81.8%	45.4%
Horn et al,[6] 2020	32	US	Late March 2020	PAH	13	NR	53.8%	7.7%
Scuri et al,[7] 2020	1	Italy	NR	PAH	4	NR	100%	0%
Nuche et al,[8] 2020	1	Spain	Until 10 April 2020	PAH	10	2.9%	70%	0%
Belge et al,[10] 2020	47	28 countries worldwide	17 April 2020–10 May 2020	PAH + CTEPH	70	NR	70%	19%
Lee et al,[11] 2020	58	US	17–24 April 2020	PAH + CTEPH	50	0.29%	30%	12%
Farmakis et al,[12] 2022	9	Greece	February 2020-August 2021	PAH + CTEPH	18	3.6%	44.4%	22.2%
Badagliacca et al,[13] 2022	25	Italy	1 March 2020–1 May 2020	PAH	20	0.46%	45%	45%
Godinas et al,[29] 2021	Patient survey	52 countries worldwide	May–June 2020	PAH + CTEPH	9	1%	NR	NR
Montani et al,[9] 2022	26	France	February 2020-April 2021	Precapillary PH	211	2.7%	59.7%	24.6%

Abbreviations: PAH, pulmonary arterial hypertension; CTEPH, chronic thromboembolic pulmonary hypertension.

Two large surveys conducted early in the pandemic, one led by European investigators and one from the US, provide more evidence and confirm such findings regarding the outcomes of COVID-19 in patients with PAH. In the survey of 47 PH centers from 28 countries worldwide (including 18 European countries), 70 COVID-19 cases were reported among PAH or chronic thromboembolic pulmonary hypertension (CTEPH) patients from 17 April 2020 to 10 May 2020.[10] The median age of the cohort was 50 to 59 years and most patients (59%) were under a combination of targeted PAH therapies. The outcomes were not favorable for this PH cohort, since 46% were hospitalized in general wards, and 17% required ICU admission, while mortality was high (20%) for patients with PAH.

The US survey was conducted from 17 April 2020 to 1 May 2020 among 58 center directors of expert PH clinics. A total of 50 patients with PAH or CTEPH with recognized COVID-19 were reported; the cumulative incidence of COVID-19 among this population was similar to the concurrent at the time CDC population estimate of COVID-19 cumulative incidence in the general US population. The results were similar to the European cohort, since 30% of patients were hospitalized (22% in an ICU) and 12% of patients died.[11]

We have recently conducted a study among 9 expert PH centers in Greece, cumulatively for 499 patients with PAH or CTEPH, covering a larger period of the pandemic, from late February 2020 (beginning of the pandemic in Greece) to late August 2021.[12] We reported 18 cases with PAH or CTEPH and COVID-19, and among them 12 cases with PAH. The incidence risk of COVID-19 among the PH population was 3.6%, lower than the concurrent incidence risk of 4.8% among the Greek general population. In the PAH subgroup, the hospitalization rate was 33.3% and the mortality rate was 16.7% (2/12 patients). Of the 2 patients who died, one was greater than 75 years old with a history of cancer, while the other one had significant comorbidities. Both required long-term oxygen therapy at home, indicating the severity of the underlying disease.

Lastly, in an Italian nationwide multicenter survey, the incidence of COVID-19 during the first peak of the pandemic (March–May 2020) was comparable to the general population, however, mortality was 45% (9 patients out of 20 patients with confirmed SARS-CoV-2 infection in total).[13]

Collectively, the aforementioned results indicate that the earlier data and the more recent observations do not match and that PAH is significant comorbidity that can lead to unfavorable outcomes during COVID-19 (see **Table 1**). In our opinion,

additional comorbidities among patients with PAH (such as diabetes mellitus, obesity, and cardiopulmonary comorbidities), as well as advanced age, play an important role in the severity of the underlying pulmonary vascular pathology, perhaps even a larger one. Frailty has been shown to be a better predictor of disease outcomes in COVID-19 than age and comorbidities alone[14] and we suggest that this also applies to the PAH population, whereby age, comorbidities, functional status, as well as the inherent PAH disease characteristics act synergistically to define prognosis. However, we must bear in mind that all of these studies were conducted during the prevaccination era, and also do not concern the Omicron variants. Thus, the characteristics of the pandemic are now changed and, therefore, different case fatality and hospitalization rates may apply to the PAH population as well.

MANAGEMENT OF SARS-CoV-2 INFECTION IN PULMONARY ARTERIAL HYPERTENSION

In general, SARS-CoV-2 infection in the context of PAH should be managed according to the current SARS-CoV-2 treatment guidelines; however, several considerations must be accounted for, especially when it comes to drug–drug interactions.[15] All experts and societies agree that PAH-targeted medication should be continued in patients with PAH during the course of infection with SARS-CoV-2. Drug treatment should be continued irrespective of the severity of COVID-19 in patients with PAH to maintain clinical stability and avoid right heart decompensation.

Although patients with PAH are particularly vulnerable and comorbid, postexposure prophylaxis to SARS-CoV-2 with monoclonal antibodies is no longer recommended because the Omicron variant, which is now predominant in most countries, is not susceptible to them. The introduction of new antiviral therapies changed the landscape of the nonsevere (no need for oxygen or hospitalization) COVID-19 management for the general population, since drugs such as molnupiravir, nirmatrelvir-ritonavir, but also remdesivir, have received a conditional recommendation for patients who are at risk for progressing to severe COVID-19. However, nirmatrelvir-ritonavir is a strong CYP3A inhibitor and, therefore, coadministration with PDE5 inhibitors is prohibited and must be avoided because it increases the concentration of these PAH drugs. In addition, bosentan, riociguat, and calcium channel blockers may also have potential interactions and the coadministration is not recommended. On the other hand, no significant interactions are expected with the use of molnupiravir and PAH-targeted therapy.

The management of hospitalized and unstable patients with PAH and concomitant COVID-19 is particularly challenging as hypoxia and the systemic inflammatory response are difficult to treat.[16] PAH-targeted drug treatment should be continued, although its composition or route of administration (for example i.v. for patients who cannot tolerate oral treatment or intubated patients) must be discussed with the PH expert team. The management of ventilation is difficult. In general, efforts must be concentrated to maintain an oxygen saturation greater than 90% and high-flow nasal cannula is an important ally toward that goal. However, in case of persistent hypercapnia, noninvasive ventilation may benefit patients, but it must be used with caution because it can further impair right ventricular function. Intubation should be discouraged in patients with PAH because of the high risk of death during the induction of general anesthesia. Maintaining a stable blood pressure (with systemic vasopressors), optimizing the fluid status (removal of excess fluids with diuretics or hemofiltration), and supporting the cardiac output (with careful use of inotropes) is of particular importance.[16] Concerning COVID-19 specific treatment its use in patients with PAH and severe or critical COVID-19 is recommended. From September 2020 using data from the SOLIDARITY and RECOVERY trials systemic corticosteroids are strongly recommended for patients with severe or critical COVID-19.[15] In addition, there is a strong recommendation for the use of interleukin-6 inhibitors (tocilizumab or sarilumab) in this group of patients.[15]

The use of PAH-targeted medication in the treatment of COVID-19 in patients without baseline PAH has a theoretic basis due to the proven anti-inflammatory effects and reduction effects on pulmonary artery blood pressure, lung edema, and remodeling of drugs such as endothelin receptor antagonists, phosphodiesterase 5 inhibitors, riociguat and prostacyclin.[17] However, their use could also be dangerous since a drop in pulmonary blood pressure in patients with lung lesions might result in an increase in ventilation/perfusion mismatch and a decrease in blood oxygenation. Some clinical studies showed positive results for the use of inhaled vasodilators (inhaled epoprostenol, iloprost, or nitric oxide) or iloprost in Pao_2/Fio_2; however, their use is not yet studied in randomized studies.[18–20] In addition, studies for the use of endothelin antagonists or PDE5 inhibitors in severe COVID-19 without baseline PAH are lacking.[21] Only recently, a noncontrolled study of 25 patients with COVID-19 pneumonitis showed suggested good toleration of sildenafil, without hemodynamic, oxygenation, or dead space

deterioration and amelioration in echocardiography and biomarkers.[22]

Lastly, we should bear in mind that vaccination is the most effective way to prevent infection with SARS-CoV-2 and the potentially fatal and disabling complications of COVID-19. All patients with PAH should receive a primary and booster vaccination and follow the general vaccination planning recommendations as these will form in the future. Significant efforts should be made by the treating physicians to reassure patients and reduce their anxiety regarding the potential adverse events of vaccines. No safety concerns in this particular subgroup of patients have been reported.[23]

PULMONARY ARTERIAL HYPERTENSION AMBULATORY TREATMENT DURING THE PANDEMIC

Similar to other chronic diseases, the management of patients with PH in general, and PAH in particular, has been considerably challenging during the pandemic. The "exposure risk" of these vulnerable patients for routine follow-up, diagnostic or laboratory testing was high, especially in the earlier phases of the pandemic. In addition, the diagnostic pathway of incident PAH cases, as well as the initiation and up-titration of new PAH-targeted therapies during the pandemic was particularly challenging.

In a large survey among Italian centers, Badagliacca and colleagues observed a 71.4% reduction of in-person visits during the first 2 months of the pandemic (March–April 2020) compared with the same period in 2019 with a similar reduction to conducted paraclinical tests.[13] A similar decline in patients visits, diagnostic testing, and overall clinic staffing was observed in a multicenter survey from the US.[11] The most common reason for declining visits was a hospital/health system mandate, as well as the fear of patients and physicians for the contraction of COVID-19. In another worldwide survey conducted from 17 April 2020 to 10 May 2020, 8 out of 10 patients with either PAH or CTEPH were provided with a remote consultation (either by video- or teleconferencing), whereas only 3% of them did not receive any consultation at all during this pandemic period.[10]

COVID-19 has imposed a significant burden on the health care system and has subsequently caused a disruption of clinical care pathways for chronic diseases such as PAH. In PAH, it is important to maintain a close relationship between the patient and the caring PAH expert center, since tight monitoring and treatment titration is mandated to achieve stratification in the low-risk category and avoid hazardous clinical outcomes.[24] Especially in the earlier phases of the pandemic, it was important to streamline chronic outpatient care to achieve 2 goals: (i) offload physicians who dealt with the increasing workload in the inpatient service and (ii) protect patients from an environment of increased infection risk such as the outpatient health services. Telehealth programs exploit the advantage of video conference and have been introduced during the pandemic to remotely evaluate and monitor the symptoms and functional status of patients.[25] Although telemonitoring does not permit a comprehensive physical examination or extensive diagnostic tests, it has been increasingly used, and according to our experience they help expert centers reach medical decisions regarding interventions and therapy titration.[26] In a study from a Japanese referral PH center, telemedicine was effective in reducing travel distances and suggested that social networking-video calls may be useful, especially for patients who need advanced care, such as patients receiving parenteral prostanoids.[27] However, older patients may experience difficulties adjusting to the new technologies and therefore more frequent, telephone visits, rather than video-call visits, would be desirable to reduce anxiety. The overall impact of the first waves of the pandemic on depression and anxiety in patients with PAH has been substantial, with problems stemming mostly from the fear of contracting COVID-19 and the difficulties in specialized care access.[28,29]

Lately, in the new phases of the pandemic, which are characterized by vaccination coverage, including boosters, and also the dominance of the Omicron variant with subsequent milder forms of COVID-19, chronic care is gradually returning to prepandemic levels. It is to acknowledge though that the merits of telehealth may and should remain for particularly stable, low-risk patients and also when local outbreaks appear.

LONG-TERM COMPLICATIONS OF COVID-19 IN RELATION TO PULMONARY VASCULAR DISEASE IN PATIENTS WITHOUT BASELINE PULMONARY HYPERTENSION

The SARS-CoV-2 is a virus that shows great affinity to the endothelium and significant vascular changes have been described in patients with COVID-19. These vascular changes can affect both the macro-as well as the microvasculature, and are evident in the whole vascular wall, from the lumen to the perivascular regions, as a result of thrombotic in situ microangiopathy and a complex immune-inflammatory cascade.[30] Some patients continue to experience symptoms following the acute phase of COVID-19, the so-called "long COVID" syndrome, pertaining to persistent damage in several organs, including the pulmonary vasculature.[31] The changes observed in the lung vessels of patients with COVID-19 share many common features with the ones observed in patients with PH; namely, medial hypertrophy and smooth muscle cell proliferation.[32] The prevalence of PH during the acute phase of COVID-19 is also high.[33,34] In a study of 21 mechanically ventilated patients with COVID-19 who underwent right heart catheterization, low pulmonary vascular resistance, coherent with a blunted hypoxic vasoconstriction, high cardiac output and postcapillary pulmonary hypertension characterized the hemodynamic profile.[35] In addition, there is a known increased incidence of pulmonary embolism, as well as in situ pulmonary thrombosis, in patients with COVID-19, as well as in those recovering from COVID-19, which could theoretically predispose to an increased incidence of chronic thromboembolic disease in the future.[36-38] Taken together, these data have sparkled the hypothesis that COVID-19 could predispose to the development of chronic PH. However, this is a subject of future investigation since long-term cohort studies are still lacking.

SUMMARY

PAH is serious comorbidity that can have a negative impact on the clinical outcomes related to COVID-19. Prognosis is determined by a combination of the underlying PAH disease features and risk stratification, along with other factors such as age, functional status, and comorbidities. The treatment of mild and severe COVID-19 in patients with PAH should follow the general recommendations, and PAH-targeted treatments should not be interrupted during the course of the disease. The epidemic has placed significant stress on PAH chronic care, prompting a move toward telemedicine. Finally, COVID-19 may increase the risk of developing chronic PH in patients without baseline PH; however, long-term evidence is currently scarce.

CLINICS CARE POINTS

- Nirmatrelvir-ritonavir is a strong CYP3A inhibitor and, therefore, coadministration with PAH drugs is prohibited and must be avoided.

- PAH-targeted drug treatment should be continued, although its composition or route of administration must be discussed with the PH expert team.

- High-flow nasal cannula is an important ally toward maintaining oxygen saturation in severe COVID-19. In case of persistent hypercapnia, noninvasive ventilation may benefit patients, but it must be used with caution. Intubation should be discouraged in patients with PAH because of the high risk of death.

- Limitation of care is a case-by-case decision and not categorical.

FUNDING

None to declare.
  Conflicts of interest.

AUTHORS' CONTRIBUTION

I.T. Farmakis and G. Giannakoulas contributed to the conception or design of the work. IF and GG contributed to the acquisition, analysis, or interpretation of data for the work. IF drafted the article. GG critically revised the article. Both gave final approval and agreed to be accountable for all aspects of the work ensuring integrity and accuracy.

ACKNOWLEDGMENTS

None to declare.

REFERENCES

1. COVID-19 Excess Mortality Collaborators. Estimating excess mortality due to the COVID-19 pandemic: a systematic analysis of COVID-19-related mortality, 2020-21. Lancet Lond Engl 2022; S0140-6736(21):02796–2803.

2. Honardoost M, Janani L, Aghili R, et al. The Association between Presence of Comorbidities and COVID-19 Severity: A Systematic Review and Meta-Analysis. Cerebrovasc Dis Basel Switz 2021; 50(2):132–40.

3. Hobohm L, Sagoschen I, Barco S, et al. Trends and Risk Factors of In-Hospital Mortality of Patients with COVID-19 in Germany: Results of a Large Nationwide Inpatient Sample. Viruses 2022 Jan 28;14(2): 275.

4. Chaturvedi A, Kanwar M, Chandrika P, et al. National trends and inpatient outcomes of pulmonary arterial hypertension related hospitalizations - Analysis of the National Inpatient Sample Database. Int J Cardiol 2020;319:131–8.

5. Harder EM, Small AM, Fares WH. Primary cardiac hospitalizations in pulmonary arterial hypertension:

6. Horn EM, Chakinala M, Oudiz R, et al. Could pulmonary arterial hypertension patients be at a lower risk from severe COVID-19? Pulm Circ 2020;10(2). 204589402092279.

7. Scuri P, Iacovoni A, Abete R, et al. An unexpected recovery of patients with pulmonary arterial hypertension and SARS-CoV-2 pneumonia: a case series. Pulm Circ 2020 Jul;10(3). 204589402095658.

8. Nuche J, Pérez-Olivares C, Segura de la Cal T, et al. Clinical course of COVID-19 in pulmonary arterial hypertension patients. Rev Esp Cardiol Engl Ed 2020;73(9):775–8.

9. Montani D, Certain MC, Weatherald J, et al. COVID-19 in Patients with Pulmonary Hypertension: A National Prospective Cohort Study. Am J Respir Crit Care Med 2022.

10. Belge C, Quarck R, Godinas L, et al. COVID-19 in pulmonary arterial hypertension and chronic thromboembolic pulmonary hypertension: a reference centre survey. ERJ Open Res 2020;6(4): 00520–2020.

11. Lee JD, Burger CD, Delossantos GB, et al. A Survey-based Estimate of COVID-19 Incidence and Outcomes among Patients with Pulmonary Arterial Hypertension or Chronic Thromboembolic Pulmonary Hypertension and Impact on the Process of Care. Ann Am Thorac Soc 2020;17(12):1576–82.

12. Farmakis IT, Karyofyllis P, Frantzeskaki F, et al. Incidence and outcomes of COVID-19 in patients with pulmonary arterial hypertension and chronic thromboembolic pulmonary hypertension: Data from the Hellenic pulmOnary hyPertension rEgistry (HOPE). Hell J Cardiol HJC Hell Kardiologike Epitheorese 2022;64:93–6.

13. Badagliacca R, Papa S, D'Alto M, et al. The paradox of pulmonary arterial hypertension in Italy in the COVID-19 era: is risk of disease progression around the corner? Eur Respir J 2022;2102276.

14. Hewitt J, Carter B, Vilches-Moraga A, et al. The effect of frailty on survival in patients with COVID-19 (COPE): a multicentre, European, observational cohort study. Lancet Public Health 2020;5(8): e444–51.

15.. Therapeutics and COVID-19: living guideline [Internet]. 2020. https://www.who.int/publications/i/item/therapeutics-and-covid-19-living-guideline. [Accessed 25 February 2022].

16. Hoeper MM, Benza RL, Corris P, et al. Intensive care, right ventricular support and lung transplantation in patients with pulmonary hypertension. Eur Respir J 2019;53(1):1801906.

17. Puk O, Nowacka A, Smulewicz K, et al. Pulmonary artery targeted therapy in treatment of COVID-19 related ARDS. Literature review. Biomed Pharmacother 2022;146:112592.

Trends and outcomes from 2001 to 2014. Respir Med 2020;161:105850.

18. Moezinia CJ, Ji-Xu A, Azari A, et al. Iloprost for COVID-19-related vasculopathy. Lancet Rheumatol 2020;2(10):e582–3.

19. Sonti R, Pike CW, Cobb N. Responsiveness of Inhaled Epoprostenol in Respiratory Failure due to COVID-19. J Intensive Care Med 2021;36(3):327–33.

20. Matthews L, Baker L, Ferrari M, et al. Compassionate use of Pulmonary Vasodilators in Acute Severe Hypoxic Respiratory Failure due to COVID-19. J Intensive Care Med 2022. 8850666221086521.

21. Castiglione L, Droppa M. Pulmonary Hypertension and COVID-19. Hamostaseologie 2021.

22. McFadyen C, Garfield B, Mancio J, et al. Use of sildenafil in patients with severe COVID-19 pneumonitis. Br J Anaesth 2022;(22):S0007–912, 00186-6.

23. Wieteska-Miłek M, Szmit S, Florczyk M, et al. COVID-19 Vaccination in Patients with Pulmonary Arterial Hypertension and Chronic Thromboembolic Pulmonary Hypertension: Safety Profile and Reasons for Opting against Vaccination. Vaccines 2021;9(12):1395.

24. Galiè N, Humbert M, Vachiery JL, et al. 2015 ESC/ERS Guidelines for the diagnosis and treatment of pulmonary hypertension: The Joint Task Force for the Diagnosis and Treatment of Pulmonary Hypertension of the European Society of Cardiology (ESC) and the European Respiratory Society (ERS): Endorsed by: Association for European Paediatric and Congenital Cardiology (AEPC), International Society for Heart and Lung Transplantation (ISHLT). Eur Heart J 2016;37(1):67–119.

25. Wesley Milks M, Sahay S, Benza RL, et al. Risk assessment in patients with pulmonary arterial hypertension in the era of COVID 19 pandemic and the telehealth revolution: State of the art review. J Heart Lung Transplant 2021;40(3):172–82.

26. Ryan JJ, Melendres-Groves L, Zamanian RT, et al. Care of patients with pulmonary arterial hypertension during the coronavirus (COVID-19) pandemic. Pulm Circ 2020;10(2). 204589402092015.

27. Tamura Y, Takeyasu R, Furukawa A, et al. How COVID-19 Affected the Introduction of Telemedicine and Patient Reported Outcomes Among Patients With Pulmonary Hypertension — A Report From a Referral Center in Japan. Circ Rep 2020;2(9):526–30.

28. Wieteska-Miłek M, Szmit S, Florczyk M, et al. Fear of COVID-19, Anxiety and Depression in Patients with Pulmonary Arterial Hypertension and Chronic Thromboembolic Pulmonary Hypertension during the Pandemic. J Clin Med 2021;10(18):4195.

29. Godinas L, Iyer K, Meszaros G, et al. PH CARE COVID survey: an international patient survey on the care for pulmonary hypertension patients during the early phase of the COVID-19 pandemic. Orphanet J Rare Dis 2021;16(1):196.

30. Halawa S, Pullamsetti SS, Bangham CRM, et al. Potential long-term effects of SARS-CoV-2 infection on the pulmonary vasculature: a global perspective. Nat Rev Cardiol 2022;19(5):314–31.

31. Nalbandian A, Sehgal K, Gupta A, et al. Post-acute COVID-19 syndrome. Nat Med 2021;27(4):601–15.

32. Suzuki YJ, Nikolaienko SI, Shults NV, et al. COVID-19 patients may become predisposed to pulmonary arterial hypertension. Med Hypotheses 2021;147:110483.

33. Pagnesi M, Baldetti L, Beneduce A, et al. Pulmonary hypertension and right ventricular involvement in hospitalised patients with COVID-19. Heart Br Card Soc 2020;106(17):1324–31.

34. Norderfeldt J, Liliequist A, Frostell C, et al. Acute pulmonary hypertension and short-term outcomes in severe Covid-19 patients needing intensive care. Acta Anaesthesiol Scand 2021;65(6):761–9.

35. Caravita S, Baratto C, Di Marco F, et al. Haemodynamic characteristics of COVID-19 patients with acute respiratory distress syndrome requiring mechanical ventilation. An invasive assessment using right heart catheterization. Eur J Heart Fail 2020;22(12):2228–37.

36. Xie Y, Xu E, Bowe B, et al. Long-term cardiovascular outcomes of COVID-19. Nat Med 2022;28(3):583–90.

37. Katsoularis I, Fonseca-Rodríguez O, Farrington P, et al. Risks of deep vein thrombosis, pulmonary embolism, and bleeding after covid-19: nationwide self-controlled cases series and matched cohort study. BMJ 2022;377:e069590.

38. Bikdeli B, Madhavan MV, Jimenez D, et al. COVID-19 and Thrombotic or Thromboembolic Disease: Implications for Prevention, Antithrombotic Therapy, and Follow-Up: JACC State-of-the-Art Review. J Am Coll Cardiol 2020;75(23):2950–73.

39. Sulica R, Cefali F, Motschwiller C, et al. COVID-19 in Pulmonary Artery Hypertension (PAH) Patients: Observations from a Large PAH Center in New York City. Diagnostics 2021;11(1):128.

Impact of Hormonal-Anabolic Deficiencies in Idiopathic Pulmonary Arterial Hypertension

Alberto M. Marra, MD, PhD[a,b,1,*], Anna D'Agostino, PhD[c,1],
Andrea Salzano, MD, PhD[c], Stefania Basili, MD[d], Michele D'Alto, MD, PhD[e],
Eduardo Bossone, MD, PhD[f], Antonio Cittadini, MD[a,b],
Carmine Dario Vizza, MD[d], Roberto Badagliacca, MD, PhD[d]

KEYWORDS

- Pulmonary arterial hypertension • Anabolic deficiencies • Hormones

KEY POINTS

- The presence of multiple hormone deficiencies is associated with a worse WHO functional class and exercise capacity in patients with PAH and this is the first study that systematically analyses an extended panel of hormone axes in this pathology.
- Multiple hormonal deficits characterize a subgroup of patients with worse exercise capacity, pulmonary hemodynamics, right ventricular remodeling, and function. These parameters were even more impaired when the hormone deficit was of greater severity.
- Our study could be considered the first step for paving the way for a series of studies on the impact and involvement of anabolic deficiencies in PAH.

INTRODUCTION

Pulmonary hypertension (PH) is a clinical condition defined by an increased resting mean pulmonary artery pressure (mPAP) with values greater than or equal to 20 mm Hg, invasively measured through right heart catheterization.[1]

The most common consequence of this condition is an increase in right ventricular afterload, which may lead to right heart failure and patient death.[2] Indeed, clinical manifestations and survival are closely associated with the ability of the right heart to adapt to the increasing pressures in the pulmonary circulation.[3] Because of this adaptation process a progressive structural and functional deterioration of the right heart occurs.[2] Several conditions might cause pulmonary hypertension. Chiefs among these are left-sided heart failure, lung parenchymal or interstitial diseases, and chronic thromboembolic disease.

Pulmonary arterial hypertension (PAH) is a rare but well-characterized form of PH whose hallmark is a pulmonary vasculopathy.[4] Usually, PAH is further divided into different subgroups: idiopathic

[a] Department of Translational Medical Sciences, "Federico II" University of Naples, Via Pansini 5, 80131, Napoli, Italy; [b] Interdepartmental Center for Biomaterials (CRIB), "Federico II" University of Naples, Piazzale Tecchio, 80 - 80125 - Napoli, Italy; [c] IRCCS SYNLAB SDN, Via Emanuele Gianturco, 113, 80143 Napoli, Italy; [d] Department of Translational and Precision Medicine, Sapienza University of Rome, Policlinico Umberto I, Viale Regina Elena 324, Rome 00161, Italy; [e] Department of Cardiology, Monaldi Hospital - University "L. Vanvitelli", Via Leonardo Bianchi, 80131 Napoli, Italy; [f] Cardiology Division, Antonio Cardarelli Hospital, Via Antonio Cardarelli, 9 - 80131, Naples, Italy

[1] These authors contributed equally.

* Corresponding author. Department of Translational Medical Sciences, University of Naples "Federico II", Via Pansini 5, Napoli 80131, Italy.

E-mail address: albertomaria.marra@unina.it

Heart Failure Clin 19 (2023) 115–123
https://doi.org/10.1016/j.hfc.2022.09.001
1551-7136/23/© 2022 Elsevier Inc. All rights reserved.

forms, hereditary forms, forms related to drug intake or exposure to toxins, forms associated with systemic diseases such as connective tissue disease, HIV infection, forms related to portal hypertension or, albeit less frequently, schistosomiasis. Although PAH can be defined as a rare disease, with an estimated prevalence of 15 to 50 cases per million, the prevalence of this condition in at-risk groups is considerably higher.[5] Hence, the need to identify subgroups of patients with pulmonary hypertension that need more attention and deeper investigation for closer clinical follow-up and more aggressive treatment strategies.[5]

In the last two decades, a growing interest has been given to the anabolic/catabolic imbalance in cardiovascular diseases, especially in chronic left heart failure,[6–10] which is the leading cause of pulmonary hypertension. The anabolic hormone axes (testosterone, dehydroepiandrosterone, growth hormone/insulin-like growth factor 1, insulin resistance) are commonly depressed in left heart failure and associated with compromised clinical conditions and increased mortality.[11–13] Notably, preliminary studies have shown that hormone replacement therapy could improve surrogate prognostic markers in patients with this condition.[14–17] Anabolic hormone deficiencies (AD) are probably also present in PAH for several reasons. Firstly, the presence of clear myopathy in patients with PAH,[18] considering that skeletal muscle is a target tissue for anabolic hormones. Secondly, the central role played by inflammatory activation in PAH could ultimately result in anabolic damage.[18,19] However, the prevalence, association with clinical variables, and impact on outcomes of hormone-anabolic deficits in PAH has not been studied so far. Therefore, the aim of this study was to assess the role of multiple hormone-metabolic deficits in idiopathic pulmonary arterial hypertension.

MATERIAL AND METHODS
Study Design

This analysis was conducted retrospectively on patients with idiopathic pulmonary arterial hypertension who were consecutively admitted from 1 January 2009 to 1 January 2013, to the Departmental Operative Unit of the Umberto I Polyclinic Hospital-University of Rome. All consecutive patients with a diagnosis of pulmonary arterial hypertension according to current European guidelines,[20] who had undergone a six-minute walk test (6MWT), cardiac magnetic resonance imaging, and functional class assessment according to World Health Organization criteria were included in the analysis.

Patients with significant left heart disease, significant respiratory disease, presence of ventilatory/perfusion scintigraphy suggestive of thrombo-embolic disease were excluded from the analysis. Patients who did not have values of the 5 hormones that were chosen for the study were also excluded, specifically: -Testosterone -Dehydroepiandrostenedione sulfate (DHEA-S) -Insulin-like growth factor 1 (IGF-1) -Insulin and blood glucose -Thyroid hormones (t3, t4 and TSH).

Right Cardiac Catheterization

The resting examination was performed as previously described[21] in the supine position using transjugular access with an 7F introducer set (MXI100, MEDEX, Smiths Group PLC, UK). Catheterization was performed with triple-lumen 7F-Swan-Ganz thermodilution catheters from Edwards Lifesciences (REF:131F7, Edwards Lifesciences LLC, Irvine, CA, USA). Pressures were continuously recorded and averaged over several respiratory cycles during spontaneous breathing. Cardiac output (CO) was measured by thermodilution by averaging 3 measurements with less than 10% variation between measured values. The zero-reference point for pressure recordings was set at mid-thoracic level according to the 2015 ESC/ERS guidelines.[1] Pulmonary vascular resistance (PVR) was calculated using the formula PVR=(mPAP-PWP)/CO. Pulmonary artery compliance was calculated as the ratio of stroke volume to pulse pressure (SV/PP): SV/PP (mL/mm Hg) = (stroke volume)/(pulmonary systolic pressure - diastolic pressure).

Cardiac Magnetic Resonance

All CMR studies were performed with a 1.5-T unit (Avanto Siemens, Erlangen, Germany) using dedicated cardiac software, phase array surface receiver coil, and ECG activation, within 1 week of RHC performance. Biventricular masses and volumes were determined using a cine free-precession, steady-state CMR technique at constant breath-hold, acquired in both horizontal and short-axis planes fully embracing both ventricles with a stack of contiguous slices. All CMR studies were analyzed off-line with the consent of 2 experienced observers using a dedicated workstation with cardiac software. (CMR 42, Circle Canada). Cine CMR was used to quantify RV and left ventricular (LV) volumes (using 4-chamber stacks), RV and ejection fraction (EF), and RV and LV masses. Image contours were plotted semiautomatically at end-diastole and end-systole from horizontal long axis planes, corresponding measurements with short axis images when necessary. For the measurement of RV mass, we considered the RV free wall thickness and 1/3 of the RV interventricular septum free wall thickness. Papillary muscle and trabeculations were included in the cavity, while special care was taken to exclude the atrium from the contours in base slices.

Hormonal Analysis

Blood samples were collected by venipuncture after overnight fasting. To obtain serum and plasma, samples were centrifuged within 1 hour, frozen, and stored at −80°C until analysis. Serum hormones were analyzed in a dedicated core-lab (IRCSS-SDN, Naples, Italy) in collaboration with the Clinical Coordination Center. Insulin and insulin growth factor-1 (IGF1) were analyzed with an enzyme-labeled chemiluminescent immunoassay (IMMULITE 2000; IGF-1, inter-test variation = 5, 7% CV, Siemens Medical Solutions Diagnostics). Total testosterone was measured with a DPC Coat-ACount RIA kit. DHEA-S was measured with a competitive solid-phase chemiluminescent immunoassay. Hormonal deficits were defined as follows: i) IGF-1 deficiency: serum IGF-1 levels below the 33rd percentile of a healthy control population: 122 ng/mL (age < 55 years); 109 ng/mL (55 years < age < 64.9 years); 102 ng/dL (65 years < age < 74 years). 9 years; 99 ng/dL (age > 75 years) [8]; (ii) testosterone deficiency (TD): serum testosterone levels below 300 ng/dL in male and below 25 ng/dL in female; DHEA-S deficiency: serum DHEAS levels below 80 µg/dL; low T3: serum free T3 below 2 pg/mL (3.).1 mmol/L); insulin resistance (IR): the presence of type 2 diabetes mellitus or HomeOstasis Model Assessment (HOMA-Index) greater than 2.5 (according to the formula: IR = insulin (mcU/mL) x glucose (mmol/L)/22.5). Patients were further divided into 2 groups reflecting the subsequent number of anabolic deficiencies: (1) patients with one anabolic deficiency or no deficit (MHDS-) and (2) patients with 2 or more anabolic deficiencies (ie,: MHDS)

Statistical Analysis

Normally distributed continuous variables were expressed as mean ± Standard Deviation (SD), while continuous data with nonnormal distributions were expressed as the median and interquartile range [IQR]. Categorical variables were expressed as counts and percentages. The distribution of the variables was tested with the Kolmogorov–Smirnov test. Student's t-test for unpaired data was used to assess the difference in clinical parametric between patients with MHDS-

and MHDS + . MHDS + PATIENTS. Associations between the analyzed variables and survival were established using Cox proportional hazards regression analyses. Both univariate and multivariable linear models were used to evaluate potential predictors of survival. In univariate analyses, demographic, biochemical, disease-related, clinical, and instrumental parameters were included. Regarding the anabolic status, we considered the single deficiency, the sum of deficiencies (from 0 = no deficiency to 5 = deficiency in all 5 axes), or the presence of an MHDS (0 = no MDHS, 1 = presence of MHDS). In addition, the severity of MHDS was assessed and classified as follows: (1 deficit = mild MHDS, 2 deficits = medium MDHS, 3 or more deficits = severe MHDS). Statistical analyses were performed using R version 3.0 (http://www.rproject.org) and version 25.0 (SPSS Inc, Chicago, Illinois, USA). A value of $P < 0.05$ was considered statistically significant.

RESULTS

A total of 46 patients were considered. After excluding 16 patients as not measuring all hormonal axes, the final population consisted of 30 patients. The mean age of the patients was 56.6 ± 13.7 years (47.0 ± 14.6 in men and 61.4 ± 10.6 in women). **Table 1** describes the general characteristics of this patient population.

Prevalence of Hormone Deficiency in Idiopathic Pulmonary Hypertension

According to the previously defined cut-offs, 1 patient presented no deficit (3.3%), 16 patients a single deficit (53.3%), 5 patients 2 deficits (16.7%), 6 patients had 3 deficits (20.0%), 1 patient had 4 deficits (3.3%) and finally, 1 patient had 5 deficits (3.3%) (**Fig. 1** panel A).

Regarding individual deficits, 5 (16.7%) patients had IGF-1 deficiency, 23 (76.7%) patients had DHEA-S deficiency, 12 patients had testosterone deficiency (40%), 6 (20%) patients were insulin resistant, and low t3 syndrome was present in 7 (23.3%) patients (**Fig. 1** panel B-F).

Multiple Hormone Deficits and Clinical Parameters in Pulmonary Arterial Hypertension Pulmonary Arterial Hypertension

Table 1 shows the differences in the main clinical parameters examined between patients with no hormone deficits or with a single deficit (MHDS-) plus concomitant hormone deficits (≥2, MHDS + deficits). MHDS + showed worse WHO

Table 1
Baseline characteristics of patients with PAH divided according to the number of deficiencies

Parametro		MHDS−	MHDS+	P value
BMI	(Kg/mq)	26.6 ± 5.0	26.3 ± 6.6	ns
WHO class	(II,III,IV)	10,6,1	2,9,1	0.03
6MWD	(m)	456.9 ± 70.4	380.1 ± 66.1	0.012
sPAP	(mm Hg)	64.9 ± 22.7	80.6 ± 17.1	ns
mPAP	(mm Hg)	40.8 ± 12.8	57.4 ± 9.3	0.012
dPAP	(mm Hg)	25.1 ± 8.5	40.6 ± 4.8	0.0001
Cardiac Index	(l/mq)	2.6 ± 0.5	2.1 ± 0.6	0.04
wedge	(mm Hg)	9.0 ± 3.5	11.6 ± 2.7	ns
PAC	(mL/mm Hg)	1.8 ± 0.7	1.37 ± 0.8	ns
RV-EDV	(mL)	172.0 ± 48.8	214.5 ± 51.9	ns
RV-ESV	(mL)	93.7 ± 48.9	153.3 ± 51.3	0.01
RV-EF	(%)	37.3 ± 10.1	26.8 ± 16.1	0.05
RV-massa	(g)	80.3 ± 20.8	100.3 ± 18.2	0.03

Abbreviations: 6MWD, six-minutes walking distance; BMI, body mass index; dPAP, diastolic pulmonary arterial pressure; EDV, end-diastolic volume; EF, ejection fraction; ESV, end-systolic volume; MHDS, multiple hormonal deficiencies syndrome; mPAP, mean pulmonary arterial pressure; ns, nonsignificant; PAC, pulmonary arterial compliance; RV, right ventricular; sPAP, systolic pulmonary arterial pressure.

Class ($P = 0.03$). Regarding the hemodynamics of the pulmonary circulation, patients with MHDS + had worse mean and diastolic pressures, a reduced cardiac index. In addition, the difference in pulmonary vascular resistance was highly significant ($P < .001$), with a difference of about 5 WU between the 2 groups. Regarding the data from the cardiac MRI examination, patients with multiple deficits were found to have increased right ventricular volumes, slightly reduced pump function, and a greater degree of right ventricular hypertrophy. Dividing according to the severity of the hormone deficits (1 deficit = mild MHDS, 2 = moderate MDHS, 3 or more deficits = severe MHDS) a statistically significant difference was found for the distance covered in the six-minute walking distance test (467.9 ± 70.6 vs 419.4 ± 61.3 vs 380.1 ± 66.1 in mild, moderate, and severe, respectively, p:0.02) **(Fig. 2**A)

A similar difference was found with regard to pulmonary vascular resistance **(Fig. 2**B) (7.3 ± 2.9 vs 8.6 ± 4.4 vs 14.2 ± 0.5 in mild moderate and severe, respectively, p:0.003) and end-diastolic **(Fig. 2**C) (170.4 ± 53.9 vs 178.2 ± 30.3 vs 249.9 ± 43.5, p:0.02) as well as end-systolic **(Fig. 2**D) (91.1 ± 48.1 vs 111.0 ± 53.6 vs 186.5 ± 10.9, in mild, moderate and severe, respectively, p:0.007) volumes, as well as right ventricular ejection fraction **(Fig. 2**E) (37.8 ± 8.9 vs 34.3 ± 14.9 vs 20.7 ± 14.6, in mild moderate and severe, respectively, p:0.05) measured by MRI.

Impact on Outcomes of MHDS in Pulmonary Arterial Hypertension

A total of 14 events were recorded during follow-up, including 10 deaths and 4 hospitalizations. Specifically, among patients in the group with no or single deficiency (n:22), 6 (27%) died and 3 were hospitalized (a total of 9 events). In the multiple-deficiency group (n:8), on the other hand, 4 patients died (50%) while 1 patient was hospitalized. Despite a difference in the combined endpoint of about 20% between the 2 groups and a 23% difference in the occurrence of the death event, the low sample size did not allow statistical significance to be reached (p: 0.278 for the composite of mortality and hospitalization, p:0.237 for mortality, **Fig. 3**).

DISCUSSION

To our knowledge, this is the first study that systematically analyses an extended panel of hormone axes in PAH. According to our data, the presence of multiple hormone deficiencies is associated with a worse WHO functional class and exercise capacity in patients with PAH. In addition, patients with multiple hormone deficiencies have a worse hemodynamic profile characterized by higher pulmonary pressures and reduced cardiac output, translating into higher pulmonary resistances. Another relevant finding is the presence of larger volumes and reduced right ventricular

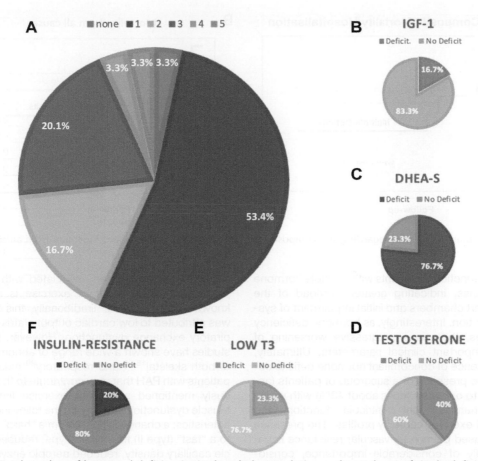

Fig. 1. Total number of hormonal deficiencies in the whole population and prevalence of single deficiency.

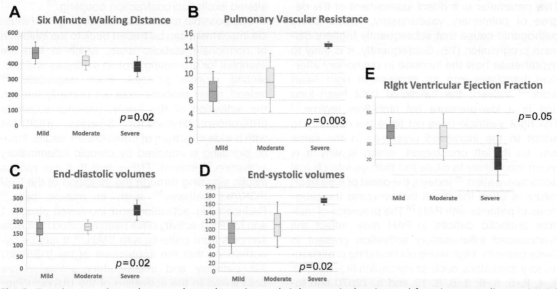

Fig. 2. Exercise capacity, pulmonary hemodynamics, and right ventricular size and function according to MHDS severity.

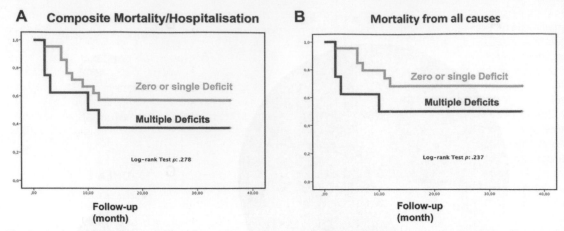

Fig. 3. Kaplan–Meier plot regarding the composite of mortality/hospitalization and mortality from all causes.

systolic function in patients with multiple hormone deficiencies, indicating greater overload of the right heart chambers and initial impairment of systolic function. Interestingly, as hormone deficiency increases, there is a progressive worsening of these important clinical parameters. Ultimately, the presence of concomitant hormone deficits denotes the presence of a subgroup of patients (according to our case series about 43%) with worse hemodynamics, right ventricular function, and reduced exercise capacity profiles. The presence of increased pulmonary vascular resistance is undoubtedly of considerable importance, considering that it is the strongest independent predictor of mortality according to the data from the American REVEAL registry, the registry with the largest number of patients in the world.[22] This parameter is a direct assessment of the degree of pulmonary vasculopathy, which is the pathogenic cause that subsequently triggers disease progression (12). Subsequently, it is easy to hypothesise how the increase in pulmonary afterload translates into an increase in right heart work.[23] Indeed, the functional right heart–lung unit is a low-pressure but high-flow regime.[24] The right ventricle does not have the capacity to adapt to the increased pressures in the same way as its left counterpart, which is why it is much more likely to dilate and then go into clinical decompensation.[25] Indeed, the onset of right heart failure is often the event that worsens the prognosis of patients with PAH.[26] The presence of multiple anabolic deficits in PAH may reflect the pronounced inflammatory activation present in these patients. High levels of circulating proinflammatory mediators, such as interleukin (IL)-1b, IL-2, IL-4, IL-5, IL-6, IL-8, IL-10, and IL-12p70 and tumor necrosis factor (TNF)-a, have been found both in animal models and in patients with

PAH[27,28] and have been associated with worse prognosis.[27] Impairment of exercise is a well-known feature of PAH. Traditionally, this feature was attributed to low cardiac output status or respiratory exchange dysfunction. However, several studies have shown a wide range of abnormalities of both skeletal[18,29] and respiratory[29] muscles in patients with PAH that may contribute to the previously mentioned significant exercise limitation. Muscle dysfunction in PAH has the following characteristics: a change in fibers from a "hard" (type I) to a "fast" (type II) fiber phenotype, reduced muscle capillary density, reduced aerobic enzyme activity, altered mitochondrial biogenesis/function, and increased muscle protein degradation mediated by the ubiquitin/proteasome protection system (UPS), mitochondrial abnormalities, and altered excitation/contraction coupling.[29]

One possible mechanism underlying PAH muscle impairment can be traced back to the inhibition of hormonal/metabolic axes, which in turn are essential for promoting protein synthesis and protecting muscle proteins from degradation.[30] Indeed, many anabolic axes act primarily through the activation of the insulin receptor substrate (IRS)/phosphatidylinositol 3-kinase (PI3K)/Akt with a wide spectrum of downstream results. Insulin signaling is impaired by chronic inflammatory activation.[31] Indeed, TNF-α and IL-6 can reduce insulin signaling through the inhibition of the IRS/PI3K/Akt pathway[32] even in muscle cells.[18] Reduced Akt activation and increased atrogin-1 and MURF-1 activity have been reported in muscle samples from patients with IPAH.[29] It can be hypothesized that the impairment of the IRS/PI3K/Akt pathway and inflammatory activation are both linked to the activation of the Ubiquitin/Proteasome system in PAH that contributes to muscle consumption in PAH.

Data regarding anabolic and hormonal abnormalities in PAH are scanty. Type 2 Diabetes Mellitus seems to be a negative prognostic factor in patients with PAH.[33] An interesting finding also comes from animal studies showing that IGF-1 through the induction of iNOS plays a protective role on pulmonary vascularization in animal models of PAH.[34] One of the most studied mediators in PAH is DHEA. Recently, a study has unequivocally shown that low DHEA-S levels are associated with a poorer prognosis in patients with PAH secondary to connective tissue disease and associated congenital heart disease.[35] Similarly, a protective role on the pulmonary vascular bed has been shown in animal models.[36] Recently, the role of thyroid disease in PAH has also been postulated. Recently, the role of thyroid diseases in PAH has also been postulated, but there are no data on the so-called Low t3 syndrome.[37]

Over the past 2 decades, the scientific community has given considerable attention to the relationship between hormones and the cardiovascular system. The first evidence dates back to the early 1990s when it was shown that patients with hypopituitary died more frequently of cardiovascular diseases. Great efforts have been directed at studying multiple hormonal deficiencies in Chronic Heart Failure (CHF) and one of the suggested hypotheses is that heart failure is not only secondary to the overexpression of biologically active molecules belonging to the adrenergic system, renin-angiotensin, and cytokines but also to the down-regulation of the cardinal hormonal axes.[9] Indeed, it has been shown that the lack of several hormones may be associated with impaired physical performance, but also with reduced survival. Various preliminary studies have been conducted to study the role of individual hormone abnormalities or deficits in CHF. Indeed, according to a recent Italian multicenter registry, the presence of two or more anabolic deficiencies is associated with increased all-cause mortality and cardiovascular hospitalization.[38] Actually, it has been demonstrated that low serum IGF-1 levels are associated with increased inflammatory activation, increased sarcopenia,[15] reduced functional class, reduced exercise capacity, and reduced survival rates.[11] Similarly, it has been shown that testosterone deficiency is also associated with a significant impairment of skeletal muscle function, exercise capacity and poor performance in patients with CHF.[39,40]

Unlike many other biomarkers routinely used and proposed in the daily management of PAH,[41-43] hormone deficiencies have the added advantage of potentially also being a valid therapeutic target, through the clinical application of hormone replacement therapy. This hypothesis has been already tested in left-sided chronic heart failure, whereby several independent groups have demonstrated that GH[14,15] or Testosterone[16] replacement therapy is associated with a significant improvement in some robust surrogate endpoints such as peak V_{O_2}. Our study could be considered the first step for the implementation of similar studies in PAH as well.

SUMMARY

According to our observations, hormonal deficits are very common in idiopathic pulmonary arterial hypertension. Multiple hormonal deficits characterize a subgroup of patients with worse exercise capacity, pulmonary hemodynamics, right ventricular remodeling, and function. These parameters were even more impaired when the hormone deficit was of greater severity. Future studies will have to confirm these data on larger patient samples, possibly trying to assess the possible association between multiple hormone deficits and mortality.

LIMITATIONS

The main limitation of this study is certainly the retrospective nature of the observation. Furthermore, the study is severely limited by the low sample size. However, PAH is a rare disease and the sample presented is the one usually presented in many studies. The sample size limitation also made it impossible to try to assess differences in the clinical outcomes evaluated. Another limitation is that no dynamic tests were performed to assess the hormonal status of the patients. In addition, there were no hormonal evaluations repeated over time. Furthermore, this study was performed only on patients with idiopathic PAH; therefore, the results cannot be generalized to the other forms of PAH associated with other conditions (such as systemic sclerosis, HIV, congenital heart diseases, porto-pulmonary hypertension, schistosomiasis). Finally, there were no measurements such as cytokines, mediators of inflammation, or muscle function that could have better clarified the pathophysiological role of multiple hormone deficits in PAH. However, the aim of this study was to generate a hypothesis regarding the role of hormone deficits in PAH, without the aim of finding any mechanistic link to explain this clinical phenomenon. Future prospective studies involving a larger number of patients may be conducted based on this evidence.

CLINICS CARE POINTS

- The impact of hormonal-anabolic deficiencies on PAH is often overlooked and requires further investigation. Patients with iPAH with multiple hormone deficiencies have a worse hemodynamic profile characterized by higher pulmonary pressures and reduced cardiac output, translating into higher pulmonary resistances.

- It would be advisable to assess the levels of anabolic hormones as multiple hormonal deficits characterize a subgroup of patients with worse exercise capacity, right ventricular remodeling, and function.

DISCLOSURE

The authors have nothing to disclose.

REFERENCES

1. Galiè N, Humbert M, Vachiery JL, et al. [2015 ESC/ERS Guidelines for the diagnosis and treatment of pulmonary hypertension]. Kardiol Pol 2015;73(12):1127–206.

2. Rudski LG, Gargani L, Armstrong WF, et al. Stressing the Cardiopulmonary Vascular System: The Role of Echocardiography. J Am Soc Echocardiogr 2018;31(5):527–50.e11.

3. Harjola VP, Mebazaa A, Čelutkienė J, et al. Contemporary management of acute right ventricular failure: a statement from the Heart Failure Association and the Working Group on Pulmonary Circulation and Right Ventricular Function of the European Society of Cardiology. Eur J Heart Fail 2016;18(3):226–41.

4. Tuder RM, Archer SL, Dorfmüller P, et al. Relevant issues in the pathology and pathobiology of pulmonary hypertension. J Am Coll Cardiol 2013;62(25 Suppl):D4–12.

5. Ling Y, Johnson MK, Kiely DG, et al. Changing demographics, epidemiology, and survival of incident pulmonary arterial hypertension: results from the pulmonary hypertension registry of the United Kingdom and Ireland. Am J Respir Crit Care Med 2012;186(8):790–6.

6. Cittadini A, Bossone E, Marra AM, et al. [Anabolic/catabolic imbalance in chronic heart failure]. Monaldi Arch Chest Dis 2010;74(2):53–6.

7. Bossone E, Arcopinto M, Iacoviello M, et al. Multiple hormonal and metabolic deficiency syndrome in chronic heart failure: rationale, design, and demographic characteristics of the T.O.S.CA. Registry. Intern Emerg Med 2018;13(5):661–71.

8. Merola B, Cittadini A, Colao A, et al. Cardiac structural and functional abnormalities in adult patients with growth hormone deficiency. J Clin Endocrinol Metab 1993;77(6):1658–61.

9. Salzano A, Marra AM, Ferrara F, et al. Multiple hormone deficiency syndrome in heart failure with preserved ejection fraction. Int J Cardiol 2016;225:1–3.

10. Salzano A, De Luca M, Israr MZ, et al. Exercise Intolerance in Heart Failure with Preserved Ejection Fraction. Heart Failure Clin 2021;17(3):397–413.

11. Arcopinto M, Bobbio E, Bossone E, et al. The GH/IGF-1 axis in chronic heart failure. Endocr Metab Immune Disord Drug Targets 2013;13(1):76–91.

12. Arcopinto M, Isgaard J, Marra AM, et al. IGF-1 predicts survival in chronic heart failure. Insights from the T.O.S.CA. (Trattamento Ormonale Nello Scompenso CArdiaco) registry. Int J Cardiol 2014;176(3):1006–8.

13. Salzano A, Cittadini A, Bossone E, et al. Multiple hormone deficiency syndrome: a novel topic in chronic heart failure. Future Sci 2018;4(6):FSO311.

14. Cittadini A, Marra AM, Arcopinto M, et al. Growth hormone replacement delays the progression of chronic heart failure combined with growth hormone deficiency: an extension of a randomized controlled single-blind study. JACC Heart Fail 2013;1(4):325–30.

15. Cittadini A, Saldamarco L, Marra AM, et al. Growth hormone deficiency in patients with chronic heart failure and beneficial effects of its correction. J Clin Endocrinol Metab 2009;94(9):3329–36.

16. Iellamo F, Volterrani M, Caminiti G, et al. Testosterone therapy in women with chronic heart failure: a pilot double-blind, randomized, placebo-controlled study. J Am Coll Cardiol 2010;56(16):1310–6.

17. Xanthouli P, Theobald V, Benjamin N, et al. Prognostic impact of hypochromic erythrocytes in patients with pulmonary arterial hypertension. Respir Res 2021;22(1):288.

18. Marra AM, Arcopinto M, Bossone E, et al. Pulmonary arterial hypertension-related myopathy: an overview of current data and future perspectives. Nutr Metab Cardiovasc Dis 2015;25(2):131–9.

19. Argiento P, Chesler N, Mulè M, et al. Exercise stress echocardiography for the study of the pulmonary circulation. Eur Respir J 2010;35(6):1273–8.

20. Galiè N, Humbert M, Vachiery JL, et al. 2015 ESC/ERS Guidelines for the diagnosis and treatment of pulmonary hypertension: The Joint Task Force for the Diagnosis and Treatment of Pulmonary Hypertension of the European Society of Cardiology (ESC) and the European Respiratory Society (ERS): Endorsed by: Association for European Paediatric and Congenital Cardiology (AEPC), International Society for Heart and Lung Transplantation (ISHLT). Eur Heart J 2016;37(1):67–119.

21. Condliffe R, Kiely DG, Peacock AJ, et al. Connective tissue disease-associated pulmonary arterial hypertension in the modern treatment era. Am J Respir Crit Care Med 2009;179(2):151–7.

22. Farber HW, Miller DP, Poms AD, et al. Five-Year outcomes of patients enrolled in the REVEAL Registry. Chest 2015;148(4):1043–54.

23. Grünig E, Peacock AJ. Imaging the heart in pulmonary hypertension: an update. Eur Respir Rev 2015;24(138):653–64.

24. Amsallem M, Sternbach JM, Adigopula S, et al. Addressing the Controversy of Estimating Pulmonary Arterial Pressure by Echocardiography. J Am Soc Echocardiogr 2016;29(2):93–102.

25. Vonk Noordegraaf A, Westerhof BE, Westerhof N. The Relationship Between the Right Ventricle and its Load in Pulmonary Hypertension. J Am Coll Cardiol 2017;69(2):236–43.

26. Yamada Y, Okuda S, Kataoka M, et al. Prognostic value of cardiac magnetic resonance imaging for idiopathic pulmonary arterial hypertension before initiating intravenous prostacyclin therapy. Circ J 2012;76(7):1737–43.

27. Soon E, Holmes AM, Treacy CM, et al. Elevated levels of inflammatory cytokines predict survival in idiopathic and familial pulmonary arterial hypertension. Circulation 2010;122(9):920–7.

28. Al-Naamani N, Palevsky HI, Lederer DJ, et al. Prognostic Significance of Biomarkers in Pulmonary Arterial Hypertension. Ann Am Thorac Soc 2016;13(1):25–30.

29. Batt J, Ahmed SS, Correa J, et al. Skeletal muscle dysfunction in idiopathic pulmonary arterial hypertension. Am J Respir Cell Mol Biol 2014;50(1):74–86.

30. Pagan J, Seto T, Pagano M, et al. Role of the ubiquitin proteasome system in the heart. Circ Res 2013;112(7):1046–58.

31. Wei Y, Chen K, Whaley-Connell AT, et al. Skeletal muscle insulin resistance: role of inflammatory cytokines and reactive oxygen species. Am J Physiol Regul Integr Comp Physiol 2008;294(3):R673–80.

32. Michell BJ, Griffiths JE, Mitchelhill KI, et al. The Akt kinase signals directly to endothelial nitric oxide synthase. Curr Biol 1999;9(15):845–8.

33. Grinnan D, Farr G, Fox A, et al. The Role of Hyperglycemia and Insulin Resistance in the Development and Progression of Pulmonary Arterial Hypertension. J Diabetes Res 2016;2016:2481659.

34. Jin C, Guo J, Qiu X, et al. IGF-1 induces iNOS expression via the p38 MAPK signal pathway in the anti-apoptotic process in pulmonary artery smooth muscle cells during PAH. J Recept Signal Transduct Res 2014;34(4):325–31.

35. Baird GL, Archer-Chicko C, Barr RG, et al. Lower DHEA-S levels predict disease and worse outcomes in post-menopausal women with idiopathic, connective tissue disease- and congenital heart disease-associated pulmonary arterial hypertension. Eur Respir J 2018;51(6). https://doi.org/10.1183/13993003.00467-2018.

36. Smith AM, Bennett RT, Jones TH, et al. Characterization of the vasodilatory action of testosterone in the human pulmonary circulation. Vasc Health Risk Manag 2008;4(6):1459–66.

37. Sweeney L, Voelkel NF. Estrogen exposure, obesity and thyroid disease in women with severe pulmonary hypertension. Eur J Med Res 2009;14(10):433–42.

38. Cittadini A, Salzano A, Iacoviello M, et al. Multiple hormonal and metabolic deficiency syndrome predicts outcome in heart failure: the T.O.S.C.A. Registry. Eur J Prev Cardiol 2021. https://doi.org/10.1093/eurjpc/zwab020.

39. Jones RD, English KM, Pugh PJ, et al. Pulmonary vasodilatory action of testosterone: evidence of a calcium antagonistic action. J Cardiovasc Pharmacol 2002;39(6):814–23.

40. Arcopinto M, Salzano A, Giallauria F, et al. Growth Hormone Deficiency Is Associated with Worse Cardiac Function, Physical Performance, and Outcome in Chronic Heart Failure: Insights from the T.O.S.C.A. GHD Study. PLoS One 2017;12(1):e0170058.

41. Salzano A, Arcopinto M, Marra AM, et al. Klinefelter syndrome, cardiovascular system, and thromboembolic disease: review of literature and clinical perspectives. Eur J Endocrinol 2016;175(1):R27–40.

42. Kostis JB, Sanders M. The association of heart failure with insulin resistance and the development of type 2 diabetes. Am J Hypertens 2005;18(5 Pt 1):731–7.

43. Doehner W, Frenneaux M, Anker SD. Metabolic impairment in heart failure: the myocardial and systemic perspective. J Am Coll Cardiol 2014;64(13):1388–400.

How to Treat Right Heart Failure. Tips for Clinicians in Everyday Practice

Giulia Crisci, MD[a,b], Roberta D'Assante, PhD[a,b], Valeria Valente, MD[a,b],
Federica Giardino, MD[a,b], Anna D'Agostino, PhD[c], Brigida Ranieri, PhD[c],
Michele Arcopinto, MD, PhD[a,b], Alberto M. Marra, MD, PhD[a,b],
Carmen Rainone, MD[a,b], Michele Modestino, MD[a,b], Salvatore Rega, MD[a],
Ludovica Fulgione, MD[d], Chiara Sepe[e], Giuseppe Caruso, MD[e],
Eduardo Bossone, MD, PhD[e], Andrea Salzano, MD, PhD, MRCP(London)[c,*,1],
Antonio Cittadini, MD[a,b,f,*,1]

KEYWORDS

• Heart failure • Right ventricle • Right ventricle heart failure • Diagnosis • Prognosis • Treatment

KEY POINTS

- In recent years, it has been demonstrated that intolerance of physical exertion and other cardinal symptoms in heart failure (HF) are closely related to the functionality of the right ventricular (RV), regardless of left heart.
- RV dysfunction complicates the course, aggravates the quality of life, and increases the mortality of patients.
- RV functional changes have an important role in driving pharmacotherapy titration and in considering eventually the need for transplantation in HF patients.
- Right HF (RHF) is a heterogeneous syndrome, caused by several different conditions, which requires specific etiologic treatment.
- The clinical management of RHF differs about the diagnosis of an acute or a chronic RHF condition.
- For clinicians, it is now possible to assess RHF characteristics and clinical features, with the use of specific imaging techniques (able to study RV function and arterial pulmonary pressure with relative "coupling") that together with the dosage of circulating biomarkers, allows a precise diagnosis of RHF anticipating the possibility of an effective management.

INTRODUCTION

The left ventricular (LV) morphology and performance have been classically considered as the undisputed protagonist of heart failure (HF) pathophysiology, clinic, and prognosis. For several decades, the right heart has always been taken backseat as responsible of the wide range of HF symptoms, considering left heart as the key player in the disease. As a result, this consideration has strongly limited the study and the knowledge of right heart, determining, until recently, a lack of interest and of evidence-based treatment on right HF; for instance, to date, even the proper definition of right HF is still missing.

[a] Department of Translational Medical Sciences, Federico II University, Via S Pansini, 5 - Naples, 80131, Italy; [b] Italian Clinical Outcome Research and Reporting Program (I-CORRP); [c] IRCCS Synlab SDN, Diagnostic and Nuclear Research Institute, Via E Gianturco 113, Naples 80143, Italy; [d] Department of Advanced Biomedical Sciences, Federico II University, Via S Pansini, 5 - Naples, 80131, Italy; [e] AORN Antonio Cardarelli Hospital, Via A Cardarelli, 9 - Naples, 80131, Italy; [f] Division of Internal Medicine and Metabolism and Rehabilitation, Federico II University of Naples, Via S. Pansini 5, Bld.18, 1stfloor, Naples 80131, Italy

[1] Equally contributed.
* Corresponding authors.
E-mail addresses: andrea.salzano@leicester.ac.uk (A.S.); antonio.cittadini@unina.it (A.C.)

Heart Failure Clin 19 (2023) 125–135
https://doi.org/10.1016/j.hfc.2022.08.022

Indeed, the current classification of HF is according to LV ejection fraction (LVEF), with no role for right HF (RHF) or RH parameters.[1] However, in recent years, several observations reported that intolerance of physical exertion and other cardinal symptoms in HF are closely related to the functionality of the right ventricular (RV), regardless of LV.[2,3] Furthermore, it has been shown that RV involvement has a detrimental impact on HF prognosis, as independent prognostic factor, especially through coupling between pulmonary artery pressure and RV function, that showed to be an important indicator in the prognostic stratification of HF.[4–8]

To date, it has been demonstrated that the RV dysfunction complicates the course, aggravate quality of life, and increase the mortality of patients, with an important role in multiple diseases, as pulmonary hypertension, ischemic and nonischemic cardiomyopathy, valvular diseases, heart congenital diseases, sepsis and, finally, HF. In addition, the evaluation of RV functional changes has an important role in driving pharmacotherapy titration and to consider eventually the need for transplantation.[9]

Despite these crucial findings, knowledge on RHF clinic, diagnostic methods, general management, and specific therapies is limited and incomparable respect LV. However, the development of strategies for the treatment and prevention may be the keys to change the natural history of disease and is therefore a clinical unmet need.[10]

Considering these premises, the present review is aimed to report tips to physicians about the current therapeutic management of right HF during acute stage and chronic phase. After a brief description of RHF pathophysiology (useful to better understand the possible therapeutic strategy) and of available diagnostic tools, acute and chronic RHF treatment strategy will be separately discussed. The present review will help to shed light on the RV and its failure (RHF), providing physicians with essential information for everyday clinical practice.

Pathophysiology

To understand the complex pathophysiology of RV, the classic considerations that right chambers are undivided units from left ventricle must be overcome. The human circulatory system is a close system where the ventricular functions are interdependent.[5] Notably, the articulated structure of the right chambers is radically different from left side because of differences in embryologic origins. These anatomic disparities are responsible of the different hemodynamic response. The RV volume

is 10% to 15% larger than the left one; however, RV displayed a thinner free wall (about 3–5 mm) and one-third to one-sixth smaller mass.[11,12]

In the complex geometry of RV recognizes 3 areas: (1) the inlet, which includes the tricuspid valve, tendinous chords, and papillary muscles; (2) the trabeculated apex; and (3) the outlet or infundibulum; crista supraventricularis divides the inlet and outlet portions.

In addition, the RV is in direct connection with pulmonary circulation, a system characterized by high-flow and low-pressure; RV and LV have similar cardiac output but RV has lower afterload and lower pulmonary vascular resistance (PVR).

The most important characteristic of RV is its capacity of managing venous returns, of whatever entity it is, maintaining constant stroke volume. The RV pump function is exerted into the pulmonary circulation. For all these reasons, RH structures respond more to increase of preload rather than the rapid increase of pressure. When pathologic conditions lead to an increase in PVR, muscular contractility increase—a phenomenon known as "ventricular-arterial coupling" (coupling RV-PA). The adaptation of RV to the increase of contractility as response to an increase of afterload depends on end-systolic elastance (E_{es}) and arterial elastance (E_a). The ventricular-arterial coupling consists in energy transfer from ventricle to the arterial system, exemplified as ratio E_{es}/E_a.[13]

As a first attempt to counteract a chronic pressure overload, the ventricular increases RV wall muscular thickness, resulting in RV concentric hypertrophy. During this adapted stage, the functionality of ventricular chamber is preserved thanks to compensatory maneuvers.

In the second step, the adaptation is deranged with consequent dilatation of cavity, leading to tricuspid regurgitation, with an increase in heart rate to consent maintaining cardiac output. When injury persists, the increase of myocardial metabolic demands of RV, similarly the increase of RV wall stress, realizing a progressive dilatation of chamber, in combination with RV mechanical desynchrony.[14] The succession of such mechanisms determines "uncoupling RV-PA," with consequent emergence of right dysfunction and RHF.

The increase in PVR is mainly due to pulmonary hypertension (PH), related by alterations in the pulmonary vasculature; the underlying mechanisms are various, with implication of different molecular pathways. Historically, PH is related to precapillary or postcapillary causes, indicating 5 groups of PH.[15]

As principal clinical manifestation, right-side dysfunction is responsible of multisystemic organ failure consisting in protein-losing enteropathy, cardiorenal syndrome, and cardiac cachexia.[16–18] Signs and symptoms are related mostly to 2 mechanisms: systemic congestion and/or reduction of cardiac output. To date a proper definition of RHF is missing; therefore, it is strongly needed a unique and broad definition that encompasses numerous aspects of syndrome. Recently, an expert consensus identified in the RV-PA coupling a major point to define RHF.[19]

Diagnosis

The lack of a unique and standardized definition of RHF leads to an underestimation of RHF with delays in the clinical practice; several proposal are available, and together they define the right HF as a clinical syndrome with evidence of systemic venous congestion associated or not to lower cardiac output,[20] the presence of possible structural and/or functional abnormalities of right heart, in environment of uncoupling RV-PA.

Complex syndrome in RHF is related to the reduction of right cardiac output and clinical evidence of systemic congestion, of which signs and symptoms are namely effort intolerance, jugular venous distension, abdominal ascites, and lower extremities edema. This clinic picture must be supported by imaging and/or invasive hemodynamics procedures.

Electrocardiographic features showing right heart involvement are enlarged P wave in leads II, III, and aVF and qR in lead V1; in addition, typical anomalies of RV hypertrophy could be present.

First tool to assess right functionality is the echocardiography; many parameters are evaluated in two-dimensional analysis, including RV index of myocardial performance, tricuspid annular plane systolic excursion (TAPSE), fractional area change (FAC), S′ of the tricuspid annulus and longitudinal speckle-tracking echocardiographic strain, and three-dimensional (3D) EF.[21] In accordance with American Society of Echocardiography guidelines recommendations of right heart, it is considered abnormal: FAC greater than 35%, TAPSE less than 17 mm, and/or tissue Doppler lateral tricuspid annular systolic velocity (<10 cm/s). The reduction of FAC is an independent predictor of death and various cardiovascular events in patients after myocardial infarction.[22] Role of TAPSE is prognostic: lower value of TAPSE is impairment of RV performance regardless of LVEF.[23] In addition, the measure of peak tricuspid regurgitation velocity and estimated central venous pressure allow to estimate a level of probability of PH.

Among noninvasive evaluation of RV function, measurement of RV 3D ejection fraction allows an accurate assessment of RV volumes studying the RV shape; technique is compared with gold standard MRI in health heart.[9] Notably, the MRI represents the gold standard for assessing RV function, allows to obtain information of structure and functionality of right heart and great vessels[24]; novels application of tools are hemodynamic measurements as mean pulmonary pressure, until now a prerogative of invasive right heart catheterization.

Regarding circulating biomarkers, especially natriuretic peptides related to myocardial stress, us brain natriuretic peptide (BNP) and NT-proBNP are useful tool to diagnosis, disease progression, and so management and prognosis of RHF.[25–27] However, several studies showed limited value of these biomarkers in group I, II, and IV of PH.[25]

Right failure has many causes, determining pressure and/or volume overload or myocardial dysfunction. Most common causes of RVD are left-sided heart disease (with reduced or preserved ejection fraction; valvulopathy), pulmonary thromboembolic disease, lung disease, and pulmonary arterial hypertension.[28]

The impairment of RV function occurs in acute or chronic form; for the characteristics listed above the response of right heart is different, as well as the management of patients.

Clinical Management of Right Heart Failure

The clinical management of RHF differs with regard to the diagnosis of an acute or a chronic RHF condition.[3,29,30] This distinction closely reflects the different pathophysiological characteristics of the 2 conditions, as briefly discussed in the previous paragraphs. Therefore, in this section, the 2 conditions will be treated separately. Further, RHF is a heterogeneous syndrome, caused by several different conditions, which require specific etiologic treatment; aim of the present section is to provide updated and evidence-based notions about general management of RHF, referring the readers to focused guidelines with regard to the specific treatment of the underlining causes (eg, pulmonary embolisms, myocardial infarction).

Acute Right Heart Failure

Acute right heart failure (ARHF) is a clinical syndrome characterized by a sudden development of systemic congestion, derived from a rapid impairment of RV filling and or/reduction of RV flow output.[30] Therefore, clinical presentation of RH failure is mostly characterized by the presence of signs of systemic congestion.[31] Impairment of RV output and increased filling pressure lead to peripheral edema, anasarca, pericardial effusion, and ascites are all hallmarks of RH failure. Increase in RA pressure leads to pulmonary edema, through a reduction of lung fluid reabsorption. Renal sodium/water retention complicates the volume overload. Severe RV failure may also lead to a general low cardiac output state with hypotension, signs of tissue hypoperfusion up to altered cognitive function and coma.[30] The most common specific causes are pulmonary embolism, pulmonary hypertension, RV infarction, and tricuspid regurgitation; the different underlying causes influence clinical presentation of syndrome and require specific treatment.

Schematically, 4 are the main general objectives in the management of ARHF: (1) management of volume and preload, (2) management of RV afterload, (3) increase of RV contractility, and (4) maintenance of systemic perfusion (**Box 1**). As a result, ARHF therapeutic options can be classified in 2 main categories: treatment volume management (ie, diuretics, renal replacement treatment, saline, and ringer lactate) and vasoactive drugs (ie, vasodilators, inotropes, and vasopressor).

On hospital admission, together with physical examination, laboratory, and electrocardiogram (EKG) findings, a primary tool is a complete echocardiographic study, which easily and rapidly allows to obtain information about RV function, contractility, congestion status, and is useful to identify specific causes and to exclude extrinsic causes. Nonetheless, in unknown diagnosis or in patients with resistance to treatment, invasive hemodynamic assessment must be used, even if for the shortest time as needed.

Schematically, based on the evaluation of the congestion state (congested = wet; noncongested = dry) and on the assessment of the perfusion status (adequate = warm; not adequate = cold), 4 phenotypes can be identified, helping in targeting the patients' management and treatment (**Fig. 1**).

The first critical point in management of ARHF is to obtain a correct volume optimization, driven by the assessment of central venous pressure and arterial pressure. When signs of volume overload and venous congestion are present (ie, wet patient), the reduction of volume overload is aimed to decrease RV wall tension with consequent impairment of contractility, and to improve tricuspid regurgitation, preventing the final compromission of cardiac output.

Therefore, in patients with normal blood pressure, the use of intravenous loop diuretics (furosemide or torasemide) to reduce systemic congestion (recommendation class I level B) often provide prompt improvement of symptoms.[1,30,32] The intravenous dose should be at least equivalent (or twice) to the oral dose taken by the patients.[30]

Box 1
Pharmacologic management and dosage in acute right heart failure

Volume Management

Wet:

Diuretics dosage diuretics-naïve patients: furosemide 20 to 40 mg or torasemide 10 to 20 mg iv

Patients already on oral diuretics: iv dose at least equivalent to the oral dose

Assessment each 24 hours of urine output and urinary sodium extraction. If no response or diuretic resistance add another class of diuretics (thiazides, spironolactone, Sodium-GLUcose Transporter [SGLT]-1 inhibitors)

If no response, consider continuous venovenous hemofiltration or ultrafiltration

Initiation of Renal Replacement therapy if oliguria unresponsive to fluid resuscitation measures, severe hyperkalemia (K+ >6.5 mmol/L), severe acidaemia (pH < 7.2), serum urea level greater than 25 mmol/L (150 mg/dL), and serum creatinine greater than 300 mmol/L (>3.4 mg/dL)

Dry

Hypotensive with normal central venous pressure → cautious volume loading saline or ringer lactate (>200 mL/15–30 min)

Afterload reduction

Warm (systolic blood pressure [SBP] >90 mm Hg) → Vasodilators:

Nitroglycerine: starting dose 10 to 20 mcg/min, increase up to 200 mcg/min

Nitroprussate: start with 0.3 mcg/Kg/min, increase up to 5 mcg/Kg/min

Perfusion maintenance and Contractility support

Cold (SBP <90 mm Hg) → Vasopressors and/or inotropes:

First choice norepinephrine (infusion rate 0.2–1.0 µg/Kg/min)

If no response, add

Levosimendan: bolus 6 to 12 µg/Kg over 10 min and then infusion rate 0.1 to 0.2 µg/Kg/min

Phosphodiesterase III inhibitors (ie, milrinone: bolus 25–75 mcg/Kg over 10–20 min with infusion rate of 0.374–0.75 mcg/Kg/min; enoximone: bolus 0.5–1.0 mg/Kg over 5–10 min, infusion rate 5–20 mcg/Kg/min)

Dobutamine: infusion rate 2 to 20 µg/Kg/min*

> *To avoid if beta-blockade is a contributive cause of hypotension, and in patients with severe pulmonary hypertension due to LV diseases
>
> Adrenaline (epinephrine): bolus 1 mg ev repeated every 3 to 5 min, infusion rate 0.05 to 0.5mcg/kg/min
>
> Severely impaired RV function under vasopressors and inotropes should be considered referred to mechanical circulatory support such as ECMO or life support (ECLS)
>
> *Adapted from* Marra AM, Sherman AE, Salzano A, et al. Right Side of the Heart Pulmonary Circulation Unit Involvement in Left-Sided Heart Failure: Diagnostic, Prognostic, and Therapeutic Implications. *Chest.* 2022;161(2):535 to 551.

Observation from clinical trials suggested to use low doses and to increase when necessary. Further, whereas daily dosage in a single bolus is discouraged (for a possible rebound salt-retention), there is no evidence of superiority of 2 to 3 daily bolus versus continue infusion.

In diuretics naïve patients, a starting dose of 20 to 40 mg of furosemide or 10 to 20 mg of torasemide is suggested, with hourly evaluation of diuresis and (when available) a spot urine sodium content measurement after 2 or 6 hours. If the response remains inadequate, even after a doubling of the loop diuretics doses, addition of other diuretics acting on different sites (eg, thiazides, metolazone, acetazolamide) or and spironolactone can be used, with a careful monitoring of serum electrolytes and renal function.

If there is no response, renal replacement therapy (veno-venous hemofiltration of ultrafiltration) can be considered, specifically when severe hyperkalemia (>6.5 mmol), acidemia, and/or oliguria are present.

However, in patients with low arterial pressure and normal central venous pressure (ie, dry), a cautious volume loading (with saline or Ringer's lactate 200 mL in 15–30 minutes) is a possible therapeutic choice.

Another strategy (specifically in patients with wet-warm phenotype; ie, congestion and arterial pressure greater than 90 mm Hg), aimed to decrease RV afterload (and consequently leading to an increase in stroke volume) is the use of vasodilator therapy, possible with 2 different categories: nonselective (ie, intravenous nitroglycerin and sodium nitroprusside), or partially selective pulmonary (ie, epoprostenol and nitric oxide). Nonselective vasodilators reduce vascular

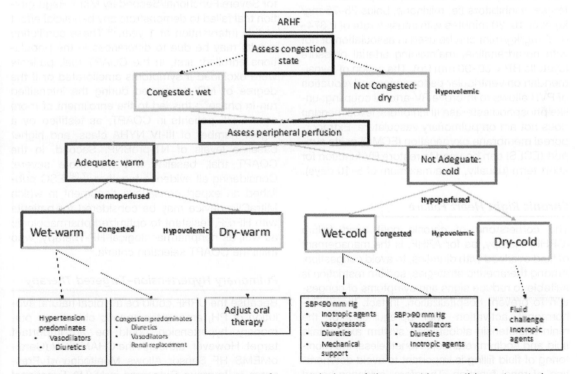

Fig. 1. Simplified algorithm for the management of acute right heart failure consider possible patients' phenotype/clinical presentation. (*From* Marra AM, Sherman AE, Salzano A, et al. Right Side of the Heart Pulmonary Circulation Unit Involvement in Left-Sided Heart Failure: Diagnostic, Prognostic, and Therapeutic Implications. *Chest.* 2022;161(2):535-551.)

resistance and PVR, with consequent improvement of biventricular cardiac output; furthermore, these drugs allow for pulmonary and systemic circulation decongestion and improvement of renal perfusion; with regard to dosages, nitroglycerine starting dose is 10 to 20 mg/min, increasable up to 200 mg/min, whereas nitroprussate starting dose is 0.3 mg/kg/min, increasable up to 5 mg/kg/min. Partially selective pulmonary vasodilators are inhaled or parenteral medications. However, in HF patients, inhaled oxide nitric determines increase of RV cardiac output and overload in LV with high risk of acute pulmonary edema.

When patients are in hemodynamic instability (ie, cold), use of vasopressors and/or inotropes may be necessary and, in advanced cases, also mechanic support. Noradrenaline is the first-choice drug (infusion rate, 0.2–1.0 mg/kg/min), consenting to increase venous returns and similarly ventricular contractility, raising arterial pressure and ensuring multisystemic perfusion (renal, cerebral, coronary). If the response is not satisfactory, levosimendan (bolus 6–12 mg/kg over 10 minutes and then infusion rate 0.1–0.2 mg/kg/min), dobutamine (infusion rate, 2–20 mg/kg/min-to avoid if b-blockade is contributing to hypotension and in patients with severe pulmonary hypertension resulting from LV disease), and phosphodiesterase III inhibitors (ie, milrinone, bolus 25–75 mg/kg over 10–20 minutes with infusion rate of 0.374–0.75 mg/kg/min) can be used in association or not with noradrenaline, maintaining arterial pressure (systolic BP < 80–90 mm Hg). The action of levosimendan on ventricular performance and reduction of PVR allows to improve RV-arterial coupling; unlike phosphodiesterase III inhibitors, levosimendan does not act on pulmonary vasculature. Extracorporeal membrane oxygenation (ECMO) or life support (ECLS) can be used to restore RV function for short term (usually, for a maximum of 5–10 days).

Chronic Right Heart Failure

The cornerstone of chronic right heart failure (CRHF) therapy, as for ARHF, is the management of fluid overload with diuretics, to avoid congestion. Among therapeutic strategies, sodium restriction is suitable to reduce signs and symptoms of congestion to prevent hospitalization. In fact, the neurohormonal activation with upregulation of the renin-angiotensin-aldosterone system axis entails fluid and sodium retention. Nonetheless, the monitoring of fluid filling is important to avoid deterioration of renal function. Therefore, evidence-based pharmacologic treatment of patients with chronic HF with reduced LVEF is appropriate where this coexists with RV failure, as well as implantable

cardioverter-defibrillator (ICD) and cardiac resynchronization therapy (CRT) indications. For the purpose of the paragraph, briefly we will focus on nonpharmacological treatment for which new or specific evidence are available (MitraClip, exercise training, interplay between RH and left ventricular assist device [LVAD]) or PH-targeted treatment, referring to the specific guidelines with regard to pharmacologic treatment of CHF.[1,33]

MitraClip

A correct assessment and treatment of functional mitral regurgitation (MR) is particularly important in patients with CRHF, especially in patients with concomitant dilated LV and HFrEF phenotype. Indeed, functional MR is strongly associated with PH and then with reduced survival rates.[34] Transcatheter percutaneous mitral valve repair showed conflicting results in 2 large clinical trials. Specifically, the Cardiovascular Outcomes Assessment of the MitraClip Percutaneous Therapy for Heart Failure Patients with Functional Mitral Regurgitation (COAPT) trial reported a reduction of HF-related hospitalization and all-cause mortality in patients treated with MitraClip on top of maximal optimal medical therapy, at 2 years,[35] whereas the Percutaneous Repair with the MitraClip Device for Severe Functional/Secondary Mitral Regurgitation trial failed to demonstrate any beneficial effect of this intervention at 1 year.[36] These conflicting results may be due to differences in the populations enrolled: first, in the COAPT trial, patients were excluded if symptoms ameliorated or if the degree of MR decreased during the intensified run-in phase[35]; this led to the enrollment of more severe HF patients in COAPT, as testified by a higher number of III-IV NYHA class, and higher baseline levels of NT-proBNP. Second, in the COAPT trial, baseline MR was more severe. Considering all evidence together,[37,38] ESC published an expert consensus document in which MitraClip device may be considered for patients with HFrEF, resistant to optimized pharmacologic as well as nonpharmacological HF-Therapy, who fulfill the COAPT selection criteria.[39]

Pulmonary Hypertension–Targeted Therapy

Because the CRHF could be a typical natural evolution of PH, among therapeutic objectives, pulmonary hypertension could be an important target. However, although the CHAMPION (CardioMEMS HF Sensor Allows Monitoring of Pressures to Improve Outcomes in NYHA Functional Class III Heart Failure Patients) trial reported a reduction in HF-hospitalization when pulmonary pressures are considered a target of therapy,[40] most interventions with PAH-targeted treatment have so far failed to demonstrate a beneficial effect in HF patients[41,42] or have reported harm associated with this approach[43,44]; however, a single pilot study performed in 44 HFpEF patients showed positive results in terms of cardiopulmonary exercise performance associated with sildenafil.[45] To date, PAH-targeted drugs are not indicated in patients with PH due to left heart disease.[15,46] When PH is not associated to LV dysfunction, possible therapeutic strategy comprises the use of pulmonary vasodilators. Riociguat is indicated in patients with chronic thromboembolism (group IV) in refractory cases; moreover, long-term treatment with riociguat significantly reduced right heart size and improved RV function in PAH and Chronic Thrombo-Embolic Pulmonary Hypertension (CTEPH).[47] Prostanoids improve exercise tolerance and Health-Related-Quality of Life (HRQoL) in group I but the use is related to advanced cases. Phosphodiesterasis 5-inhibitors are indicated in group I of PH with or not in combination with other vasodilators, aging on contractility, vascular remodeling and tolerance of physical exertion.[48-56] Current research is focusing on the search for new biomarkers that may be a fast and practical tool to assess not only prognosis but also the appropriateness/response to these therapies.[57]

Notably, similar to patients with PAH,[58,59] in patients with HFpEF exercise training is associated with exercise capacity improvement and survival[60-62] and is currently recommended by HF guidelines.[29]

Mechanical Circulatory Support

In clinical case refractory to optimal medical management of ARHF or CRHF, the therapeutic choice is mechanical circulatory support (MCS) device with temporary or long-term use.

Different types of MCS device are available (ie, right ventricular assist device [RVAD]; LVAD; ECMO: extracorporeal membrane oxygenation; biventricular assist device). Notably, the assessment of specific dysfunction (eg, RV alone, LV and RV together) drives the choice of the device; for instance, when RV involvement is secondary to LHF, the support for only LV (LVAD) allows an improvement also of the RV function. Meanwhile, when a primary RV involvement is present, an LVAD is contraindicated, with the need of a biventricular support. In addition, LVAD is contraindicated in advanced HF with RV dysfunction, preferred by biventricular support.

Notably, it has been described that from 10% to 40% of LVAD implants are complicated by RV

failure,[63,64] both early after LVAD implantation or weeks after.[63] This is caused by the change in the interplay among LV and RV that occurs after LVAD implantation. Indeed, LVAD causes an increase in LV output, resulting in an increase in venous return to RV. The result may be exacerbation of established RV dysfunction, or unmasking of hitherto unrecognized RH disease.[63] To date, a growing body of evidence identifies the necessity of assessing RH function risk in patients before LVAD implantation. In this context, a relatively simple risk score has been proposed,[64] based on severe RV dysfunction (2 points), ratio of RA/PCWP 0.54 or greater (2 points), advanced INTERMACS class 1 through 3 (2 points), need for 3 or greater intravenous inotropes (2.5 points), and hemoglobin 10 g/dL or less (1 point); indeed, the European Registry for Patients with Mechanical Circulatory Support Right-Sided Heart Failure Risk Score[64] predicts the development of early right HF right HF mortality after continuous-flow LVAD implantation. Finally, a recent systematic review and meta-analysis identified several parameters associated with the development of RV failure after LVAD implantation[65]: female sex; need for ventilatory support or dialysis; INR; RV stroke work index; high central venous pressure (specifically in patients undergoing continuous flow LVAD); and echocardiographic parameters such as moderate-to-severe RVD, high RV/LV ratio, and low longitudinal systolic strain.

Finally, when pulmonary vasculature diseases are present, ECMO rather than RVAD is preferred, to avoid the increase of PAPs, typical of RVAD.[66]

SUMMARY AND FUTURE CLINICAL PERSPECTIVES

Despite being considered for a long time as a mere passive spectator in HF pathophysiology, clinic, and natural history, to date a growing body of evidence is shedding light on the relevance of RH as a distinct entity from LH, with own rules and dignity. Pathophysiologic mechanism driving to right dysfunction before and RHF after have been now almost elucidated, with the partial understanding of the mechanisms underpinning the chronic overload in pulmonary circulation resulting in changes of the morphology of right chambers with RV hypertrophy, atrial and ventricular dilatation, and impaired function, with both RV diastole and systole involvement; in addition, the novel concept of a central role of RV-PA coupling, and the novel evidence about the role of RV-PA impairment in HF patients clinic, led to an increase of our insights on right side, leading to the current research of new management strategies and treatment of HF disease more focused on RH.

For clinicians, it is now possible to assess RHF characteristics and clinical features, with the use of specific imaging techniques (able to study RV function and arterial pulmonary pressure with relative "coupling") that together with the dosage of circulating biomarkers, allows a precise diagnosis of RHF anticipating the possibility of an effective management. However, evidence-based management strategies are still lacking, and targeting RH dysfunction in HF should be an objective of future investigations, specifically considering the detrimental impact of RH in prognosis of HF, particularly in advanced stage of the disease.

CLINICS CARE POINTS

- In the diagnosis of right heart failure (RHF), remind to carefully investigate the ventricular-arterial coupling.

- When a diagnosis of RHF has been performed, check for specific cause, for which a targeted treatment is mandatory.

- In the management of acute RHF, a key issue is to evaluate the congestion state and the peripheral perfusion of your patient.

- A correct volume optimization is the first objective to obtain; if congested, the patient needs to be decongested, mainly with the use of diuretics; if not, a cautious volume loading could be considered as a therapeutic option.

- A correct peripheral perfusion state is the second objective to obtain; if the patient is hypoperfused, remind to adequately correct with inotropic agents and vasopressors.

- For the perfusion maintenance, norepinephrine is the first choice, followed by levosimendan, phosphodiesterase III inhibitors, and dobutamine.

- Use vasodilators (nitroglycerine or nitroprussate) to obtain afterload reduction when necessary.

- In the management of chronic RHF, evidence-based pharmacologic treatment of patients with chronic heart failure with reduced left ventricular ejection fraction are appropriate where this coexists with RV failure.

- Novel nonpharmacological treatment is available for the management of chronic RHF: MitraClip, exercise training, and mechanical circulatory support.

- Pulmonary hypertension represents a possible target in the management of chronic RHF and should be treated with a targeted therapy.

ACKNOWLEDGMENTS

None.

REFERENCES

1. McDonagh TA, Metra M, Adamo M, et al. 2021 ESC Guidelines for the diagnosis and treatment of acute and chronic heart failure: Developed by the Task Force for the diagnosis and treatment of acute and chronic heart failure of the European Society of Cardiology (ESC). With the special contribution of the Heart Failure Association (HFA) of the ESC. Eur J Heart Fail 2022;24:4–131.

2. Haddad F, Doyle R, Murphy DJ, et al. Right ventricular function in cardiovascular disease, Part II - Pathophysiology, clinical importance, and management of right ventricular failure. Circulation 2008;117: 1717–31.

3. Konstam MA, Kiernan MS, Bernstein D, et al. Evaluation and Management of Right-Sided Heart Failure: A Scientific Statement From the American Heart Association. Circulation 2018;137:e578–622.

4. Ghio S, Guazzi M, Scardovi AB, et al. Different correlates but similar prognostic implications for right ventricular dysfunction in heart failure patients with reduced or preserved ejection fraction. Eur J Heart Fail 2017;19:873–9.

5. Disalvo TG, Mathier M, Semigran MJ, et al. Preserved right-ventricular ejection fraction predicts exercise capacity and survival in advanced heart-failure. J Am Coll Cardiol 1995;25:1143–53.

6. de Groote P, Millaire A, Foucher-Hossein C, et al. Right ventricular ejection fraction is an independent predictor of survival in patients with moderate heart failure. J Am Coll Cardiol 1998;32:948–54.

7. Polak JF, Holman BL, Wynne J, et al. Right ventricular ejection fraction: an indicator of increased mortality in patients with congestive heart failure associated with coronary artery disease. J Am Coll Cardiol 1983;2:217–24.

8. Salzano A, D'Assante R, Iacoviello M, et al. Progressive right ventricular dysfunction and exercise impairment in patients with heart failure and diabetes mellitus: insights from the T.O.S.CA. Registry. Cardiovasc Diabetol 2022;21(1):108.

9. Ramani GV, Gurm G, Dilsizian V, et al. Noninvasive assessment of right ventricular function: will there be resurgence in radionuclide imaging techniques? Curr Cardiol Rep 2010;12:162–9.

10. Obokata M, Reddy YNV, Melenovsky V, et al. Deterioration in right ventricular structure and function over time in patients with heart failure and preserved ejection fraction. Eur Heart J 2019;40:689.

11. Dellitalia LJ. THE RIGHT VENTRICLE - ANATOMY, PHYSIOLOGY, AND CLINICAL IMPORTANCE. Curr Probl Cardiol 1991;16:659–720.

12. Kawel-Boehm N, Maceira A, Valsangiacomo-Buechel ER, et al. Normal values for cardiovascular magnetic resonance in adults and children. J Cardiovasc Magn Reson 2015;17. https://doi.org/10.1186/s12968-015-0111-7.

13. Noordegraaf AV, Chin KM, Haddad F, et al. Pathophysiology of the right ventricle and of the pulmonary circulation in pulmonary hypertension: an update. Eur Respir J 2019;53. https://doi.org/10.1183/13993003.01900-2018.

14. Badagliacca R, Reali M, Poscia R, et al. Right Intraventricular Dyssynchrony in Idiopathic, Heritable, and Anorexigen-Induced Pulmonary Arterial Hypertension Clinical Impact and Reversibility. Jacc-Cardiovascular Imaging 2015;8:642–52.

15. Galiè N, Humbert M, Vachiery JL, et al. 2015 ESC/ERS Guidelines for the diagnosis and treatment of pulmonary hypertension: The Joint Task Force for the Diagnosis and Treatment of Pulmonary Hypertension of the European Society of Cardiology (ESC) and the European Respiratory Society (ERS): Endorsed by: Association for European Paediatric and Congenital Cardiology (AEPC), International Society for Heart and Lung Transplantation (ISHLT). Eur Heart J 2016;37:67–119.

16. Tang WHW, Mullens W. Cardiorenal syndrome in decompensated heart failure. Heart 2010;96:255–60.

17. Johnson JN, Driscoll DJ, O'Leary PW. Protein-Losing Enteropathy and the Fontan Operation. Nutr Clin Pract 2012;27:375–84.

18. Mehra MR. Fat, cachexia, and the right ventricle in heart failure: a web of complicity. J Am Coll Cardiol 2013;62:1671–3, 20130731.

19. Marra AM, Sherman AE, Salzano A, et al. Right Side of the Heart Pulmonary Circulation Unit Involvement in Left-Sided Heart Failure: Diagnostic, Prognostic, and Therapeutic Implications. Chest 2021;20210927.

20. Gorter TM, van Veldhuisen DJ, Bauersachs J, et al. Right heart dysfunction and failure in heart failure with preserved ejection fraction: mechanisms and management. Position statement on behalf of the Heart Failure Association of the European Society of Cardiology. Eur J Heart Fail 2018;20:16–37.

21. Lang RM, Badano LP, Mor-Avi V, et al. Recommendations for Cardiac Chamber Quantification by Echocardiography in Adults: An Update from the American Society of Echocardiography and the European Association of Cardiovascular Imaging. Eur Heart Journal-Cardiovascular Imaging 2015;16:233–71.

22. Anavekar NS, Skali H, Bourgoun M, et al. Usefulness of right ventricular fractional area change to predict death, heart failure, and stroke following myocardial infarction (from the VALIANT ECHO study). Am J Cardiol 2008;101:607–12.

23. Mohammed SF, Hussain I, Abou Ezzeddine OF, et al. Right Ventricular Function in Heart Failure With Preserved Ejection Fraction A Community-Based Study. Circulation 2014;130. 2310-U2186.

24. Contaldi C, Dellegrottaglie S, Mauro C, et al. Role of Cardiac Magnetic Resonance Imaging in Heart Failure. Heart Failure Clin 2021;17:207–21, 20210203.

25. Salzano A, D'Assante R, Israr MZ, et al. Biomarkers in Heart Failure: Clinical Insights. Heart Failure Clin 2021;17:223–43, 20210210.

26. Suzuki T, Lyon A, Saggar R, et al. Editor's Choice-Biomarkers of acute cardiovascular and pulmonary diseases. Eur Heart Journal-Acute Cardiovasc Care 2016;5:416–33.

27. Salzano A, Marra AM, D'Assante R, et al. Biomarkers and Imaging: Complementary or Subtractive? Heart Fail Clin 2019;15:321–31.

28. Padang R, Chandrashekar N, Indrabhinduwat M, et al. Aetiology and outcomes of severe right ventricular dysfunction. Eur Heart J 2020;41:1273.

29. Ponikowski P, Voors AA, Anker SD, et al. 2016 ESC Guidelines for the diagnosis and treatment of acute and chronic heart failure: The Task Force for the diagnosis and treatment of acute and chronic heart failure of the European Society of Cardiology (ESC). Developed with the special contribution of the Heart Failure Association (HFA) of the ESC. Eur J Heart Fail 2016;18:891–975.

30. Harjola VP, Mebazaa A, Čelutkienė J, et al. Contemporary management of acute right ventricular failure: a statement from the Heart Failure Association and the Working Group on Pulmonary Circulation and Right Ventricular Function of the European Society of Cardiology. Eur J Heart Fail 2016;18:226–41.

31. Simon MA. Assessment and treatment of right ventricular failure. Nat Rev Cardiol 2013;10:204–18.

32. Maddox TM, Januzzi JL, Allen LA, et al. 2021 Update to the 2017 ACC Expert Consensus Decision Pathway for Optimization of Heart Failure Treatment: Answers to 10 Pivotal Issues About Heart Failure With Reduced Ejection Fraction: A Report of the American College of Cardiology Solution Set Oversight Committee. J Am Coll Cardiol 2021;77:772–810, 20220111.

33. Heidenreich PA, Bozkurt B, Aguilar D, et al. 2022 AHA/ACC/HFSA Guideline for the Management of Heart Failure: Executive Summary: A Report of the American College of Cardiology/American Heart Association Joint Committee on Clinical Practice Guidelines. J Am Coll Cardiol 2022;79:1757–80, 20220401.

34. Bursi F, Barbieri A, Grigioni F, et al. Prognostic implications of functional mitral regurgitation according to the severity of the underlying chronic heart failure: a long-term outcome study. Eur J Heart Fail 2010;12:382–8.

35. Stone GW, Lindenfeld J, Abraham WT, et al. Transcatheter Mitral-Valve Repair in Patients with Heart Failure. N Engl J Med 2018;379:2307–18.

36. Obadia JF, Messika-Zeitoun D, Leurent G, et al. Percutaneous Repair or Medical Treatment for Secondary Mitral Regurgitation. N Engl J Med 2018; 379:2297–306.

37. Bertaina M, Galluzzo A, D'Ascenzo F, et al. Prognostic impact of MitraClip in patients with left ventricular dysfunction and functional mitral valve regurgitation: A comprehensive meta-analysis of RCTs and adjusted observational studies. Int J Cardiol 2019;290:70–6.

38. Nishimura RA, Bonow RO. Percutaneous Repair of Secondary Mitral Regurgitation - A Tale of Two Trials. N Engl J Med 2018;379:2374–6.

39. Seferovic PM, Ponikowski P, Anker SD, et al. Clinical practice update on heart failure 2019: pharmacotherapy, procedures, devices and patient management. An expert consensus meeting report of the Heart Failure Association of the European Society of Cardiology. Eur J Heart Fail 2019;21:1169–86.

40. Abraham WT, Adamson PB, Bourge RC, et al. Wireless pulmonary artery haemodynamic monitoring in chronic heart failure: a randomised controlled trial. Lancet 2011;377:658–66.

41. Hoendermis ES, Liu LC, Hummel YM, et al. Effects of sildenafil on invasive haemodynamics and exercise capacity in heart failure patients with preserved ejection fraction and pulmonary hypertension: a randomized controlled trial. Eur Heart J 2015;36: 2565–73.

42. Bonderman D, Ghio S, Felix SB, et al. Riociguat for patients with pulmonary hypertension caused by systolic left ventricular dysfunction: a phase IIb double-blind, randomized, placebo-controlled, dose-ranging hemodynamic study. Circulation 2013;128:502–11.

43. Vachiéry JL, Delcroix M, Al-Hiti H, et al. Macitentan in pulmonary hypertension due to left ventricular dysfunction. Eur Respir J 2018;51. https://doi.org/ 10.1183/13993003.01886-2017.

44. Bermejo J, Yotti R, García-Orta R, et al. Sildenafil for improving outcomes in patients with corrected valvular heart disease and persistent pulmonary hypertension: a multicenter, double-blind, randomized clinical trial. Eur Heart J 2018;39:1255–64. https:// doi.org/10.1093/eurheartj/ehx700.

45. Guazzi M, Vicenzi M, Arena R, et al. PDE5 inhibition with sildenafil improves left ventricular diastolic function, cardiac geometry, and clinical status in patients with stable systolic heart failure: results of a 1-year, prospective, randomized, placebo-controlled study. Circ Heart Fail 2011;4:8–17.

46. Vachiéry JL, Tedford RJ, Rosenkranz S, et al. Pulmonary hypertension due to left heart disease. Eur Respir J 2019;53. https://doi.org/10.1183/13993003. 01897-2018.

47. Marra AM, Egenlauf B, Ehlken N, et al. Change of right heart size and function by long-term therapy with riociguat in patients with pulmonary arterial hypertension and chronic thromboembolic pulmonary hypertension. Int J Cardiol 2015;195:19–26.

48. Frey MK, Lang I. Tadalafil for the treatment of pulmonary arterial hypertension. Expert Opin Pharmacother 2012;13:747–55, 20120223.

49. Galie N, Barbera JA, Frost AE, et al. Initial Use of Ambrisentan plus Tadalafil in Pulmonary Arterial Hypertension. N Engl J Med 2015;373:834–44.

50. Prasad S, Wilkinson J, Gatzoulis MA. Sildenafil in primary pulmonary hypertension. N Engl J Med 2000; 343:1342.

51. Samarzija M, Zuljevic E, Jakopovic M, et al. One Year Efficacy and Safety of Oral Sildenafil Treatment in Severe Pulmonary Hypertension. Coll Antropol 2009;33:799–803.

52. Galie N, Ghofrani HA, Torbicki A, et al. Sildenafil citrate therapy for pulmonary arterial hypertension. N Engl J Med 2005;353:2148–57.

53. Sastry BKS, Narasimhan C, Reddy NK, et al. Clinical efficacy of sildenafil in primary pulmonary hypertension - A randomized, placebo-controlled, double-blind, crossover study. J Am Coll Cardiol 2004;43: 1149–53.

54. De Santo LS, Buonocore M, Agrusta F, et al. Pattern of resolution of pulmonary hypertension, long-term allograft right ventricular function, and exercise capacity in high-risk heart transplant recipients listed under oral sildenafil. Clin Transplant 2014;28:837–43.

55. Galie N, Brundage BH, Ghofrani HA, et al. Tadalafil Therapy for Pulmonary Arterial Hypertension. Circulation 2009;119. 2894-U2865.

56. Simonneau G, Rubin LJ, Galie N, et al. Addition of Sildenafil to Long-Term Intravenous Epoprostenol Therapy in Patients with Pulmonary Arterial Hypertension A Randomized Trial. Ann Intern Med 2008; 149. 521-W102.

57. Marra AM, Bossone E, Salzano A, et al. Biomarkers in Pulmonary Hypertension. Heart Fail Clin 2018;14: 393.

58. Marra AM, Egenlauf B, Bossone E, et al. Principles of rehabilitation and reactivation: pulmonary hypertension. Respiration 2015;89:265–73.

59. Grünig E, Eichstaedt C, Barberà JA, et al. ERS statement on exercise training and rehabilitation in patients with severe chronic pulmonary hypertension. Eur Respir J 2019;53:2019–20102/28.

60. Kitzman DW, Brubaker P, Morgan T, et al. Effect of Caloric Restriction or Aerobic Exercise Training on Peak Oxygen Consumption and Quality of Life in Obese Older Patients With Heart Failure With Preserved Ejection Fraction: A Randomized Clinical Trial. JAMA 2016;315:36–46. https://doi.org/10. 1001/jama.2015.17346.

61. Salzano A, De Luca M, Israr MZ, et al. Exercise Intolerance in Heart Failure with Preserved Ejection Fraction. Heart Fail Clin 2021;17:397–413.

62. Crisci G, De Luca M, D'Assante R, et al. Effects of exercise on heart failure with preserved ejection fraction. An updated review of literature. J Cardiovasc Development Dis 2022;9(8):241.

63. Lampert BC, Teuteberg JJ. Right ventricular failure after left ventricular assist devices. J Heart Lung Transplant 2015;34:1123–30.

64. Soliman OII, Akin S, Muslem R, et al. Derivation and Validation of a Novel Right-Sided Heart Failure Model After Implantation of Continuous Flow Left Ventricular Assist Devices: The EUROMACS (European Registry for Patients with Mechanical Circulatory Support) Right-Sided Heart Failure Risk Score. Circulation 2018;137:891–906.

65. Bellavia D, Iacovoni A, Scardulla C, et al. Prediction of right ventricular failure after ventricular assist device implant: systematic review and meta-analysis of observational studies. Eur J Heart Fail 2017;19: 926–46.

66. Verbelen T, Verhoeven J, Goda M, et al. Mechanical support of the pressure overloaded right ventricle: an acute feasibility study comparing low and high flow support. Am J Physiology-Heart Circulatory Physiol 2015;309:H615–24.

Noncoding RNAs in Pulmonary Arterial Hypertension
Current Knowledge and Translational Perspectives

Nadia Bernardi, MSc[a], Eva Bianconi, PhD[b], Andrea Vecchi, MD[a],
Pietro Ameri, MD, PhD, FHFA[a,b,*]

KEYWORDS

- Pulmonary arterial hypertension • Pathogenesis • Mechanisms • RNA • microRNA
- Long noncoding RNA

KEY POINTS

- Experimental evidence indicates that noncoding RNAs (ncRNAs), including microRNA and long noncoding RNAs, contribute to the pathogenesis of pulmonary arterial hypertension (PAH).
- Altered levels of several ncRNAs have been associated with decreased nitric oxide production, proliferation and resistance to apoptosis of smooth muscle cells, and endothelial-to-mesenchymal transition in pulmonary arteries.
- In principle, ncRNAs may be measured in peripheral blood and used as biomarkers, and may be targeted for treatment of PAH.
- However, current gaps in knowledge and major technical issues must be overcome to bring ncRNA-based diagnostic and therapeutic approaches into the clinical arena.

BACKGROUND

Pulmonary arterial hypertension (PAH) is the type of pulmonary hypertension (PH) for which the pathogenesis has been characterized most extensively. Seminal studies revealed that three pathways are deregulated in pulmonary arteries of subjects with PAH: nitric oxide (NO) is deficient, endothelin is hyperactive, and prostacyclin signaling is defective. Therefore, the core of contemporary PAH pharmacotherapy aims at restoring NO and prostacyclin effects and at antagonizing endothelin activities.[1] This strategy is certainly effective, with the best proof being the remarkable improvement in PAH outcomes observed after the introduction of combination therapies modulating two or three of these pathways.[2]

Yet, a significant proportion of patients still face clinical worsening, indicating that other cellular and molecular events contribute to PAH development and progression in addition to the imbalance in NO, endothelin, and prostacyclin. These events may be initiated by specific ligands, such as serotonin or the ligands of activin receptor type IIA, which are indeed targeted by drugs that are being tested in clinical trials (NCT04712669, NCT04576988). Alternatively, pathologic changes in pulmonary arteries may be caused by intracellular, noncoding ribonucleic acids (ncRNAs), including microRNA (miRNAs) and long noncoding RNAs (lncRNAs) (**Fig. 1**).

[a] Department of Internal Medicine, University of Genova, Viale Benedetto XV, 6, Genova 16132, Italy;
[b] Cardiovascular Disease Unit, Cardiac, Thoracic and Vascular Department, IRCCS Ospedale Policlinico San Martino – IRCCS Italian Cardiology Network, Largo Rosanna Benzi 10, Genova 16132, Italy
* Corresponding author. Viale Benedetto XV, 6, Genova 16132, Italy.
E-mail address: pietroameri@unige.it

Heart Failure Clin 19 (2023) 137–152
https://doi.org/10.1016/j.hfc.2022.08.020

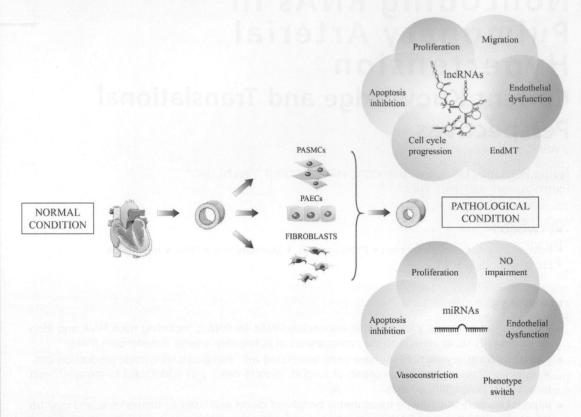

Fig. 1. Main effects of long noncoding RNAs (lncRNAs) and microRNA (miRNAs) implicated in the pathogenesis of pulmonary arterial hypertension. EndMT, endothelial-to-mesenchymal transition; NO, nitric oxide; PAECs, pulmonary artery endothelial cells; PASMCs, pulmonary artery smooth muscle cells.

Here, we provide a narrative review of the data regarding the role of miRNAs and lncRNAs in PAH, followed by key considerations about the possibility of exploiting such evidence for biomarker or therapeutic discovery.

MicroRNAs IN PULMONARY ARTERIAL HYPERTENSION

miRNAs are single-strand RNAs of approximately 22 nucleotides and can be produced in two different ways, so-called canonical and noncanonical pathways.

The former begins in the nucleus, where RNA polymerase II transcribes a miRNA-encoding gene into a hairpin-like structure of approximately 1000 nucleotides.[3] The primary immature miRNA is then cleaved by the microprocessor complex, including the RNA-binding protein DiGeorge Syndrome Critical Region 8, a ribonuclease enzyme (Drosha), and other cofactors, to create a shorter hairpin of 70 nucleotides. This precursor is translocated by exportin-5 from the nucleus to the cytoplasm to be further processed by the ribonuclease Dicer into a short double-stranded

immature miRNA. Finally, the two strands are separated to form the mature single-strand miRNA that is incorporated into a specific conserved site of Argonaut proteins, a crucial step for subsequent interaction with its targets.

In the noncanonical pathway, the primary immature miRNA is processed by enzymes different from those aforementioned.[4]

To date, it is thought that miRNAs can regulate approximately 50% to 60% of all protein-coding messenger RNAs (mRNAs), by binding partially complementary binding sites located on the 3′ untranslated regions (UTR) of mRNAs, impairing their stability and, thus, promoting their degradation.[5,6] In this way, miRNAs down-regulate protein expression. A specific mRNA can be targeted by different miRNAs having different miRNA binding sites in its 3′ UTR region, and the same miRNA can bind several mRNAs ("divergent pathway"). Moreover, several miRNAs can modulate a single intracellular signaling pathway at multiple levels, through the "convergent pathway."

miRNA clusters contain more than one miRNA, are transcribed in a polycistronic way, and have high-sequence similarity. Thus, these miRNAs act on the same target genes or on different genes encoding proteins within the same pathway.[7]

miRNAs are involved in cellular homeostasis and in multiple diseases,[5,8,9] among which PAH.[10,11]

For the purpose of this review, we classify miR-NAs as acting in pulmonary artery endothelial cells (PAECs), pulmonary artery smooth muscle cells (PASMCs), or multiple pulmonary artery cell populations. The main miRNAs implicated in PAH development are listed in **Table 1**.

MicroRNAs Acting in Pulmonary Artery Endothelial Cells

The pulmonary artery endothelium is constantly exposed to shear stress and stretch generated by blood flow. These stimuli are sensed and integrated into PAECs by mechano-miRNAs, which control the expression of genes implicated in EC function and proliferation.[12,13] Among these miR-NAs, the most relevant in PAH are miR-21, and miR-143/145.[14]

Numerous studies have established that NO production by ECs is influenced by miRNAs, such as miR-24, miR-27b, miR-122, miR-155, miR-182, and miR-221/222.

miR-24 has recently been shown to inhibit endothelial NO synthase (eNOS) expression in ECs and promote EC proliferation by targeting Sp1 that recognizes a specific high-affinity binding site located on cis-acting elements.[15] miR-27b and miR122 were also linked to impaired NO synthesis in ECs. By using both the monocrotaline (MCT) rat model of PH (hereafter abbreviated to MCT-PH) and human PAECs (hPAECs), it was shown that miR-27b down-regulates peroxisome proliferator-activated receptor (PPAR)-γ and this results in disruption of Hsp90-eNOS coupling, leading to decreased NO.[15] Instead, miR-122 may alter L-arginine and NO metabolism, targeting the 3′ UTR of the Solute Carrier Family 7 Member 1 gene (SLC7A1).[16] Interestingly, NO levels may be diminished by SLC7A1 polymorphisms.[17]

miR-155 also affects eNOS expression by decreasing eNOS mRNA stability, although the molecular mechanism remains elusive.[18]

Finally, miR-221 and miR-222 regulate eNOS via both translational and posttranslational modifications.[19]

MicroRNAs Acting in Pulmonary Artery Smooth Muscle Cells

Bone morphogenetic protein (BMP) receptor type 2 (BMPR2) is a serine/threonine receptor kinase that halts PASMC proliferation and is central to

prevent pathologic modifications resulting in PAH. Indeed, inactivating mutations in the BMPR2 gene have been associated with familial PAH.[20] In HEK293 T cells, overexpression of the miR-17/92 cluster causes BMPR2 downregulation via c-myc and Signal Transducer and Activator of Transcription 3 (STAT3)/IL-6.[21] In addition, miR-17/92 induces an increase in hypoxia-induced factor-1α (HIF-1α) via p53 leading to hypoxia-mediated apoptosis.

Specific inhibition of miR-17 and miR-20a, which are part of the miR-17/92 cluster, by means of RNA oligonucleotides (antagomiRs) restored BMPR2 levels and signaling and reduced proliferation in human PASMCs (hPASMCs), and blunted pulmonary vasculopathy and right ventricular hypertrophy in mice with MCT-PH or hypoxia-induced PH (hypoxia-PH).[22,23]

miR-130/301 is another cluster associated with PASMC proliferation, which was investigated in both animal models (SU5416 mouse, MCT-PH, and sheep with shunt-induced PH) and in vitro (hPASMCs and hPAECs). These miRNAs are upregulated via HIF-2α and POU5F1/OCT4 and control proliferation of hPASMCs through PPAR-γ. At the molecular level, the miR-130/301 cluster elicits miR-204 downregulation, which in turn triggers the overexpression of STAT3. STAT3 then further decreases miR-204.[24] In PASMCs, the down-regulation of miR-204 promotes the activation of Src kinase, nuclear factor of activated T cells (NFAT), HIF-1α, and RUNX2 leading to PASMC proliferation and resistance to apoptosis.[25,26] Of note, miR-204 down-regulation was confirmed in MCT-PH and hypoxia-PH, as well as in the lungs of patients with PAH.[27]

The data for miR-206 are contradictory. On one side, the up-regulation of miR-206 was reported to enhance PASMC differentiation and block both their proliferation and migration by targeting Notch3.[28] On the other hand, it was shown that miR-206 can regulate PASMC proliferation through the modulation of HIF-1α/Fhl-1, with HIF-1α being increased as a consequence of the competition among miR-206 and other miRNAs at the 3′ UTR of the HIF1A gene, as well as for miRNA processing enzyme.[29]

MicroRNAs Acting in Multiple Pulmonary Artery Cell Types

In vitro studies indicate that miR-21 acts both in PASMCs and PAECs. PASMCs cultured under hypoxia conditions showed the up-regulation of miR-21 and, consequently, reduced levels of BMPR2 and a higher proliferation rate.[30,31] As the promoter region of miR-21 contains a HIF

Table 1
microRNAs involved in pulmonary arterial hypertension

miRNA	Model	Target	Main Findings	Reference
miRNAs acting in PAECs				
Cluster miR-143/145	PAECs	Hexokinase II Integrin β8	SMC de-differentiation and inhibition of EC proliferation	37,38
miR-24	ECs	Sp1 protein	Inhibition of eNOS expression and promotion of proliferation	15
miR-27b	MCT-PH and hPAEC	PPAR-γ	Impairment of NO production	15
miR-122	PAH patients	SLC7A1 (3′-UTR)	Impairment of L-arginine and NO metabolism	16
miRNAs acting in PASMCs				
miR-145	PASMCs of PAH patients and lungs of BMPR2-deficient mice; Hypoxic mouse model and plexiform lesion; Patients with idiopathic PAH and congenital PH	KLF4, KLF5 and myocardin	BMP4 mutation causes an increase in miR-145; increased miR-145 and its targets; decreased miR-145 and its targets	39,40
Cluster miR-17-92	HEK293 T; MCT-PH and PASMCs	BMPR2; HIF-1α; SMAD5; p21	Regulation of c-myc transcription factor via STAT3/IL6; Hypoxia mediated apoptosis; Antagomir against miR-20a restores BMPR2 signal pathway; Antagomir against miR-17 reduces muscularization of pulmonary arteries	21,22; 23
Cluster miR-130/131	SU5416 mouse, MCT-PH, sheep with shunt-induced PH models; hPASMCs, PAECs	miR-204	Regulation of PASMCs proliferation	24
miR-204	Chronic hypoxia rat model, MCT-PH, PAH patient lung and PASMCs	Src kinases/NFAT/HIF-1α/RUNX2 axis	PASMC proliferation and reduction in apoptosis	27
miR-206	PASMCs	Notch3; HIF-1α (3′ UTR)	Enhanced differentiation, blockade of proliferation and migration; Regulation of proliferation	28; 29

miRNAs with versatile effects

miRNA	Model/condition	Targets	Effect	
miR-21	MCT-PH, hypoxia-mouse model, human serum and lung samples of patients with idiopathic PAH	BMPR2, WWP1, SATB1 and YOD1	Different pathobiology in PH process according to the model in use	14,30,32,33
	PASMCs cultured in hypoxic condition		Increased proliferation and decreased BMPR2 expression	
	PAECs cultured in hypoxic condition	RhoB	Suppression of angiogenesis and vasodilatation	
miR-124	PASMCs	NFAT	Inhibition of proliferation	41
	Fibroblasts	NFAT, NFATc1 and CAMTA1	Increased proliferation, migration, inflammation and MCP-1 expression	
		PTBP1 (3′ UTR)	Regulation of Notch1/PTEN/FOXO3/p21Cip1 and p27Kip1 axes	42
miR-138	PASMCs	Mst1	Anti-apoptotic effect	34
	ECs	SA100A1	Vasoconstriction effect	35
miR-424	PAECs	FGF2 and FGFR1	Proliferative effect	36
miR-503	PAECs and PASMCs			

Abbreviations: BMPR2, bone morphogenetic protein receptor type 2; EC, endothelial cells; eNOS, endothelial nitric oxide synthase; FGF2, fibroblast growth factor 2; FGFR1, fibroblast growth factor receptor 1; hPAECs, human pulmonary artery endothelial cells; hPASMCs, human pulmonary artery smooth muscle cells; MCT-PH, monocrotaline rat model of pulmonary hypertension; miR/miRNA, microRNA; Mst1, serine/threonine kinase metastasis 1; NO, nitric oxide; PAEC, pulmonary artery endothelial cells; PAH, pulmonary arterial hypertension; PASMCs, pulmonary artery smooth muscle cells; PH, pulmonary hypertension; PPARγ, peroxisome proliferator activated receptor γ.

(From Marra AM, Sherman AE, Salzano A, et al. Right Side of the Heart Pulmonary Circulation Unit Involvement in Left-Sided Heart Failure: Diagnostic, Prognostic, and Therapeutic Implications. Chest. 2022;161(2):535-551.)

response element, HIF-1α induction is at least partly driven by miR-21. However, it is now known that miR-21 expression may be also promoted in a HIF-independent manner.[14] In PAECs exposed to both hypoxia and BMPR2 activation, Parikh and colleagues[32] found that the up-regulation of miR-21 was associated with inhibition of *RhoB* expression and Rho-Kinase activity, which in turn led to molecular alterations favoring the suppression of angiogenesis and vasodilatation. The diverse effects of miR-21 are due to its numerous targets that include PDCD4, SPRY2, and PPAR-α, besides BMP, BMPR2, and the Rho/Rho kinase signaling pathway.[14] Even though miR-21 has been consistently implicated in PAH pathogenesis, some data are conflicting and further investigations are essential. For example, miR-21 appears to be down-regulated in MCT-PH, but upregulated in hypoxia-PH. Remarkably, miR-21 downregulation was also observed in serum and lung samples of patients with idiopathic PAH.[33]

By targeting the serine/threonine kinase metastasis-1 (Mst1), a well-known modulator of cell death, miR-138 is anti-apoptotic in PASMCs.[34] Upon induction by endothelin-1, TNF-α and angiotensin II, the same miRNA downregulates S100A1 in PAECs impairing the production of NO and, therefore, causing vasoconstriction of pulmonary arterioles.[35]

Other miRNAs with dual activity in both PAECs and PASMCs are miR-424 and miR-503. Loss of apelin in PAECs results in reduced levels of miR-424 and miR-503 and an increase in both fibroblast growth factor 2 and its receptor, FGFR1. On the other hand, the overexpression of miR-424 and miR-503 in PAECs and PASMCs has antiproliferative effects.[36]

miRNA may also mediate the communication between PAECs and PASMCs. As an example, miR-143/145 can be mutually transferred from ECs to SMCs *via* extracellular vesicles or microparticles, leading to SMC de-differentiation and blunted EC proliferation and angiogenesis, respectively.[37,38] Expression of miR-143/145 has been repeatedly assessed in specimens from PAH patients or animals with PH, but the overall evidence is inconsistent so far. On one hand, miR-143/145 was overexpressed in PASMCs from subjects with PAH and a mutation in *BMPR2*, in lungs of BMPR2-deficient mice, in plexiform lesions of PAH patients, and in lungs of wild-type mice exposed to hypoxia.[39,40] On the other hand, it was decreased in lung samples of subjects with idiopathic and congenital PAH.

miR-124 was found to be down-regulated in PASMCs, as well as in fibroblasts, under hypoxic conditions. In PASMCs, the down-regulation of miR-124 suppresses NFAT expression, with the functional effects being a reduction in proliferation and enhancement of differentiation.[41] Furthermore, miR-124 controls the proliferative, migratory and inflammatory phenotype of fibroblasts; the depletion of miR-124 through anti-miR-124 elicits an increase in proliferation, migration, and expression of MCP-1 by fibroblasts, whereas transfection of fibroblasts with a construct expressing miR-124 leads to opposite effects. Mechanistically, miR-124 affects the Notch1/PTEN/FOXO3/p21Cip1 and p27Kip1 axes by binding the 3′ UTR of *PTBP1*.[42]

LONG NONCODING RNAs IN PULMONARY ARTERIAL HYPERTENSION

lncRNAs are made of approximately 200 nucleotides and are characterized by long introns and relatively short exons. By definition, they do not encode proteins.

The lncRNAs gene sequences fall within protein-coding genes and the activation of specific lncRNA promoter sequences is responsible for the tissue-specific pattern of expression of lncRNAs.[43] Like mRNAs, lncRNAs can be transcribed by RNA polymerase II and undergo polyadenylation process, splicing, and alternative splicing, allowing the generation of different lncRNAs starting from the same sequence.[44] Another mechanism for lncRNAs generation involves RNA polymerase III. The lncRNAs produced in this way do not undergo polyadenylation.[44,45]

lncRNAs regulation occurs through post-transcriptional modifications such as N6-methyl-Adenosine (m6A), which is responsible for altering the lncRNAs structure or m6A protein recruitment.[46]

Again, similarly to mRNAs, lncRNAs are degraded by several enzymes. The degradation begins in the nucleus, implies 5′-decapping operated by Dpc2, is followed by RAT1 action, and is influenced by the recognition of specific nucleotide sequences with the lncRNAs by RBP.[47–49] Recently, some miRNAs (miR-let-7b, miR-9, miR-34a, miR-211, miR-547-5p, and miR-124) have also been reported to alter lncRNA stability.[49]

The activity of lncRNAs depends on their intracellular localization. In the nucleus, lncRNAs mainly regulate gene expression, whereas in the cytoplasm they are generally involved in post-transcriptional regulatory processes. Interestingly, lncRNAs can also act as miRNA-sponges through multiple binding sites for miRNAs in their sequence.[8]

The main lncRNAs that have been related to PAH development are listed in **Tables 2** and **3**.

Table 2
lncRNAs mentioned in the article

Abbreviation	Full name
ANRIL	Antisense Noncoding RNA in the INK4 Locus
CASC2	Cancer Susceptibility Candidate 2
GAS5	Growth arrest specific 5
GATA6-AS1	GATA6 antisense RNA 1
H19	H19 imprinted maternally expressed transcript
HOXA-AS3	HOXA cluster antisense RNA 3
LincRNA-COX2	Long intergenic noncoding RNA-COX2
lncAng362	miR222/221 cluster host gene
LnRTP	–
MALAT1	Metastasis Associated Lung Adenocarcinoma Transcript 1
MANTIS	LOC107985770
MEG3	Maternally Express Gene 3
NONRATT015587.2	–
PAHRF	NONHSAT169231.1 or surfactant associated 3
PAXIP1-AS1	PAXIP1 Antisense RNA
RPS4L	Ribosomal protein S4-Like
SMILR	Smooth Muscle Enriched Long Noncoding RNA
TCONS_00034812	–
TUG1	Taurine up-regulated 1
TYKRIL	Tyrosine Kinase Receptor Inducing
UCA1	Urothelial carcinoma associated 1

Long Noncoding RNAs Acting in Pulmonary Artery Endothelial Cells

Three lncRNAs have been shown to act in PAECs: MANTIS, GATA6-AS1, and MALAT1.

MANTIS stimulates angiogenesis *via* still unknown mechanisms.[50] It is controlled by the histone deacetylase JARID1B and is downregulated in lung tissue samples from patients with idiopathic PAH and in MCT-PH.[50]

GATA6-AS1 suppresses the expression of two angiogenesis-related genes, *PTGS2* and *POSTN*, by inhibiting the deaminase function of lysyl oxidase-like 2; hence, it favors endothelial-to-mesenchymal transition (EndMT), an event contributing to PAH pathogenesis.[51]

Overexpression of MALAT1 also results in EndMT *via* ox-LDL regulation and activation of the Wnt/beta-catenin pathway. In fact, MALAT1 knockdown prevents EndMT. In addition, in endothelial progenitor cells MALAT1 is up-regulated by transforming growth factor β1 (TGF-β1) and acts as miRNA sponge for miR-145, which would inhibit TGF-β1-induced EndMT by targeting the TGF-β receptor and its downstream mediator SMAD3.[52]

Long Noncoding RNAs Acting in Pulmonary Artery Smooth Muscle Cells

Experiments in which lncRNAs were down- and/or up-regulated have shown that lncRNAs can promote the proliferation of PASMCs by sponging off miRNAs that, in turn, curb proliferation by inhibiting mitogenic factors or intracellular pathways. In some cases, apoptosis is also blocked. MALAT1 binds miR-124-3b, GAS5 miR-23b-3p, and TUG1 miR-374c, with ensuing increased activity of KLF5, KCNK3, and Foxc1/Notch, respectively.[53–55] Similarly, H19 indirectly and negatively regulates angiotensin II receptor by sponging off let-7b, SMILR halts the RhoA/ROCK pathway by sponging off miR-141, and PAHRF (also known as NONHSAT169231.1) decreases MST1 by sponging off miR-23a-3p.[56–58] Furthermore, when up-regulated in response to hypoxia through histone 3 lysine 9 (H3L9) acetylation, HOXA-AS3 sponges off miR-675-3p, leading to greater availability of PDE5A and, therefore, enhanced proliferation and migration and diminished apoptosis.[59,60] Consistently, upregulation of HOXA-AS3 was reported *in vivo* in MCT-PH and hypoxia-PH and *in vitro* in hypoxic-PASMCs, as well as in lung samples from PAH patients.[61]

For some of these lncRNAs, additional mechanisms of action exist. TUG1 knockdown inhibits proliferation and migration and initiates apoptosis of PASMCs through the expression of both HIF-1α and vascular endothelial growth factor,[62] and has also been implicated in cell cycle progression via miR-328 inhibition.[63] In MCT-PH, melatonin up-regulated H19 and miR-675-3p, whereas miR-200a was down-regulated, causing a decrease in insulin-like growth factor 1 receptor (IGF1R) and an increase in PDCD4, which eventually blocked proliferation and triggered apoptosis.[64]

Table 3
lncRNAs involved in pulmonary arterial hypertension

lncRNAs	Model	Target	Main Findings	Reference
lncRNAs affecting PAECs and EndMT				
GATA6-AS1	HUVEC and hEC-based xenograft model	LOXL2	Epigenetic regulation of endothelial gene expression	51
MANTIS	MCT-PH and lung tissue samples from patients with idiopathic PAH	BRG1	Regulation of angiogenesis	50
MALAT1	PAECs	ox-LDL Wnt/β-catenin pathway miR-145	EndMT by increasing β-catenin EndMT by releasing TGF-β receptor type II and SMAD3	52
lncRNAs affecting PASMCs: cell-cycle progression, proliferation, and migration				
MALAT1	PASMCs	miR-124-3b	Regulation of cell cycle progression and migration	53
MEG3	PAH patients and hypoxia-induced PASMCs PAH patients and hPASMCs	miR-328-3p miR-21	Promotes cell cycle progression Promotes PTEN liberation; cell proliferation and migration	58,75 76
LnRTP	MCT-PH	PI3K	Promotes cell proliferation	66
ANRIL	Hypoxic PASMCs	unknown	Migration and cell cycle progression	78
LincRNA-COX2	PASMCs	miR-let-7a/STAT3 pathway	Inhibition of cell cycle progression and migration	79
GAS5	Hypoxia-induced pulmonary rat model and PASMCs	miR-23b-3p	Regulation of cell proliferation	55
lncRNAs affecting PASMCs: proliferation, migration and apoptosis inhibition				
lncAng362	PAH patients	miR-221 miR-222	Increased proliferation, migration, and NF-kB; reduced apoptosis	65

lncRNA	Model/cells	Target	Function	Reference
TUG1	Hypoxic-pulmonary hypertension mouse model and hypoxic-PASMCs	miR-374c	Pulmonary arterial remodeling	54
	PASMCs	miR-328	Regulation of cell cycle progression	63
	PASMCs	HIF-1α and VEGF	Inhibition of cell proliferation and migration; promotion of apoptosis	62
lncRNAs affecting PASMCs: proliferation and cell cycle progression				
HOXA-AS3	MCT-PH, hypoxia-induced PH mouse model and PAH patients	Ki67 and Cyclin A	Enhancement of cell cycle progression and cell proliferation	59,61
	PASMCs	miR-675-3p	Inhibition of cell proliferation, migration and apoptosis	60
RPS4L	Hypoxia-induced PH mice and hypoxic PASMCs	HIF-1α	Cell proliferation, cell cycle progression and migration Encodes for RPS4XL peptide	68
lncRNAs affecting PASMCs: proliferation and apoptosis inhibition				
CASC2	Hypoxia-induced PH rat model and PASMCs	Unknown	Promotion of cell proliferation and inhibition of apoptosis	77
NONRATT015587.2	MCT-PH and PASMCs	p21	Cell proliferation	70
	MCT-PH		Cell proliferation and apoptosis inhibition	69
PAHRF	Hypoxic PASMCs Samples from PAH patients	miR-23a-3p	Increased proliferation and decreased apoptosis of PASMCs	57
PAXIP1-AS1	Small pulmonary arteries, adventitial fibroblast and PAH-PASMCs	Paxillin and FAK	Inhibition of cell proliferation and migration, cytoskeletal disruption, increase of apoptosis secondary	72,73
	MCT-PH and hypoxic-PASMCs	WIPF1	Cell proliferation and migration	
TCONS_00034812	Sprague rat model and hypoxic-PASMCs	Stox1	Proliferation of PASMCs and inhibition of apoptosis	74

(continued on next page)

Table 3
(continued)

lncRNAs	Model	Target	Main Findings	Reference
TYKRIL	Ex-vivo studies (lung slice samples) and PASMCs	p53 N-terminal region	Promotes proliferation and inhibits apoptosis	71
UCA1	Hypoxic-PASMCs	HnRNP-I	Increases proliferation and inhibits apoptosis	84
lncRNA generally involved in pulmonary vascular remodeling				
H19	MCT-PH	miR-let-7b	Increases PASMCs proliferation	64,85
	MCT-PH treated with melatonin	miR-675-3p/IGFR1 miR-200a/PDCD4	Inhibition of cell proliferation and promotion of apoptosis	
SMILR	PASMCs and MCT-PH	miR-141	Proliferation PASMCs (in vitro) and vascular remodeling (in vivo)	56

Abbreviations: EndMT, endothelial-to-mesenchymal transition; hEC, human endothelial cells; HIF-1, hypoxia-induced factor-1; hPASMCs, human pulmonary artery smooth muscle cells; HUVEC, human umbilical vein endothelial cells; MCT-PH, monocrotaline rat model of pulmonary hypertension; PAECs, pulmonary artery endothelial cells; PAH, pulmonary arterial hypertension; PASMCs, pulmonary artery smooth muscle cells; PH, pulmonary hypertension.

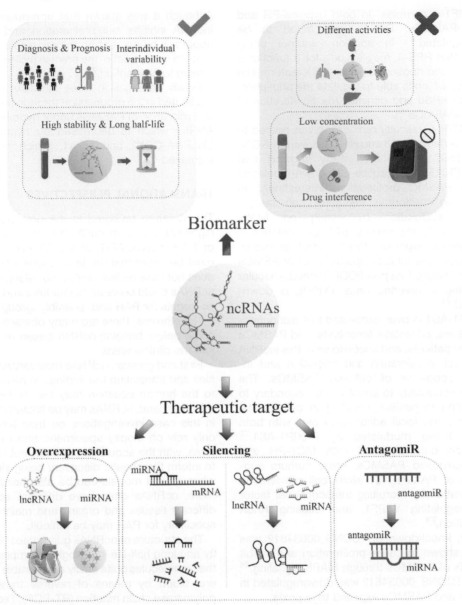

Fig. 2. Potential clinical use of noncoding RNAs (ncRNAs). The upper panels depict the advantages and limitations of ncRNAs as biomarkers for diagnosis and prognostic stratification of pulmonary arterial hypertension, whereas the lower panel shows how ncRNAs can be targeted for treatment. lncRNA: long noncoding RNA; miRNA: microRNA.

Conversely, lnc-Ang362, which was found to be elevated in lung tissues from PAH patients, is transcribed with and positively regulates miR-221 and miR-222, thus sustaining NF-kB signaling, proliferation and migration, and preventing apoptosis.[65]

Modulation of intracellular pathways governing proliferation of PASMCs by lncRNAs can also be non-miRNA-dependent.

LnRTP is regulated by platelet-derived growth factor (PDGF) and TGF-β and it was detected in

pulmonary arteries of MCT-treated rats. It was shown that LnRTP is down-regulated in response to PDGF-BB and that this is followed by enhanced expression of Notch3 and JAG1 and, as a consequence, proliferation. In contrast, the up-regulation of LnRTP inhibits rat PASMC proliferation.[66]

RPS4L affects cell cycle progression, proliferation, and migration in hypoxic-PASMCs by stabilizing the interleukin enhancer-binding factor 3

(ILF3)/HIF1-α complex. In both hypoxia-PH and hypoxic-PASMCs, RPS4L was found to be down-regulated.[67] In addition, another study showed that RPS4L may encode for a functional peptide called ribosomal protein S4X isoform-like (RPS4XL), which is able to regulate the phosphorylation of RPS6 and diminish the proliferation of hypoxic-PASMCs.[68]

In MCT-PH, vascular remodeling was related to the involvement of p53 and HIF-1α driven by NON-RATT015587.2.[69] Another study showed that NONRATT015587.2 causes p21 down-regulation allowing PASMC proliferation. Interestingly, in this setting metformin treatment can restore PASMC proliferation by acting on NON-RATT015587.2 and causing p21 up-regulation.[70] p53 is also a target of TYKRIL, which promotes proliferation and inhibits apoptosis of hPASMCs when upregulated via p53/PDGF. Indeed, vascular remodeling is reverted once TYKRIL is down-regulated.[71]

PAXIP1-AS1 is over-expressed in small pulmonary arteries, adventitial fibroblasts, and PASMCs from PAH patients, and knockdown of this lncRNA inhibits cell proliferation and migration and increases apoptosis of cultured PASMCs. The higher susceptibility to apoptosis is secondary to a reduction in paxillin, resulting in cytoskeletal disruption, and focal adhesion kinase, with both proteins being modulated by PAXIP1-AS1.[72] Based on data obtained with MCT-PH and hypoxia-exposed PASMCs, other authors suggested that PAXIP1-AS1 elicits cell proliferation and migration by recruiting transcriptional factor ETS1, regulating WIPF1, and causing RhoA upregulation.[73]

Finally, knockdown of TCONS_00034812 was recently shown to cause proliferation and inhibit apoptosis of PASMCs through MAPK signaling.[74] Indeed, TCONS_00034812 was downregulated in both rats and PASMCs exposed to hypoxia.

MEG3 is another lncRNA that promotes PASMC proliferation; however, it uniquely does so when it is both up- and down-regulated. On one side, MEG3 elicits an increase in IGF1R levels by sponging off miR-328-3p. Consistently, silencing of MEG3 inhibited cell cycle progression in PASMCs from idiopathic PAH patients and mice with hypoxia-PH.[75] On the other side, MEG3 was found to be downregulated in lungs and pulmonary arteries, and to promote proliferation and migration of PASMCs through the p53 pathway.[58] MEG3 down-regulation allows the PTEN liberation by sponging off miR-21.[76]

Some lncRNAs act in PASMCs by modalities yet to be characterized. Levels of CASC were reported to be reduced in both hypoxia-PH and PASMCs.

Although it was shown that upregulation of this lncRNA inhibits cell proliferation and promotes apoptosis by decreasing the expression of alpha-smooth muscle actin, the precise molecular events remain to be clarified.[77]

Finally, changes in three lncRNAs have been implicated in the progression through the cell cycle and migration of PASMCs under hypoxic stimulus: ANRIL, which is decreased by hypoxia,[78] and LincRNA-COX2 and UCA1, which are instead increased.[79]

TRANSLATIONAL PERSPECTIVES

The literature reviewed in the previous sections highlights a role of ncRNAs in the development of PAH, hypoxia-PH, and MCT-PH, although it must be noted that the latter experimental model does not have a clear clinical correlate. Therefore, ncRNAs could serve as biomarkers and therapeutic targets for PAH and, possibly, group 3 PH.

Nonetheless, there are many obstacles to overcome before bringing ncRNA-based technologies into the clinical arena.

First and general, ncRNAs may vary across species and translating the findings in animal models to the human situation may be challenging. On the other hand, ncRNAs may be limited to humans: in this case investigations on their function can only rely on biopsy specimens and cellular cultures, with the acquisition of sufficient knowledge to inform therapeutic discovery being slower than when animal models can be also used. Furthermore, ncRNAs often have different activities in different tissues and organs and maintaining the specificity for PAH may be difficult.

The structure of ncRNAs guarantees high stability and long half-life in biological samples, making these molecules quite easily measurable in peripheral blood by means of reverse transcriptase-polymerase chain reaction (RT-PCR). Technical issues that can impact the reproducibility of the measurements are related to the way ncRNAs are extracted for subsequent RT-PCR and to the criteria adopted to normalize ncRNA expression. In this regard, standardization of protocols is of utmost importance. The possible interference of concomitant drugs with RT-PCR should be also kept in mind: for instance, heparin is known to alter miRNA expression levels.[14]

Several microRNAs have been proposed as biomarkers to diagnose PAH or stratify the prognosis of PAH patients.[80] The combination of multiple miRNAs and the identification of candidate miRNAs by unbiased, artificial intelligence-guided analysis may improve the diagnostic or prognostic yield of miRNA panels.[80] The simultaneous assessment of several miRNAs may also account for interindividual variability and for the fact that one miRNA may be increased in the circulation because of an unrelated disease or even a physiologic process. The specificity of miRNA arrays may be also increased by evaluating the gradients across the right ventricle or the pulmonary circulation.[81]

Data about lncRNAs as biomarkers for PAH are less than those about miRNA. It was recently reported that circulating H19 concentrations discriminate PAH patients from controls, as well as PAH subgroups with different prognosis when added to N-terminal pro-B-type natriuretic peptide or clinical risk scores. Furthermore, plasma levels of H19 predict survival in PAH.[82] Importantly, the amounts of lncRNAs are often very low in tissues and even more so in plasma, to the point that they are undetectable or only occasionally detectable despite being convincingly identified in cellular studies.[83]

miRNA expression can be modulated by two opposite approaches: miRNA mimic, by which the expression of miRNAs with desirable effects is forced in pulmonary artery cells, and anti-miRNA, by which instead oligonucleotides called miRNA antagonists or antagomiRs are used to inhibit the expression of miRNAs with unwanted effects that are responsible for pulmonary artery cell pathobiology[14] (Fig. 2). Like for any therapeutics, an essential feature of either strategy is that the miRNA mimic or antagomiR is delivered specifically into the pulmonary vessels, so that off-target actions are avoided. In this regard, topical administration, for example, by the intranasal route[36] or by aerosol[27] is preferable over systemic administration. Especially for antagomiRs, there is the risk that intracellular pathways are perturbed even though they are not the primary target of the therapeutic intervention, with possible side effects. Another present limitation to the application of miRNA-based treatments is that no antidote currently exists.[14]

SUMMARY

A large body of experimental evidence indicates that miRNAs and lncRNAs participate in PAH pathogenesis by acting at the transcriptional and post transcriptional levels and by influencing gene and protein expression, as well as pulmonary artery cell fate. This wealth of knowledge has broadened the understanding of the mechanisms of PAH and has laid the foundations for the development of novel biomarkers and therapies for this condition. Although there are still open questions about the role of ncRNAs in PAH and unsolved problems hindering the implementation of ncRNA-based tools for diagnosis, prognostication, and treatment of PAH, the study of ncRNAs represents a promising field in PAH research.

DISCLOSURE

P. Ameri received personal fees from Janssen and MSD for speaker or advisor activity related to the topic of PAH; the other authors have no conflicts of interest to disclose.

ACKNOWLEDGMENTS

The authors thank David Hollingworth for his helpful assistance with proofreading this article. The figures were made by using Smart Servier Medical Art (available at https://smart.servier.com/), BioRender (available at https://biorender.com/) and StockAdobe (available at https://stock.adobe.com/).

REFERENCES

1. Sommer N, Ghofrani HA, Pak O, et al. Current and future treatments of pulmonary arterial hypertension. Br J Pharmacol 2021;178(1):6–30.
2. Vizza CD, Lang IM, Badagliacca R, et al. Aggressive Afterload Lowering to Improve the Right Ventricle: A New Target for Medical Therapy in Pulmonary Arterial Hypertension? Am J Respir Crit Care Med 2022;205(7):751–60.
3. Dueck A, Meister G. Assembly and function of small RNA - argonaute protein complexes. Biol Chem 2014;395(6):611–29.
4. O'Brien J, Hayder H, Zayed Y, et al. Overview of MicroRNA Biogenesis, Mechanisms of Actions, and Circulation. Front Endocrinol (Lausanne) 2018;9. https://doi.org/10.3389/FENDO.2018.00402.
5. Condorelli G, Latronico MVG, Cavarretta E. MicroRNAs in cardiovascular diseases: Current knowledge and the road ahead. J Am Coll Cardiol 2014; 63(21):2177–87.
6. Romaine SPR, Tomaszewski M, Condorelli G, et al. MicroRNAs in cardiovascular disease: an introduction for clinicians. Heart 2015;101(12):921–8.
7. Kabekkodu SP, Shukla V, Varghese VK, et al. Cluster miRNAs and cancer: Diagnostic, prognostic and therapeutic opportunities. Wiley Interdiscip Rev RNA 2020,11(2).e1563.
8. Hombach S, Kretz M. Noncoding RNAs: Classification, Biology and Functioning. Adv Exp Med Biol 2016;937:3–17.
9. Sayed D, Abdellatif M. MicroRNAs in development and disease. Physiol Rev 2011;91(3):827–87.
10. Gupta S, Li L. Modulation of miRNAs in Pulmonary Hypertension. Int J Hypertens 2015;2015. https://doi.org/10.1155/2015/169069.

11. Lee A, McLean D, Choi J, et al. Therapeutic implications of microRNAs in pulmonary arterial hypertension. BMB Rep 2014;47(6):311–7.

12. Neth P, Nazari-Jahantigh M, Schober A, et al. MicroRNAs in flow-dependent vascular remodelling. Cardiovasc Res 2013;99(2):294–303.

13. Kumar S, Kim CW, Simmons RD, et al. Role of flow-sensitive microRNAs in endothelial dysfunction and atherosclerosis mechanosensitive athero-miRs. Arterioscler Thromb Vasc Biol 2014;34(10):2206–16.

14. Bienertova-Vasku J, Novak J, Vasku A. MicroRNAs in pulmonary arterial hypertension: pathogenesis, diagnosis and treatment. J Am Soc Hypertens 2015;9(3):221–34.

15. Bi R, Bao C, Jiang L, et al. MicroRNA-27b plays a role in pulmonary arterial hypertension by modulating peroxisome proliferator-activated receptor γ dependent Hsp90-eNOS signaling and nitric oxide production. Biochem Biophys Res Commun 2015; 460(2):469–75.

16. Yang Z, Kaye DM. Mechanistic insights into the link between a polymorphism of the 3'UTR of the SLC7A1 gene and hypertension. Hum Mutat 2009; 30(3):328–33.

17. Yang Z, Venardos K, Jones E, et al. Identification of a novel polymorphism in the 3'UTR of the L-arginine transporter gene SLC7A1: contribution to hypertension and endothelial dysfunction. Circulation 2007; 115(10):1269–74.

18. Sun HX, Zeng DY, Li RT, et al. Essential role of microRNA-155 in regulating endothelium-dependent vasorelaxation by targeting endothelial nitric oxide synthase. Hypertension 2012;60(6): 1407–14.

19. Suárez Y, Fernández-Hernando C, Pober JS, et al. Dicer dependent microRNAs regulate gene expression and functions in human endothelial cells. Circ Res 2007;100(8):1164–73.

20. Deng Z, Morse JH, Slager SL, et al. Familial primary pulmonary hypertension (gene PPH1) is caused by mutations in the bone morphogenetic protein receptor-II gene. Am J Hum Genet 2000;67(3): 737–44.

21. Pospisil V, Vargova K, Kokavec J, et al. Epigenetic silencing of the oncogenic miR-17-92 cluster during PU.1-directed macrophage differentiation. The EMBO J 2011;30(21):4450.

22. Brock M, Samillan VJ, Trenkmann M, et al. Antago-miR directed against miR-20a restores functional BMPR2 signalling and prevents vascular remodelling in hypoxia-induced pulmonary hypertension. Eur Heart J 2014;35(45):3203–11.

23. Pullamsetti SS, Doebele C, Fischer A, et al. Inhibition Of MicroRNA-17 Improves Lung And Heart Function In Experimental Pulmonary Hypertension. 2012: A2617-A2617. doi:10.1164/AJRCCM-CONFER-ENCE.2012.185.1_MEETINGABSTRACTS.A2617

24. Bertero T, Lu Y, Annis S, et al. Systems-level regulation of microRNA networks by miR-130/301 promotes pulmonary hypertension. J Clin Invest 2014; 124(8):3514–28.

25. Santos-Ferreira CA, Abreu MT, Marques CI, et al. Micro-RNA Analysis in Pulmonary Arterial Hypertension: Current Knowledge and Challenges. JACC Basic Transl Sci 2020;5(11):1149–62.

26. Ruffenach G, Chabot S, Tanguay VF, et al. Role for Runt-related Transcription Factor 2 in Proliferative and Calcified Vascular Lesions in Pulmonary Arterial Hypertension. Am J Respir Crit Care Med 2016; 194(10):1273–85.

27. Courboulin A, Paulin R, Giguère NJ, et al. Role for miR-204 in human pulmonary arterial hypertension. J Exp Med 2011;208(3):535–48.

28. Jalali S, Ramanathan GK, Parthasarathy PT, et al. Mir-206 Regulates Pulmonary Artery Smooth Muscle Cell Proliferation and Differentiation. PLoS ONE 2012;7(10). https://doi.org/10.1371/JOURNAL. PONE.0046808.

29. Yue J, Guan J, Wang X, et al. MicroRNA-206 is involved in hypoxia-induced pulmonary hypertension through targeting of the HIF-1α/Fhl-1 pathway. Lab Invest 2013;93(7):748–59.

30. Yang S, Banerjee S, de Freitas A, et al. miR-21 regulates chronic hypoxia-induced pulmonary vascular remodeling. Am J Physiol Lung Cell Mol Physiol 2012;302:521–9.

31. Davis BN, Hilyard AC, Lagna G, et al. SMAD proteins control DROSHA-mediated microRNA maturation. Nature 2008;454(7200):56–61.

32. Parikh VN, Jin RC, Rabello S, et al. MicroRNA-21 integrates pathogenic signaling to control pulmonary hypertension: results of a network bioinformatics approach. Circulation 2012;125(12):1520–32.

33. Caruso P, MacLean MR, Khanin R, et al. Dynamic changes in lung microRNA profiles during the development of pulmonary hypertension due to chronic hypoxia and monocrotaline. Arterioscler Thromb Vasc Biol 2010;30(4):716–23.

34. Li S, Ran Y, Zhang D, et al. MicroRNA-138 plays a role in hypoxic pulmonary vascular remodeling by targeting Mst1. Biochem J 2013;452(2):281–91.

35. Sen A, Most P, Peppel K. Induction of microRNA-138 by pro-inflammatory cytokines causes endothelial cell dysfunction. FEBS Lett 2014;588(6):906–14.

36. Kim J, Kang Y, Kojima Y, et al. An endothelial apelin-FGF link mediated by miR-424 and miR-503 is disrupted in pulmonary arterial hypertension. Nat Med 2012;19(1):74–82.

37. Hergenreider E, Heydt S, Tréguer K, et al. Athero-protective communication between endothelial cells and smooth muscle cells through miRNAs. Nat Cell Biol 2012;14(3):249–56.

38. Climent M, Quintavalle M, Miragoli M, et al. TGFβ triggers miR-143/145 transfer from smooth muscle

cells to endothelial cells, thereby modulating vessel stabilization. Circ Res 2015;116(11):1753–64.

39. Cheng Y, Liu X, Yang J, et al. MicroRNA-145, a novel smooth muscle cell phenotypic marker and modulator, controls vascular neointimal lesion formation. Circ Res 2009;105(2):158–66.

40. Caruso P, Dempsie Y, Stevens HC, et al. A role for miR-145 in pulmonary arterial hypertension: evidence from mouse models and patient samples. Circ Res 2012;111(3):290–300.

41. Kang K, Peng X, Zhang X, et al. MicroRNA-124 suppresses the transactivation of nuclear factor of activated T cells by targeting multiple genes and inhibits the proliferation of pulmonary artery smooth muscle cells. J Biol Chem 2013;288(35):25414–27.

42. Wang D, Zhang H, Li M, et al. MicroRNA-124 controls the proliferative, migratory, and inflammatory phenotype of pulmonary vascular fibroblasts. Circ Res 2014;114(1):67–78.

43. Marchese FP, Raimondi I, Huarte M. The multidimensional mechanisms of long noncoding RNA function. Genome Biol 2017;18(1).

44. Derrien T, Johnson R, Bussotti G, et al. The GENCODE v7 catalog of human long noncoding RNAs: analysis of their gene structure, evolution, and expression. Genome Res 2012;22(9):1775–89.

45. Taniue K, Akimitsu N. The Functions and Unique Features of LncRNAs in Cancer Development and Tumorigenesis. Int J Mol Sci 2021;22(2):1–20.

46. Pan T. N6-methyl-adenosine modification in messenger and long noncoding RNA. Trends Biochem Sci 2013;38(4):204–9.

47. Geisler S, Lojek L, Khalil AM, et al. Decapping of long noncoding RNAs regulates inducible genes. Mol Cell 2012;45(3):279–91.

48. Johnson AW. Rat1p and Xrn1p are functionally interchangeable exoribonucleases that are restricted to and required in the nucleus and cytoplasm, respectively. Mol Cell Biol 1997;17(10):6122–30.

49. Chen C, He Y, Feng Y, et al. Long noncoding RNA review and implications in acute lung inflammation. Life Sci 2021;269. https://doi.org/10.1016/j.lfs.2021.119044.

50. Leisegang MS, Fork C, Josipovic I, et al. Long Noncoding RNA MANTIS Facilitates Endothelial Angiogenic Function. Circulation 2017;136(1):65–79.

51. Neumann P, Jaé N, Knau A, et al. The lncRNA GATA6-AS epigenetically regulates endothelial gene expression via interaction with LOXL2. Nat Commun 2018;9(1). https://doi.org/10.1038/S41467-017-02431-1.

52. Xiang Y, Zhang Y, Tang Y, et al. MALAT1 Modulates TGF-β1-Induced Endothelial-to-Mesenchymal Transition through Downregulation of miR-145. Cell Physiol Biochem 2017;42(1):357–72.

53. Wang D, Xu H, Wu B, et al. Long noncoding RNA MALAT1 sponges miR-124-3p.1/KLF5 to promote pulmonary vascular remodeling and cell cycle progression of pulmonary artery hypertension. Int J Mol Med 2019;44(3):871–84.

54. Yang L, Liang H, Shen L, et al. LncRNA Tug1 involves in the pulmonary vascular remodeling in mice with hypoxic pulmonary hypertension via the microRNA-374c-mediated Foxc1. Life Sci 2019;237. https://doi.org/10.1016/J.LFS.2019.116769.

55. Hao X, Li H, Zhang P, et al. Down-regulation of lncRNA Gas5 promotes hypoxia-induced pulmonary arterial smooth muscle cell proliferation by regulating KCNK3 expression. Eur J Pharmacol 2020;889. https://doi.org/10.1016/J.EJPHAR.2020.173618.

56. Lei S, Peng F, Li ML, et al. LncRNA-SMILR modulates RhoA/ROCK signaling by targeting miR-141 to regulate vascular remodeling in pulmonary arterial hypertension. Am J Physiol Heart Circ Physiol 2020;319(2):H377–91.

57. Liu Y, Hu R, Zhu J, et al. The lncRNA PAHRF functions as a competing endogenous RNA to regulate MST1 expression by sponging miR-23a-3p in pulmonary arterial hypertension. Vascul Pharmacol 2021;139. https://doi.org/10.1016/J.VPH.2021.106886.

58. Sun Z, Nie X, Sun S, et al. Long Noncoding RNA MEG3 Downregulation Triggers Human Pulmonary Artery Smooth Muscle Cell Proliferation and Migration via the p53 Signaling Pathway. Cell Physiol Biochem 2017;42(6):2569–81.

59. Golpon HA, Geraci MW, Moore MD, et al. HOX genes in human lung: altered expression in primary pulmonary hypertension and emphysema. Am J Pathol 2001;158(3):955–66.

60. Li ZK, Gao LF, Zhu XA, et al. LncRNA HOXA-AS3 Promotes the Progression of Pulmonary Arterial Hypertension through Mediation of miR-675-3p/PDE5A Axis. Biochem Genet 2021;59(5):1158–72.

61. Zhang H, Liu Y, Yan L, et al. Long noncoding RNA Hoxaas3 contributes to hypoxia-induced pulmonary artery smooth muscle cell proliferation. Cardiovasc Res 2019;115(3):647–57.

62. Zhang J, Silva T, Yarovinsky T, et al. VEGF blockade inhibits lymphocyte recruitment and ameliorates immune-mediated vascular remodeling. Circ Res 2010;107(3):408–17.

63. Wang S, Cao W, Gao S, et al. TUG1 Regulates Pulmonary Arterial Smooth Muscle Cell Proliferation in Pulmonary Arterial Hypertension. Can J Cardiol 2019;35(11):1534–45.

64. Wang R, Zhou S, Wu P, et al. Identifying Involvement of H19-miR-675-3p-IGF1R and H19-miR-200a-PDCD4 in Treating Pulmonary Hypertension with Melatonin. Mol Ther Nucleic Acids 2018;13:44–54.

65. Wang H, Qin R, Cheng Y. LncRNA-Ang362 Promotes Pulmonary Arterial Hypertension by

Regulating miR-221 and miR-222. Shock 2020; 53(6):723–9.

66. Chen J, Guo J, Cui X, et al. The Long Noncoding RNA LnRPT Is Regulated by PDGF-BB and Modulates the Proliferation of Pulmonary Artery Smooth Muscle Cells. Am J Respir Cell Mol Biol 2018; 58(2):181–93.

67. Liu Y, Zhang H, Li Y, et al. Long Noncoding RNA Rps4l Mediates the Proliferation of Hypoxic Pulmonary Artery Smooth Muscle Cells. Hypertension 2020;76(4):1124–33.

68. Li Y, Zhang J, Sun H, et al. lnc-Rps4l-encoded peptide RPS4XL regulates RPS6 phosphorylation and inhibits the proliferation of PASMCs caused by hypoxia. Mol Ther 2021;29(4):1411–24.

69. Sun Z, Liu Y, Yu F, et al. Long noncoding RNA and mRNA profile analysis of metformin to reverse the pulmonary hypertension vascular remodeling induced by monocrotaline. Biomed Pharmacother 2019;115. https://doi.org/10.1016/J.BIOPHA.2019. 108933.

70. Sun Z, Liu Y, Hu R, et al. Metformin inhibits pulmonary artery smooth muscle cell proliferation by upregulating p21 via NONRATT015587.2. Int J Mol Med 2022;49(4). https://doi.org/10.3892/IJMM.2022. 5104.

71. Zehendner CM, Valasarajan C, Werner A, et al. Long Noncoding RNA TYKRIL Plays a Role in Pulmonary Hypertension via the p53-mediated Regulation of PDGFRβ. Am J Respir Crit Care Med 2020; 202(10):1445–57.

72. Jandl K, Thekkekara Puthenparampil H, Marsh LM, et al. Long noncoding RNAs influence the transcriptome in pulmonary arterial hypertension: the role of PAXIP1-AS1. J Pathol 2019;247(3):357–70.

73. Song R, Lei S, Yang S, et al. LncRNA PAXIP1-AS1 fosters the pathogenesis of pulmonary arterial hypertension via ETS1/WIPF1/RhoA axis. J Cell Mol Med 2021;25(15):7321–34.

74. Liu Y, Sun Z, Zhu J, et al. LncRNA-TCONS_ 00034812 in cell proliferation and apoptosis of pulmonary artery smooth muscle cells and its mechanism. J Cell Physiol 2018;233(6):4801–14.

75. Xing Y, Zheng X, Fu Y, et al. Long Noncoding RNA-Maternally Expressed Gene 3 Contributes to Hypoxic Pulmonary Hypertension. Mol Ther 2019;27(12). https://doi.org/10.1016/J.YMTHE.2019.07.022.

76. Zhu B, Gong Y, Yan G, et al. Down-regulation of lncRNA MEG3 promotes hypoxia-induced human pulmonary artery smooth muscle cell proliferation and migration via repressing PTEN by sponging miR-21. Biochem Biophys Res Commun 2018; 495(3):2125–32.

77. Gong J, Chen Z, Chen Y, et al. Long noncoding RNA CASC2 suppresses pulmonary artery smooth muscle cell proliferation and phenotypic switch in hypoxia-induced pulmonary hypertension. Respir Res 2019;20(1). https://doi.org/10.1186/S12931-019-1018-X.

78. Wang S, Zhang C, Zhang X. Downregulation of long noncoding RNA ANRIL promotes proliferation and migration in hypoxic human pulmonary artery smooth muscle cells. Mol Med Rep 2020;21(2): 589–96.

79. Cheng G, He L, Zhang Y. LincRNA-Cox2 promotes pulmonary arterial hypertension by regulating the let-7a-mediated STAT3 signaling pathway. Mol Cell Biochem 2020;475(1–2):239–47.

80. Wei C, Henderson H, Spradley C, et al. Circulating miRNAs as potential marker for pulmonary hypertension. PLoS One 2013;8(5). https://doi.org/10.1371/JOURNAL.PONE.0064396.

81. Chouvarine P, Geldner J, Giagnorio R, et al. Trans-Right-Ventricle and Transpulmonary MicroRNA Gradients in Human Pulmonary Arterial Hypertension. Pediatr Crit Care Med 2020;21(4):340–9.

82. Omura J, Habbout K, Shimauchi T, et al. Identification of Long Noncoding RNA H19 as a New Biomarker and Therapeutic Target in Right Ventricular Failure in Pulmonary Arterial Hypertension. Circulation 2020;142(15):1464–84.

83. Schlosser K, Hanson J, Villeneuve PJ, et al. Assessment of Circulating LncRNAs Under Physiologic and Pathologic Conditions in Humans Reveals Potential Limitations as Biomarkers. Sci Rep 2016;6. https://doi.org/10.1038/SREP36596.

84. Zhu TT, Sun RL, Yin YL, et al. Long noncoding RNA UCA1 promotes the proliferation of hypoxic human pulmonary artery smooth muscle cells. Pflugers Archiv Eur J Physiol 2019;471(2):347–55.

85. Su H, Xu X, Yan C, et al. LncRNA H19 promotes the proliferation of pulmonary artery smooth muscle cells through AT1R via sponging let-7b in monocrotaline-induced pulmonary arterial hypertension. Respir Res 2018;19(1):1–18.

Printed and bound by CPI Group (UK) Ltd, Croydon, CR0 4YY

03/10/2024

01040367-0013